ALLE ZEIT WACH

1842

Progress in Pediatric Surgery

Volume 27

Paediatric Thoracic Surgery

Volume Editors

N. A. Myers and T. A. Angerpointner

With a Foreword by A. W. Auldist

With 80 Figures
and 44 Tables

Springer-Verlag Berlin Heidelberg GmbH

Nathaniel A. Myers
AM, MD, FRCS, FRACS
Royal Children's Hospital Melbourne
Flemington Road, Parkville, Victoria, 3052
Australia

Priv.-Doz. Dr. Thomas A. Angerpointner
Zenettistraße 48/III, D-8000 Munich 2 (W)
Federal Republic of Germany

Volumes 1–17 of this series were published
by Urban & Schwarzenberg, Baltimore–Munich

ISBN 978-3-642-87769-8 ISBN 978-3-642-87767-4 (eBook)
DOI 10.1007/978-3-642-87767-4

Library of Congress Cataloging-in-Publication Data
Paediatric thoracic surgery / volume editors, N. A. Myers and T. A. Angerpointner;
with foreword by A. W. Auldist. p. cm. – (Progress in pediatric surgery; v. 27)
Includes bibliographical references and index.
(alk. paper) – (alk. paper)
1. Chest – Surgery. 2. Children – Surgery.
I. Myers, N. A. (Nathaniel A.), 1922– . II. Angerpointner, Thomas. III. Series.
[DNLM: 1. Thoracic Surgery – in infancy & childhood. W1 PR677KA v. 27 / WF 980 P126]
RD137.A1P7 vol. 27 [RD536] 617'.98 s – dc20 [617.5'4059] DNLM/DLC
for Library of Congress 91-4594 CIP

Originally published by Springer-Verlag Berlin Heidelberg New York in 1991
Softcover reprint of the hardcover 1st edition 1991

23/3145-543210 Printed on acid-free paper

Dedication

This volume is dedicated
to Russell Howard, ED, MD, FRCS, FRACS, MRCOG
in recognition of his leadership, wisdom
and surgical skill

Foreword

This volume of *Progress in Pediatric Surgery* has been produced at a time when medical progress is frequently measured in terms of technological advances. Important as they are it is essential to remember that soundly based clinical skills are necessary in order to plan all aspects of therapy, both medical and surgical. Bedside evaluation combined with the results of investigation should enable a definite diagnosis or differential diagnosis to be made and thus point the way to appropriate treatment.

In this context the articles in this volume concentrate on the clinical aspects of a variety of thoracic problems and at the same time include papers devoted to history, nursing aspects and basic science, all of which are important in understanding and planning patient management.

The contributions are largely from the clinical school of the Royal Children's Hospital, Melbourne, which is the paediatric teaching institution for the University of Melbourne and the Royal Australasian College of Surgeons. The contributors have independently presented their views and experience and the volume is richer for the additional contributions from Sydney and Denver. It is important to recognize that special training and skills are required of the paediatric surgeon who operates on babies and children with a thoracic surgical problem.

A. W. Auldist
Melbourne, Australia

Contents

Editors

Angerpointner, T. A., Priv.-Doz. Dr.
Zenettistraße 48/III, D-8000 München 2 (W)

Gauderer, Michael, W. L., MD
Rainbow Babies and Childrens Hospital, 2074 Abington Road
Cleveland, OH 44106, USA

Hecker, W. Ch., Prof. Dr.
Kinderchirurgische Klinik im Dr. von Haunerschen Kinderspital
der Universität München, Lindwurmstraße 4
D-8000 München 2 (W)

Prévot, J., Prof.
Clinique Chirurgical Pédiatrique, Hôpital d'Enfants de Nancy
F-54511 Vandœvre Cedex

Rickham, P. P., Prof. Dr.
MD, MS, FRCS, FRCSI, FRACS, DCH, FAAP
Universitätskinderklinik, Chirurgische Abteilung
Steinwiesstraße 75, CH-8032 Zürich

Spitz, L., Prof., PhD, FRCS, Nuffield Professor of Pediatric Surgery
Institute of Child Health, University of London
Hospital for Sick Children, Great Ormond Street, 30 Guilford Street
GB-London WC1N 1EH

Stauffer, U. G., Prof. Dr.
Universitätskinderklinik, Kinderchirurgische Abteilung
Steinwiesstraße 75, CH-8032 Zürich

Wurnig, P., Prof. Dr.
Facharzt für Chirurgie und Kinderchirurgie
Schellinggasse 12, A-1010 Wien

Contributors

You will find the addresses at the beginning of the respective contribution

Introduction

N. A. Myers and T. A. Angerpointner

Although various opinions are expressed regarding a special place for thoracic operations in children, no one should argue with the recognition of the increasing importance of this subspecialty. As time has passed, it has become increasingly clear that thoracic surgical problems occupy an important place within the field of paediatric surgery as a whole. The corollary of this is that the paediatric surgical trainee must be exposed to the clinical and operative management of a wide variety of conditions which affect the chest wall, the lungs, the mediastinum, the diaphragm and the oesophagus.

With the evolution of time, and the enormous progress which has been made in the surgical management of congenital cardiac malformations, it was inevitable that paediatric cardiac surgery would become a further subspecialty, and in large centres there is now a place for paediatric surgeons who have made a particular study of thoracic problems, and cardiac surgeons who devote their time to the surgery of congenital cardiac malformations. Nevertheless, it is important that both groups are familiar with the interests and techniques of both areas and, ideally, training programmes should allow exposure to thoracic non-cardiac and cardiac paediatric surgery. Each group has much to learn from the experience of the other, and the preoperative, operative and postoperative aspects of thoracotomy, regardless of the reason for the procedure, are widely applicable.

This is the background to presenting this volume devoted to a wide variety of paediatric thoracic surgical conditions. It is not meant to be all inclusive, or to replace the many published articles and standard textbooks which devote part of their space to these and other problems; but rather to highlight a miscellany of aspects and conditions which confront the paediatric thoracic surgeon with varying frequency.

It is appropriate that such a volume should include historical aspects, and that this be given pride of place. Dr. Chang, with his wide knowledge of the history of surgery, has made a very significant contribution, which I am sure will be appreciated by all who read this volume.

Some explanation may be necessary to indicate how the other contributors were selected; from the list of contributions, it will be seen that all but one of these other contributions have been provided by members of staff of the Royal Children's Hospital, Melbourne. Subjects were selected because of their frequency, or because of difficulties in diagnosis and/or management, and thus represent much of the experience in paediatric thoracic surgery in Melbourne during the past 4 decades.

Progress in Pediatric Surgery, Vol. 27
Myers and Angerpointner (Eds.)

Quite deliberately, an article entirely concerned with the clinical and operative aspects of oesophageal atresia was not included. On the one hand, there have now been many contributions describing experience with oesophageal atresia and tracheo-oesophageal fistula; and on the other hand, too few articles have looked at some of the subjects selected for this volume.

Thoracic surgery in paediatric practice encompasses a wide variety of conditions affecting children and adolescents of all ages. It follows that it was necessary to limit the number of papers in this volume of *Progress in Pediatric Surgery* to ten, and the cooperation of the authors is recognized and gratefully acknowledged. The subjects selected provide a good cross-section of thoracic surgical problems encountered in clinical practice, supplemented by a historical review and the article on nursing perspectives. These two articles are given pride of place, and Chang's masterly review cannot fail to be of interest to all paediatric surgeons, not only those involved in the surgery of the thorax. Highlights from his paper include his erudite description of the "beginnings" and the description of the early surgery of empyema thoracis, with emphasis on the classical contributions of Hippocrates. Chang has integrated scientific progress with history, and there are several delightful anecdotal episodes, not the least of which concerns Vesalius and his problems. Of particular interest to the paediatric surgeon are Chang's references to foreign bodies in the oesophagus, to Morgagni's observations and to tracheostomy. Also, he rightly highlights the three great developments of anaesthesia, aseptic surgery and blood transfusion, all of which we tend to take for granted today. Finally, he itemizes many important events in the history of the surgery, including Bauhinus and his description of Pectus excavatum in 1594, Durston and Gibson's oft-quoted papers on oesophageal atresia in the late seventeenth century, and Bochdalek's description of the diaphragmatic hernia which bears his name, in 1848. As Chang concludes, "by the latter half of the nineteenth century, paediatrics, paediatric nursing and paediatric surgical care were on the ascent".

With these words, it is appropriate that the second paper is on "Nursing Perspectives". Faced with the daunting task of summarizing the nursing care of paediatric patients before and after operation, Telfer and Willis' paper does provide, as the title implies, nursing perspectives. They have combined practical nursing techniques with recognition of the need for the practising nurse to have a sound knowledge of basic anatomy, physiology and pathology. In addition, their approach is very human, pointing out that the baby, infant or child is a family member and that care must be holistic, and include support for the family as a whole. Both Telfer and Willis have had extensive clinical and teaching experience at the Royal Children's Hospital, Melbourne, and their contribution is a direct result of their close contact with parents and staff. It is essential that surgeons work in close association with their nursing colleagues and combine a "team approach" with a system of "mutual trust".

A similar team approach has become obligatory in the field of paediatric oncology, and this is highlighted by the article presented by Simpson and Campbell on "Mediastinal Masses in Childhood". As one reads this article, one cannot fail to be impressed by the breadth of knowledge displayed by the authors, who clearly by no means restrict their approach to morbid anatomy and histology. Apart from extensive factual data, they have presented their message loudly and clearly. And that is that the surgeon must work in close collaboration with the paediatric pathologist to make possible the provision of optimal management for their patients. In turn, paediatric pathologists must be aware of the clinical and radiological significance of the specific conditions they diagnose in their laboratories. I feel sure that this article will prove to be a reference source for many years to come.

Beasley wisely points out that "anatomical and physiological considerations specific to the newborn infant affect the surgical management of many neonatal thoracic conditions". He then applies these principles to the management of the baby with oesophageal atresia, with or without tracheo-oesophageal fistula. Frequently, published articles on this subject have concentrated on anastomotic techniques with little consideration given to the merits of various surgical approaches. Not only does Beasley consider this latter aspect, he also provides data regarding long-term follow-up, which is essential if correct surgical decisions are to be made at the time of the primary operation. Combining theoretical considerations with the practicalities of patient management, Beasley has provided a thoughtful contribution which will be of value to experienced paediatric surgeons, as well as to surgical trainees. It is very appropriate that he has devoted considerable space to the vexed subject of tracheomalacia, which has emerged as a very important problem in the baby with repaired oesophageal atresia. A similar comment is applicable to the section on gastro-oesophageal reflux.

Glasson originally planned to consider the subject of mediastinocervical cystic hygroma, but wisely made a total review of cervical cystic hygroma as well. This has provided information regarding a large series of lymphangiomata from The Children's Hospital, Sydney, a sister institution to the Royal Children's Hospital, Melbourne. This information is presented in a logical manner, and highlights the point that cystic hygroma must be seen as a condition with cervical or mediastinal components, or both, and that, in paediatric surgery practice, specific problems can arise which necessitate operative intervention in the neck or the thorax, or both. If any justification were needed to include such an extensive review of cervical cystic hygroma in a volume essentially concerned with thoracic surgical problems, it is therefore provided by recognition of these facts.

Kent has given us a "position paper" on intralobar sequestration which, based upon his own personal experience as well as the experience of others in Melbourne, does a great deal to provide a straightforward approach to a subject which latterly has been clouded by attempts to provide an all-embracing classification and terminology. From the surgical point of view – and this is Kent's message – the important issues are method of presentation and treatment options, and his contributions will be of value to thoracic physicians and radiologists, as well as to his surgical colleagues.

In a similar vein, Stokes has summarized the literature on "Unusual Varieties of Diaphragmatic Herniae", and stressed that our attention should not focus only on the almost overwhelming problem of diaphragmatic hernia in the newborn. He would be the first to agree that the list he has provided may be incomplete, but in a concise manner he has described the most frequently seen "unusual varieties". As with other contributions in this issue, the material can surely be the basis for a later monograph.

Mee is a paediatric cardiac surgeon in the modern image, and he has combined clinical acumen with theoretical considerations to give those who need to know a summary of the current status of paediatric cardiac surgery. It is not difficult to define "those who need to know", because congenital cardiac defects frequently coexist with other intrathoracic anomalies, and, although there may be separate surgical disciplines, it is essential that the paediatric surgeon be aware of therapeutic possibilities available for severe congenital cardiac malformations. Previously, many of these were considered inoperable, and their presence influenced case selection. Today, the cardiac surgeon must be considered as part of a team and his involvement is frequently required. But apart from summarizing recent advances in the care of those babies who have a cardiac problem, Mee demonstrates par excellence that surgery is an all-embracing science, demanding a knowledge of basic physiology and anatomy. The reader will find much of value in his article.

The final two articles are largely a personal approach to subjects which have interested the author for 4 decades. Many may not agree with their contents, and, if they do not, hopefully they will be stimulated to write of their own experiences.

Thus, in this volume of *Progress in Pediatric Surgery* various thoracic surgical problems seen during childhood and adolescence are discussed. It is, I believe, very significant that the articles in this volume were collected in 1989, 50 years following the classic contribution by Robert Gross, which was published in 1939 in the *Journal of the American Medical Association.* This contribution, which was entitled "Ligation of the Patent Ductus Arteriosus", ushered in the era of modern cardiac surgery, and outstanding progress has been in that field in the half century which has since elapsed. But Gross's contribution can perhaps be seen in the broader light, in that it also ushered in the era of modern thoracic surgery in childhood, and it is not without interest to note that Gross also reported the first successful pneumonectomy for congenital cystic disease of the lung in 1946, and in the same year reported the first successful repair of a posterolateral diaphragmatic hernia in a baby aged less than 24 h. For this reason alone, it is appropriate to conclude these editorial comments by giving credit to Robert Gross, and a host of other pioneers in the field of paediatric thoracic surgery.

Historical Aspects

J. H. T. Chang

Summary

Although thoracic afflictions may be traced to the prehistoric age, successful thoracic surgery was a development of the late nineteenth and early twentieth centuries. From 1543 to 1661, Vesalius, Servetus, Harvey and Malpighi established the dynamic anatomy of the pulmonary system. Boyle, Hooke, Black and Lavoisier elaborated upon the respiratory gases between 1660 and 1794. Although the drainage of empyema had been known since Hippocratic times, the underwater seal drainage bottle to prevent pneumothorax was not invented until 1872. At the turn of the century, Sauerbruch delayed the development of thoracic surgery for 30 years by opposing the use of positive pressure ventilation, which had not only been known to the ancients but also in clinical practice since the mid-1800s. Once positive pressure ventilation was established, routine successful thoracic surgery still had to await the development of safe blood transfusion by Landsteiner (1900, 1940) and the availability of antibiotics discovered by Chain, Florey and Waksman in the 1940s. Techniques and instrumentation were then developed for the safe and routine surgery of specific thoracic organs.

Zusammenfassung

Obwohl Thoraxleiden bis in das prähistorische Zeitalter zurückverfolgt werden können, ist die erfolgreiche Thoraxchirurgie eine Entwicklung des späten 19. und frühen 20. Jahrhunderts. Zwischen 1543 und 1661 etablierten Vesalis, Servetus, Harvey und Malpighi die dynamische Anatomie der Lunge. Zwischen 1660 und 1794 erforschten Boyle, Hooke, Black and Lavoisier nähere Einzelheiten der Blutgase. Die Empyemdrainage war zwar schon zu Zeiten des Hippokrates bekannt, aber die Drainage mit Wasserschloß zur Prävention eines Pneumothorax wurde erst 1872 eingeführt. Um die Jahrhundertwende verzögerte Sauerbruch die Weiterentwicklung der Thoraxchirurgie durch seinen Widerstand gegenüber der Überdruckbeatmung, die nicht nur in der Antike schon bekannt war, sondern bereits seit der Mitte des 18. Jahrhunderts in die klinische Praxis eingeführt war. Nachdem die Überdruckbeatmung etabliert war, bedurfte es zu einer erfolgreichen Thoraxchirurgie noch der Entwicklung sicherer Bluttransfusionen durch Landsteiner (1900, 1940) und der Verfügbarkeit von Antibiotika, die Chain, Florey und Waksman in den 40er Jahren einführten. Operationsmethoden und Instrumentierung wurden dann zur routinemäßigen Anwendung von Operationen an den einzelnen Thoraxorganen verfeinert.

Résumé

Bien que l'on ait apporté la preuve que les affections thoraciques soient connues depuis l'ère préhistorique, ce n'est qu'à la fin du 19e siècle et au début du 20e que l'on commença à avoir recours

Pediatric Surgery Associates, PC, Suite 501, 1010 East Nineteenth Avenue, CO 80218, Denver, USA.

Progress in Pediatric Surgery, Vol. 27
Myers and Angerpointner (Eds.)

à la chirurgie thoracique avec quelque chance de succès. Entre 1543 et 1661, Vésale, Servet, Harvey et Malpighi avaient découvert l'anatomie dynamique du système pulmonaire. Boyle, Hooke, Black et Lavoisier publièrent les résultats de leurs recherches sur les gaz respiratoires entre 1660 et 1794. Bien que le drainage d'un emplyème ait déja été pratiqué à l'époque d'Hippocrate, le flacon de drainage étanche sous l'eau pour éviter un pneumothorax ne fut inventé qu'en 1872. A la fin du siècle dernier et au début de ceclui-ci. Sauerbruch fit prendre 30 ans de retard à la chirurgie thoracique en s'opposant à la ventilation à pression positive qui non seulement ètait connue elle aussi dès l'Antiquité mais était aussi utilisée en clinique depuis la moitié du 19e siècle. Une fois la ventilation à pression positive bien établie, il a encore fallu attendre de pouvoir pratiquer une transfusion sanguine en toute sécurité, donc les traveux de Landsteiner (1900, 1940) et d'avoir à sa disposition les antibiotiques découvert par Chain, Florey et Waksmann durant les années 40. Les techniques et l'instrumentation furent alors mises au point et permirent dès lors, en toute sécurité, le traitement chirurgical de routine de certains organes spécifiques du thorax.

If it is well with your belly, chest and feet,
the wealth of kings can give you nothing more.
Horace, Epistles

A historical perspective on the development of paediatric thoracic surgery, by necessity, encompasses the fields of anatomy, pathology, pulmonary physiology, paediatrics, anaesthesiology and surgery as well as the development of the underwater seal bottle, the endotracheal tube and positive pressure ventilation. The author, due to time constraints alone, has had to depend upon "authoritative" sources for much information. These include well-recognized books by Lew Hochberg [15], Richard Meade [21, 22], Fielding Garrison [12] and Arturo Castiglioni [6]. The chapter on historical development by John Perkins in the *Handbook of Physiology on Respiration* [29] and the many review articles [4, 9, 10, 13, 19, 26, 32] were most helpful. Citations, conflicts in dates and accuracy of quotes were confirmed through Leslie Morton's A Medical Bibliography [24] and researched to their origins when possible.

Although thoracic surgery was an offspring of the technological development of this present century, its roots may be traced to aboriginal times. Paleopathology has provided evidence that prehistoric man suffered many of the ills which afflict his more modern brethren. Human fossil remains showed evidence of tuberculosis of the thoracic spine (Pott's disease) as well as rib fractures (with callus formation). Unfortunately, the decomposition of the soft tissues has erased any record of intrathoracic wounds which early man was certainly capable of inflicting upon one another. It is safe to conjecture that even the most primitive mind would eventually correlate the rhythmic movement of the chest with life itself and that the cessation of movement signalled the departure of life. It is therefore not surprising that early man attributed a religious connotation to the contents of the chest and considered it the seat of the soul [15]. Egyptian hieroglyphics of the First Dynasty (ca. 3000 B.C.) demonstrated knowledge of the anatomical forms of the heart, great vessels, trachea and lungs which was gained from the practice of embalming. In the *Edwin Smith Surgical Papyrus,* remedies for fractures of the clavicle and sternum were given. While internal thoracic injuries were alluded to, they were relegated to the verdict of untreatable [5]:

If thou examinest a man having a break in the ribs of his breast, over which a wound has been inflicted; [and] thou findest that the ribs of his breast crepitate under thy finger,... Thou shouldst say concerning him: "One having a break in the ribs of his breast, over which a wound has been inflicted. An ailment not to be treated."

These accounts of examination followed by diagnosis and decision of therapy demonstrate the earliest recorded examples of deductive reasoning. Early recordings of the Far East assigned not only a physiological role to the act of breathing but also a philosophical character. The Chinese of 2000 B.C. recommended *lien chi'i* or proper breathing in order to transform the vital nature of the air into the seed of the soul [23]. Anaximenes (570-500 B.C.), of Miletus in Asia Minor of the sixth century B.C., thought that the nucleus of all living things was the air and breathing or "pneuma" was fundamental to all life: "As our soul, being air, sustain us, so pneuma and air pervade the whole world" [29].

The initial phase in man's understanding of respiration encompassed the knowledge of static and dynamic anatomy. As early as the mid-400's B.C., Empedocles (504-443 B.C.) of Sicily theorized the ebb tide of blood flow to and from the heart. Respiration was thought to take place not only in the lungs but also through the entire skin surface. As with his predecessors, philosophy was integrated with physiology and Empedocles believed that the "inner heat" or soul was distributed through the body by the blood. Matter was thought to be composed of four essential elements: earth, air, fire and water. A contemporary of Empedocles, Diogenes of Appollonia, contributed one of the first orderly descriptions of the vascular system. Even though Diogenes knew of the pulse, he thought that air was carried by the blood vessels [29].

Rudimentary knowledge of the consequences of impaired respiratory function was begun in the Hippocratic era (ca.460-360 B.C.). While classic descriptions such as phthisis and physical diagnostic signs of succussion splash and the pleural friction rub were established, superstition remained dominant. Disease was based upon the imbalance of the four humours: blood, yellow bile, black bile and phlegm. A notable exception was the drainage of empyema. At a time when surgery was looked upon with suspicion, the evacuation of pus from the chest was not only accepted, it was almost obligatory: "Patients attainted with hydropsy or empyema, who are not very promptly relieved of fluid or pus collections, will succumb, unless iron or fire [scalpel or cautery] be applied". Once the chest was opened, the wound was packed with linen or cotton cloth to allow egress of the pus and to prevent the entrance of air. The following passage is found in De morbis written after the death of Hippocrates [2]:

The patient should be seated in a chair, his arms firmly pinioned by assistants: Grasping his shoulders, his body should be vigorously shaken while the surgeon's ear is applied to the chest, so that he may judge of the location of the fluid collection from the sound induced by the displacement thereof... He must beforehand mark out the limits of the wound he intends to make, least while cutting, the skin be displaced and his hand and eye deceived. The incision should be made with a large bistouri, but when the instrument has cut through the skin, a pointed lancet is to be substituted, the better to penetrate the soft parts. The edge of the instrument should be so guarded as to lay bare no more tissue than the width of a man's thumb nail. After a certain portion of the pus has been permitted to run out, there should be introduced a tent or seton of raw flax with a thread attached. This thread must be used two or three times a day to draw out the seton, to permit exit of the retained fluid.

After two days all that remains to the contained pus must be evacuated, a plug of linen cloth placed in the opening and because the lung, long used to the presence of the fluid, must not be too rapidly relieved, the emptied cavity should be partly filled with a mixture of wine and oil, introduced through a cannula.

The drainage technique certainly antedated Hippocrates, but its origin is lost to history. Existing side by side with the analytical Hippocratic method was the belief that the heart was the seat of the inner heat and the lungs were used to cool this torrid organ. The atria acted as bellows to bring cooling air from the lungs to the ventricles via the pulmonary artery and veins. Plato (427-347 B.C.) ascribed to these views and wrote in his Timaeus: "As the heart might be easily raised to too high a temperature by hurtful irritation, the genii placed the lungs in its neighborhood, which adhere to it and fill the cavity of the thorax, in order that their air vessels might moderate the great heat of that organ, and reduce the vessels to an exact obedience". Plato's most distinguished pupil, Aristotle (384-322 B.C.) furthered the misconception of the vascular transport of air through animal experimentation. In preparing for dissection, Aristotle would starve an animal until it was literally so thin that its blood vessels stood out. The animal would then be killed by strangulation (one can safely assume there was not a Greek *Handbook of Animal Care*). The effect of asphyxia would of course cause massive venous congestion and leave the arterial vascular system nearly devoid of blood. This was thought by Aristotle to support the concept of air being carried through the arterial system.

However, it was the views of Galen (129-200 A.D.) that influenced the study of respiration far longer than any other man. Born in Pergamum, Asia Minor, Galen became physician to the gladiators at the age of 18 years. After studying medicine at Smyrna, Corinth and Alexandria, he became physician to emperor Marcus Aurelius. His writings on anatomy and physiology were prodigious, with four works specifically focused on respiration: Whether Blood Is Contained in the Arteries in Nature, On the Value of Respiration, On the Causes of Respiration, and On the Function of the Pulse. Galen's physiological-philosophical hypothesis involved the passage of blood from the right ventricle through invisible pores of the interventricular septum into the left. In the left ventricle the blood is mixed with "pneuma" or world spirit which is then conducted throughout the body. Galen showed experimentally that the vascular system contained blood only, and not air, by cutting the exposed left ventricle and a section of an artery which had been tied between ligatures. It was indeed unfortunate that Galen did not extend his reasoning to the understanding of the recirculation of blood. He was actually quite close in this realization as he wrote in The Uses of the Parts: "In the whole body the arteries communicate with the veins and exchange air and blood with them by means of extremely fine, invisible openings". However, Galen's concept of the ebb and flow of blood held sway until the sixteenth century. It should be noted that Ibn An-Nafis of the thirteenth century, without experimentation and only with the writings of Galen, deduced that blood flowed from the right side of the heart to the left via the lungs and not through "invisible" interventricular pores. Unfortunately, his thoughts as well as those of other men of science and learning were buried in the stagnant era of the Dark Ages [29].

With the fall of Constantinople to the Ottoman Turks in 1453, men of science, arts and letters fled from Asia Minor to Europe. This act coupled with the invention of printing by Gutenberg established the period of the revival of learning, the Renaissance. Of particular interest to the pulmonary sciences of this time were the works of Vesalius, Servetius and Harvey. Andreas Vesalius (1514–1564) was born in Brussels, studied medicine in Paris under Jacobus Sylvius and at the age of 23 years became professor of surgery and anatomy at Padua. His early works were a recapitulation of Galenic thought. However, through careful dissection of the human body (versus Galen who derived anatomy from animal dissections), Vesalius corrected many of the anatomical errors of Galen including Adam's missing rib, the five-lobed liver, the bicornate uterus, the seven-segmented sternum, the double bile ducts and the interventricular pores. His De Humani Corporis Fabrica Libri Septem published in 1543 contained a very accurate representation of the heart and the pulmonary vessels. Many modern anatomists consider Vesalius' anatomical plates the finest ever cut. Yet, his anti-Galenic writings were nearly considered heretic. Vesalius was condemned by his contemporaries, labelled a madman by his former teacher and driven from his academic position 1 year after the publication of the Fabrica. He then assumed the lucrative but rather boring position of physician-in-ordinary to Emperor Charles V and later to King Philip II of Spain. Tragically, Vesalius was later offered his former position at Padua (upon the death of Fallopio) but died on the island of Zante on his sea voyage home [12]. As noted earlier, Ibn An-Nafis hypothesized the passage of blood through the lungs but did little to promote his theory. The same tenet was supported by Michael Servetus (1509–1553), a fellow student of Vesalius. In 1553, Servetus privately printed 1000 copies of his book, Christianismi Restitutio, a religious book of Unitarian views containing the following passage:

> ...this communication is made not through the middle wall of the heart, as is commonly believed, but by a very ingenious arrangement the subtle blood is urged forward by a long course through the lungs;...

He made no suggestion as to what the arrangement was nor to the possibility of recirculation. Lamentably for Servetus, his Unitarian views and his book did not fare as well as Vesalius. Servetus was declared a heretic by the Catholics and Protestants and he and most copies of his work were together burned at the stake (Fig. 1). Andreas Caesalpinus, professor of medicine at Pisa, coined the term "circulation", and stated in 1571 that the blood flowed from the vena cava into the right heart then through the pulmonary artery and vein into the left heart. Unfortunately, the ebb tide concept still held sway and Caesalpinus believed that blood also flowed from the heart into the pulmonary vein and vena cava [29].

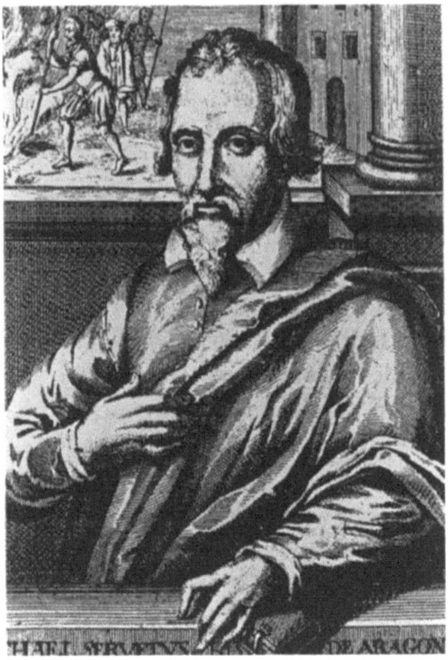

Fig. 1. Michael Servetus (1511–1553), Spanish theologian and anatomist, described the pulmonary circulation. He was burned at the stake for his Unitarian views

In 1603, Hieronymus Fabricius ab Aquapendente (1537–1619), the great Paduan anatomist, published his book, De Venarum Ostiolis, and described the venous valves. He did not fully understand their function and thought they simply slowed the flow of blood to the periphery. Fortuitously, for the 2 years prior to the publication of Fabricius' book, there was a student at Padua named William Harvey (1578–1657). After studying at Caius College, Cambridge, and at Padua with Fabricius, Harvey returned to London and established himself as a physician and later a lecturer on anatomy for the Royal College of Physicians. On 17 April, 1616, he delivered a lecture stating [29]:

It is plain from the structure of the heart that the blood is passed continuously through the lungs to the aorta as by two clacks of a water bellows to raise water. it is shown by the application of a ligature that the passage of the blood is from the arteries into the veins. Then it follows that the movement of the blood is constantly in a circle, and is brought about by the beat of the heart.

Learning quantitative methodology from his Paduan contemporary, Galileo, Harvey used mathematical proof to show that the volume ejected by the heart in 30 min exceeded the blood volume of the entire person and therefore concluded that the blood flow is not only continuous in one direction but also recirculates. Harvey formally published his theory in De Motu Cordis, in 1628, a book considered by some historians as the most important in the history of medicine [16].

Although Harvey hypothesized the passage of blood from the pulmonary artery into the pulmonary vein, he did not realize the existence of the capillaries. In addition, knowledge of chemistry and physics was exceedingly primitive and thus pulmonary function was unexaminable. By the turn of the sixteenth century, Dutch spectacle makers, particularly Hans Jansen, had constructed the compound microscope. Marcello Malpighi (1628–1694), of Bologna and Pisa, utilized the newly developed microscope and examined the tissues of the frog lung. He published his findings in 1661, which consisted of two letters sent to his friend, G. A. Borelli, professor of mathematics at Pisa, under the title, Duae Epistolae de Pulmonibus. Malpighi clearly demonstrated that the air channels from the trachea branched until it ended in the alveoli [29]:

...I have discovered that the whole mass of the lung to which are attached the excurrent vessels, is an aggregate of very thin fine membranes which, stretched and folded, form an almost infinite number of orbicular bladders... These have such partition and connection that passage is provided from the trachea into them.

In the second letter, Malpighi described the capillary system:

My doubt was changed into certainty by the dried lung of a frog... by the help of our more perfect glass, there met the eye... vessels joined together in a ring-like fashion. And such is the wandering about of these vessels, as they proceed on this side from the vein and on the other side from the artery, that the vessels no longer maintain a straight direction, but there appears a network made up of the articulations of the blood flowed away along tortuous vessels and was not poured into spaces, but was always contained within tubules...

One should bear in mind that Malpighi preceded the Micrographia of Robert Hooke by 4 years and the Ontledingen en ontdekkingen of von Leeuwenhoek by 24 years. He also described the presence of red corpuscles in the blood. Unfortunately, Malpighi never grasped the purpose of the alveoli's intimate relationship to the arborized capillaries, which was understandably due to a lack of knowledge regarding the chemistry and physics of gases.

In 1660, Robert Boyle (1627–1691) and Robert Hooke (1635–1703) initiated a series of experiments which consisted of removing air from a chamber containing a flame or various small animals. The extinguishment of the flame as well as the lives of the animals led them to the conclusion that combustion and respiration were related and the purpose of respiration was to rid the body of waste substances. Hooke dramatically demonstrated his theory by utilizing artificial respiration with bellows (a technique previously used by Leonardo da Vinci and Vesalius) in a dog whose chest was opened with its ribs and diaphragm removed [29]:

This being continued for a pretty while, the Dog, as I expected, lay still, as before, his eyes being all the time very quick, and his Heart beating very regularly. But, upon ceasing this blast, and suffering the lungs to fall and lye still, the Dog would immediately fall into Dying convulsive fits; but he as soon reviv'd again by the renewing the fulness of his Lungs with the constant blast of fresh Air...

Towards the latter end of this Experiment a piece of the Lung was cut quite off where 'twas observable, that the Blood did freely circulate, and pass thorow the Lungs, not only when the Lungs were kept thus constantly extended, but also when they were suffer'd to subside and lye still. Which seem to be Arguments, that as the bare Motion of the Lungs without fresh Air contributes nothing to the life of the Animal, he being found to survive as well, when they were not mov'd, as when they were; so it was not the subsiding or movelessness of the Lungs, that was the immediate cause of Death, or the stopping of the Circulation of the Blood through the Lungs, but the want of a sufficient supply of fresh Air.

Unfortunately, at the end of the seventeenth century, the phlogiston (Greek *phlogistos* = burnt, inflammable) theory of Georg Ernst Stahl became dominant and retarded respiratory chemistry for nearly a century. This doctrine stated that every combustible substance was a compound of phlogiston and the phenomena of combustion were due to the liberation of phlogiston with the other constituent left as a residue. For example, alkalies as quicklime were produced by heating limestone, which according to the prevailing dogma, took up phlogiston and gained weight in transformation. In 1754, Joseph Black published his MD dissertation entitled Experiments on Magnesia Alba, Quicklime, and Some Other Alkaline Substances. While studying medicine at Glasgow under Dr. William Cullen, Black found that limestone or chalk lost weight upon heating which was in opposition to the phlogiston theory. He believed the weight loss was due to the loss of air (i.e. gas) and called it "fixed air", which was, of course, carbon dioxide. He further showed that this "fixed air", which could extinguish both flame and life, was a product of respiration. In the 1770s Joseph Priestley, a Unitarian minister, produced oxygen be heating mercurius calcinatus per se (mercuric oxide) which floated on top of mercury in a glass vessel inverted in a basin of the same liquid:

But what surprised me more than I can yet well express, was that a candle burned in this air with a remarkably vigorous flame... and a piece of red-hot wood sparkled in it.

However, Priestley and his independent co-discoverer of oxygen, Carl Wilhelm Scheele, both supported the phlogiston theory.

The honor of understanding respiration and combustion, of overthrowing the phlogiston theory, of initiating the study of metabolism and of coining the term "oxygine" belonged to Antoine Laurent Lavoisier (Fig. 2). Over a period of 10 years and through a series of elegant experiments which was read in 1775 to the Paris Academy of Sciences as the Mémoire, Lavoisier carefully showed that air contained an "eminently respirable air" (oxygen), a "fixed air" (carbon dioxide) of Black and finally a "mephitic portion" (nitrogen). With his mathematician colleague, P.S. Laplace, Lavoisier used an ice calorimeter to measure heat produced by animals and related to the amount of "fixed air" collected. Using Seguin's method of gas analysis and Seguin as the experimental subject, Lavoisier showed that oxygen use was temperature, food intake and exercise dependent. In 1779, he authored the Elements of Chemistry, which included 33 elements and formed the foundation of modern chemistry. Tragically, Lavoisier had joined the Ferme Général early in his career in order to fund his work. The Ferme Général was a form of internal revenue service in which members paid the king for the right to tax the people. Abuse of the taxation privilege by some of Lavoisier's predecessors led to his being charged in common with them and in 1794, after the French Revolution, Lavoisier was beheaded by the guillotine. Of his friend, Lagrange said: "It took but a second to cut off his head; a hundred years will not suffice to produce one like it" [29].

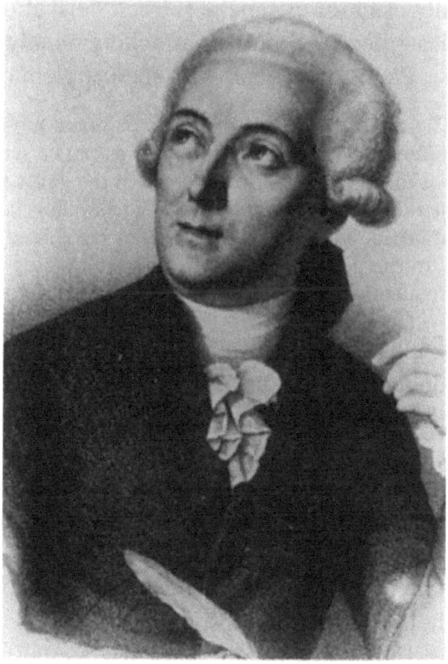

Fig. 2. Antoine Laurent Lavoisier (1743–1794), physiologist and chemist, described the component gases of respiration, coined the term "oxygine", studied metabolism, authored the Elements of Chemistry and died by the guillotine

If one views the advancements in the fields of anatomy and physiology as sluggish, progress in the thoracic surgical arena must then surely appear as a snail's pace. A representative attitude is found in the writings of Aurelius Cornelius Celsus, who lived in the times of Tiberius Caesar (ca. 14-37 A.D.): "... as soon as the knife really penetrates to the chest,... the man loses his life at once". Incidentally, Celsus was not a physician, but rather, as described by Garrison: "a private gentleman of the noble family of Cornelii who, like Cato and Varro, compiled or, more probably, translated encyclopedic treatises on medicine, agriculture, and other subjects for the benefit of the Admirable Crichtons of his own station in life" [12]. Thus, thoracic surgery remained limited to surface procedures including poultices and binding of externally displaced rib fractures and the drainage of empyemas. Of note, however, were the teachings of Antyllus, a contemporary of Galen, describing the procedure of tracheotomy:

...in inflammation about the mouth and palate, and in cases of indurated tonsils which obstruct the mouth of the windpipe as the trachea is unaffected, it will be proper to have recourse to pharyngotomy, in order to avoid the risk of suffocation. When, therefore, we engage in the operation we slit open a part of the arteria aspera (trachea) (for it is dangerous to divide the whole) below the top of the windpipe, about the third or fourth ring. For this is a convenient situation, as being free of flesh, and because the vessels are placed at a distance from the part which is divided.

Antyllus' method was quoted in the sixth book of Paulus Ægineta (625-690 A.D.), last of the Byzantine physicians. Paulus' Seven Books were translated from the Greek by Francis Adam in 1846. Adam commented that pharyngotomy was usually used for cynanche (Greek derivation – a bad kind of sore throat), which was described by Pollux as attacking mostly children, perhaps meaning croup.

Paulus also dealt with the problem of foreign bodies of the esophagus [1]:

> Thorns, or the bones of fishes, or other substances, are often swallowed in eating, and fix in different places. Wherefore, such as can be seen are to extract with the forceps for that purpose; but those which are lower down in the gullet we must manage differently. Some are of opinion that the patient ought to be made to swallow large morsels, such as the stalk of lettuces, or pieces of bread; but others direct us to bind a thread about a small piece of clean soft sponge and give it to the patient to swallow, and then taking hold of the thread to draw it up, and to do this frequently in order that the thorn may get fixed in the sponge and be brought up.

Paulus Ægineta may be looked upon as the last of the Greek and Latin school of medicine. The Dark Ages, heralded by the fall of the Roman Empire, were to inhibit the advancement of surgery and science for nearly 10 centuries. The medicine and surgery of the period were merely imitations of earlier works with minuscule original thought. Ruggiero Frugardi (Roger of Palermo) did write of attempts to remove broken sword blades which lodged in the thorax, but not aggressivley: "... if it is concealed beneath the ribs, open the intercostal space and dilate it with a wedge; if open in this way and it is not possible to extract the metal, then abandon it" [15].

Even with the dawn of the Renaissance, very little was immediately accomplished in the field of thoracic surgery and even less so in paediatric surgery or in general paediatric care. One must recall that a child's life of the fifteenth to the eighteenth centuries meant very little. Infanticide and abandonment were common. Waifs relegated to charitable institutions were often drugged. Children were purposefully deformed to advance their sympathetic appeal as beggars. Child labour laws were virtually unheard of. Paediatric surgical treatises were limited to the Cerrahiyei Ilhaniye of Sabuncuoglu written in 1465 and the The Children's Book of Felix Wurtz in 1612. The former dealt with surface procedures and the latter was little more than common sense advice in the prevention of orthopaedic deformities [7].

However, general surgery was advancing, albeit slowly, which eventually would allow progress in thoracic surgery. Of singular note was a reference to the case of Rolandus in 1499 in which lung tissue was removed [15]:

> Called to a citizen of Bologna on the sixth day after his wound, I found a portion of the lung issued between two ribs; the afflux of the spirits and humours had determined such a swelling of the part, that it was not possible to reduce it. The compression exercised by the ribs retained its nutriment from it, and it was so mortified that worms had been developed in it. They had brought together the most skillfull chirurgeons of Bologna, who, judging the death of the patient to be inevitable, had abandoned him. But I, yielding to his prayers, and to those of his parents and his friends, and having obtained the leave of the Bishop, the master, and the man himself, I yielded to the solicitations of about thirty of my pupils and made an incision through the skin, the breadth of my little finger-nail away from the wound, all round it. Then, with a cutting instrument, I removed all the portion of the lung level with my incision. The wound resulting from this resection was closed by the blood issuing from my incision, and was dressed frequently with red powder and other adjuvants. By the grace of God it cicatrised, and recovery took place. It is true that one had to wait long for it. The patient, with his master Rolandini, has since made the voyage to Jerusalem, and has returned in good health.

As any thoughtful surgeon would, Rolandus theorized what he would have done if he had seen the wound initially:

> If you ask me what I should have done in this case, if I had been called to it at once, I answer that I should have dilated the wound with a small piece of wood, keeping the lung warm with a cock or a fowl split down the back, and should then have reduced it, and kept the wound open till the portion of lung was wholly mortified.

It was fortunate for both the patient and the cock that Rolandus was not consulted until the 6th day.

From this time forward, the progression of thoracic surgery was dependent upon three mechanical problems: prevention of pneumothorax, maintenance of respiratory function during open chest procedures and technical surgical innovations.

It was well recognized from the time of Hippocrates that air introduced into the chest usually resulted in the demise of the patient. The most common situations resulting in pneumothorax were war injuries or iatrogenic injuries during empyema drainage. The greatest surgeon of the Renaissance, Ambroise Paré (1510–1590), encountered both circumstances while in Italy as master barber (army surgeon) in the ill-fated army of Francis the First of France. He carefully distinguished between the symptoms and signs of injuries to the chest wall, lung, heart and diaphragm. Paré recommended the closure of clean chest wounds which did not result in a significant haemothorax. Drainage of substantial amounts of blood in the chest was advised particularly if associated with infection. Paré also promoted the use of pleural irrigation as Syrupus de rosis siccu and mel rosarum and of pleural drainage by the use of "pipes of gold, silver or lead" in the much dreaded complication of a bronchopleural fistula. The irrigants were administered into the pleural cavity by means of a "syringe". His innovation of the use of ligature to arrest arterial haemorrhage and his condemnation of the use of boiling oil for gunshot wounds and cautery for haemorrhage founded a new school of surgery based on clinical observation and logical deduction rather than a reliance on superstition and fallacious doctrines. Paré's aphorism that war was the greatest school of surgery certainly held true over the next 350 years [14]. The use of air guns during the Napoleonic Wars (1782–1812) and the development of gunpowder-directed trajectories brought a new dimension to injuries of the chest.

Although Hippocrates had suggested the use of the trocar for the evacuation of empyemas, its use was not popularized until the 1700s. Even then, surgeons continued to argue for the use of the knife versus the cautery to accomplish thoracic drainage. However, the concept that trapped air (tension pneumothorax) may itself be an affliction was introduced. This was exemplified in the writings of Matthaeus Gothofredus Purmannus in 1694 [15]:

> Paracentesis (Greek para – through; kentein – to pierce) is an incision made with large Lancet in the hollow part of the Breast... Many as well Ancient as Modern Authors, are utterly against this Operation in any case whatsoever, and say, that it never effected any thing, but only increased the Patient's Pain and Torment;... but I suppose its only because they never experienced it, or don't understand the use and benefit of it. For my part, I can truly say, that I have had the

Tryal of it many and many times, especially in the Camp, and that with the greatest Success Imaginable; for in Wounds of the Breast, where the patient is almost suffocated and ready to yield up his Life, the Opening of the Breast, in a Minutes time will Snatch him from the Brink of the Grave.

Hermann Boerhaave perhaps recorded the first case of pneumothorax without trauma in 1724. His patient, Baron de Wassenaer, a famous Dutch admiral, died after a paroxysm of coughing. At autopsy, he was found to have a ruptured oesophagus and a large amount of air in the pleural cavity with a collapsed lung [17].

The purposeful introduction of air into the thoracic cavity dated to Hippocratic times and was used to relieve pain of pleuritic origin. By the middle of the 1700s, pneumothorax was introduced for the "rest" treatment of tuberculosis [15, 21, 22]. This was also an era rich in pathological descriptions culminating in the 1761 publication of the De Sedibus, et Causis Morborum per Anatomen Indagatis libri Quinque by Giovanni Battista Morgangni (1682–1771). Virtually every aliment known to man was described, including pneumothorax [3]:

A tailor, of twenty years of age, was wounded by a foreigner, for a reason of very little consequence, by a double-edg'd and pretty broad knife... enter'd the lower side of the right cavity of the thorax, ... after an hour, or a little more... he died... when the thorax was open'd, ſome quantity of blood was found in the cavity on that ſide; and the lobe of the lungs therein was drawn upwards to a conſiderable degree.

For this lobe was every-where unconnected to the pleura; whereas the left lobe was connected thereto anteriorly, and at the ſide, but particularly on the back-part. Beſides theſe things, there was nothing either in the thorax, or in the belly, that deſerves to be taken notice of here.

Clearly, Morgagni did not understand the significance of his observation.

Aspiration therapy, paracentesis, for pneumothorax was first advocated by Alexander Munro (1697–1767) in 1761 and published by his pupil, William Hewson (1739–1774) in 1767. Hewson produced penetrating wounds of the chest wall and lungs of animals and correctly concluded that lung collapse and not lung injury was the cause of the symptoms [27]. This was remarkable considering Laennec's stethoscope was 51 years from invention.

The term pneumothorax was first applied to a collection of gas in the thoracic cavity by Jean E. Itard in 1803. While many physicians and surgeons encountered the situation, therapy was by no means uniform. Again, war was instrumental in the direction of therapy. Barron Dominique Jean Larrey, Napoleon's surgeon, wrote in his Mémoirs [21]:

... a soldier was brought to the hospital of the Fortress of Ibrahym Bey, immediately after a wound penetrated the thorax, between the fifth and sixth true ribs. It was about 8 cm in extent. A large quantity of frothy and vermilion blood escaped from it with a hissing noise at each inspiration. His extremities were cold, pulse scarcely perceptible, countenance discoloured, and respiration short and laborous; in short, he was every moment threatened with a fatal suffocation. After having examined the wound, the divided edges of the part, I immediately approximated the two lips of the wound, and retained them by means of adhesive plaster, and a suitable bandage around the body. In adopting this plan, I intended only to hide from the sight of the patient and his comrades, the distressing spectacle of a hemorrhage, which would soon prove fatal; and I therefore thought that the effusion of blood into the cavity of the thorax, could not increase the danger. But the wound was scarcely closed, when he breathed more freely, and felt easier. The heat of the body soon returned, and the pulse rose. In a few hours, he became quite calm, and to my great surprise, grew better. He was cured in a very few days, and without difficulty.

Experimental physiology was certainly not prevalent during the early 1800s. A notable exception was the studies of James Carson starting on 27 August 1817 and reported to the Royal Society. Carson opened one side of the animal's chest and found: "As soon... as the cavity has been opened, and the external surface of the lungs exposed to the contact of the circumambient air, these organs shrink into dimensions far less extensive than those which they occupied in the living body". He discovered that opening one side of the chest resulted in restlessness but the animal survived. Simultaneous opening of both sides of the chest resulted in death. Carson concluded [15]:

...there can be no doubt...that one of the lungs of an animal may be reduced to a state of collapse with perfect impunity. This was a priori indeed to be presumed, as in all other cases in which animals are supplied with double organs, one of these organs may be removed or rendered unfit for the discharge of its function without destroying or materially injuring the animal.

By the latter part of the 1800s, the majority of chest wounds were closed but were reopened at any sign of respiratory distress from the accumulation of intrathoracic blood. Also at this time, Bromfield reported the insertion of a cannula through the chest wall to allow escape of trapped intrapleural air after a traumatic pneumothorax. It is difficult to understand why paracentesis was not widely practised as sharp-pointed trocars had been available since antiquity.

During the Civil War, John Shaw Billings, principal founder of the Library of the Surgeon General, recorded that assistant surgeon, A.H. Smith, devised a valve which allowed for the egress of blood and other fluids from the chest but prevented the entrance of air. The valve, made from a piece of intestine, was placed in the centre of a circular piece of leather. Used in cases of collapsed lung, this valve would allow for the escape of air and the re-expansion of the lung [15].

In the latter half of the nineteenth century, closed drainage of empyemas by trocar and cannula became commonplace. James Carson secundus devised a closed drainage system capable of irrigation of the chest. Airtight trocars were invented and promoted by distinguished surgeons, as reported by Henry Ingersol Bowditch (who also wrote a most learned treatise on diaphragmatic hernias): "Since my last article on Thoracentesis, I have been more confirmed than ever in my belief of the importance of this operation as a remedial measure, to be used not as a last resource, but like any other simple remedy, if necessary at any period of disease". In 1863, he reported that 21 of 26 patients with serous effusions and 7 of 24 with empyemas recovered. By 1869, the Frenchman Potain had devised a trocar and cannula which was attached to a reservoir and an aspirating syringe [31]. The negative intrapleural pressure facilitated the egress of the intrapleural fluids. Finally, in 1872, Playfair of England modified the closed intercostal system of drainage into an underwater seal apparatus [30] (Fig. 3):

The procedure is nearly as simple as ordinary paracentesis, and the necessary apparatus is so inexpensive as to be within the reach of every one. All that is required is about six inches of ordi-

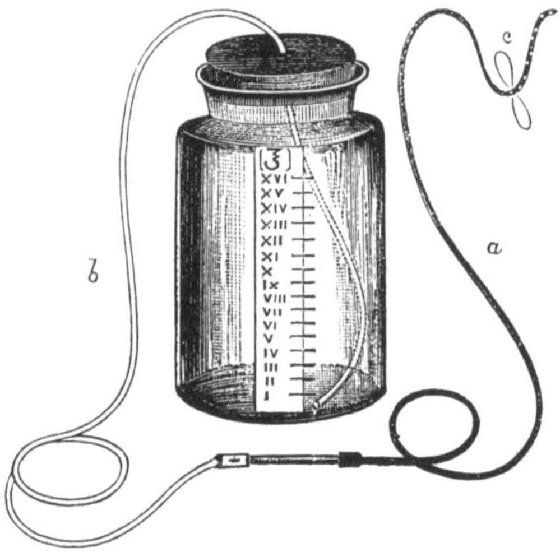

Fig. 3. W. S. Playfair's 1872 underwater drainage bottle. See text for explanation

nary fine drainage tubing (a) and about six feet of ordinary caoutchouc tubing (b). These are attached to each other by about an inch of glass tubing, over each end of which one extremity of the tube is passed. The free extremity of the drainage tube lies within the cavity of the pleura; that of the india rubber tube passes through a perforated cork into a bottle half filled with water... The mode of using the apparatus is as follows: In a case of suspected empyema a puncture is made with an exploring needle to determine the fact of the contained fluid being purulent. For this purpose nothing is better than the ordinary syringe for subcutaneous injection, which resembles a pneumatic aspirator in miniature. Should it prove to be so, a trocar is passed, the cannula of which is of sufficient size to admit of the passage of the drainage tube. As soon as there is free flow of pus this is passed into the pleural cavity through the cannula, which is then withdrawn over it. An assistant now pinches the tubing closed to its entrance into the chest to stop the flow of pus through it until the other end of the drainage tube is attached to the small piece of glass tubing. The pus is now allowed to flow into the bottle of water and the drainage tube is attached to the chest by passing around it a loop of wire (c) which is fixed by strapping. The tube remains permanently in the pleural cavity, and any pus that is formed drains away at once.

The next stage in the development of thoracic surgery, and perhaps the most impeding, was the evolution of ventilatory control of an open chest. As mentioned before, da Vinci, Vesalius as well as Hooke had maintained the respiration of animals through a tracheostomy utilizing positive pressure either by mouth or by means of a bellows. This technique was used repeatedly through the centuries in animal experiments. Its physiological principles were clearly elaborated by Meltzer's work, The Respiratory Changes of the Intrathoracic Pressure, published in 1892. Tracheostomy in humans had also been known since the time of Galen and its successful use was reported in 1546 by Musa Brasavola, in 1620 by Nicolas Habicot, in 1730 by George Martin for diphtheria, in 1743 by Vigili and in 1833 by Armand Trousseau. Endotracheal intubation, with a leather nasotracheal tube, was reported to have been used as early as 1800 by Fine, in Geneva. Dessault successfully used nasotracheal intubation for the treatment of glottic edema in 1801. A metal tube was even devised by Chaussier for the resuscitation of new-

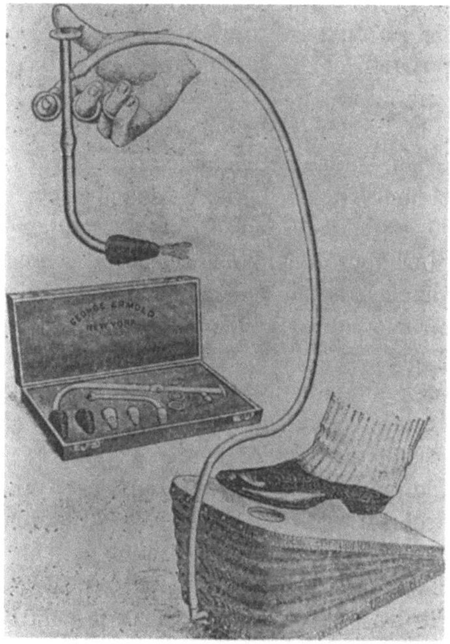

Fig. 4. Joseph O'Dwyer's 1887 laryngeal intubation apparatus. The bellow was a later addition

borns in 1806. The need to develop a means of maintaining airway patency other than tracheostomy, which carried a significant mortality, was due to the diphtheric croup epidemic of the mid-1800s. This was accomplished by the endotracheal tube through the successful therapeutic results of Bouchut in 1851, MacEwen in 1879 and O'Dwyer in 1885 [15]. Joseph O'Dwyer's article, "Fifty cases of croup in private practice treated by intubation of the larynx, with a description of the method and of the dangers incident thereto", was reported in *The Medical Record* (New York) of 1887. O'Dwyer wrote that his previous experinece of 65 operative cases resulted in 9 survivors or 14%. This report of 50 patients with intubation resulted in 12 survivors or 24%. His later intubation equipment included a bellow for positive pressure ventilation (Fig. 4) [28]. Trendelenburg, by 1871, devised an inflatable cuff on a tracheostomy cannula. In 1893, Fell, of Buffalo, devised an apparatus to maintain artificial respiration in patients with opium poisoning [10]. Yet, it was not until World War I, and even later in Germany, that the combination of endotracheal intubation and positive pressure ventilation were utilized in thoracotomies.

We shall digress for a moment to discuss the occurrence of three signal events which will impact on the development of thoracic surgery. By the end of the nineteenth century, two of the greatest developments in medical history occurred. The first was the development of anaesthesia. The techniques for the alleviation of pain were known to early man through the use of cold, wine, opium, henbane, hemlock and mandragora. Paracelsus, in 1540, while searching for such an agent, combined alcohol and sulphuric acid and noted that when the resulting mixture, which he called "sweet vitriol" (ether), was "taken in even by chickens,... they fall asleep from it for a while but awaken later without harm". Then in the finest tradition of the carnival barker, Paracelsus claimed that "it quiets all suffering without any harm, and relieves all pain, and quenches all fevers, and prevents complications in all illnesses". Humphrey Davy, in 1800, published a rather lengthy monograph entitled, Researches, chemical and philosophical; chiefly concerning nitrous oxide, or dephlogisticated nitrous air, and its respiration. Davy suggested its use in surgical operations: "As nitrous oxide in its extensive operation appears capable of destroying physical pain, it may probably be used with advantage during surgical operations in which no great effusion of blood takes place". However, the use of ether and nitrous oxide became great sport in the United States with "ether frolics" and "laughing-gas parties". The serious use of these anaesthetic agents began in January 1842 when William E. Clarke, then a student at Berkshire Medical College, administered ether on a towel to a young woman in order for dentist, Elijah Pope, to extract a tooth. Chronologically after Clarke, Crawford W. Long also used ether to painlessly remove a tumor from the neck of James A. Venable on 30 March 1842. Long did not publish his experiences with Venable and other patients until 1849. In December 1844, dentist Horace Wells used and publicized the use of nitrous oxide for tooth extractions. His attempt to anaesthetize a patient before Dr. John C. Warren of Harvard Medical School failed. However, Wells' former partner with whom he had shared his knowledge of the use of nitrous oxide was successful. On 16 October 1846, William Thomas Green Morton anaesthetized a patient for Warren, who then made a 3-inch incision and removed a tumour of the neck. Following this momentous milestone ensued a monumental melee to establish primacy and credit which even today is debated by historians [27].

The other significant event occurred in the discovery of first the antiseptic principles followed by the development of aseptic techniques and antibiotics. On 13 February 1843, Oliver Wendell Holmes (1809–1894) read his paper, On the Contagioousness of Puerperal Fever, to the Boston Society for Medical Improvement. He suggested that puerperal fever was transmitted from the dissecting room to the women in childbed by physicians' hands. Holmes did not vigorously pursue his view as did Ignaz Phillip Semmelweis (1818–1865) of Vienna. Not only did Semmelweis realize the contagiousness of puerperal fever, but he also recognized it to be a blood poisoning. Opposition to his precepts forced Semmelweis to leave Vienna for Budapest, where he became professor of obstetrics. In 1861, he published his classic work, The Cause, Concept, and prophylaxis of Puerperal Fever as well as his scathing retribution, Open Letters to Sundry Professors of Obstetrics. However, Semmelweis' constitution was not suited to controversy and resulted in his insanity and death [12]. In 1865, Joseph Lister (1827–1912), recognizing the importance of Pasteur's work, began to experiment with chemical antiseptics and fortuitously struck upon carbolic acid. It is well known that Lister was far from the first man to use carbolic acid, as it had been available on the Continent for many years. What he did was to use carbolic acid in a standardised, prescribed manner. On 12 August 1865, he employed it in a case of compound fracture with complete success. His 2 years' investigation was published in two papers, the latter of which bore the title, On the Antiseptic Principle in the Practice of Surgery [18]. While Lister's work significantly improved surgical outcomes, infection was still a very significant cause of morbidity and mortality. Visceral surgery was in its infancy and thoracic surgery was non-existent. It was not until the 1940s when Chain and Florey, and Waksman showed the effectiveness of penicillin and streptomycin, respectively, that invasive operative procedures surged in popularity [22].

The final achievement in support of successful thoracic surgery was the safe administration of blood. Bleeding by the lance or leeches had been practised since antiquity and some experimentation of animal to animal transfusions had been performed. On 15 June 1667, Jean Denys of France transfused lamb's blood into a 15-year-old boy. Five months later, Richard Lower and Edmund King of England transfused sheep's blood into a man. The complication of transfusion incompatibility was first recorded in one of Denys' adult patients: tachycardia, sweating, pain in the back and black urine. Another of Denys' later patients unfortunately died after a second transfusion. The patient's widow successfully sued Denys although it was later discovered that she had poisoned her spouse. Nevertheless, the adverse result led to the control of further transfusion by the Faculty of Medicine. An *arrèt* was then issued in 1670 forbidding transfusions altogether. The first documented man-to-man transfusion was reported by James Blundell of Guy's and St. Thomas' Hospitals in 1818. His patient, moribund from a long-standing pyloric obstruction, improved temporarily after receiving 12–14 ounces of blood. By 1829, Blundell's success rate was a remarkable 50%. However, it was not until 1900 and 1940 when Karl Landsteiner elaborated upon the presence of agglutinins, isoagglutinins and Rh factors in blood that transfusions were placed on a scientific and safe basis [22].

Returning now to the beginning of the twentieth century, the stage for the development of thoracic surgery was set. Anaesthesia, the endotracheal tube, antiseptic technique, underwater seal chest drainage and blood were available. However, the availability of thoracic surgery would wait another 30 years before erupting into its own glory. Extensive animal experimentation from the time of Vesalius and human endotracheal intubation had shown the feasibility of sustaining ventilation in an open chest. Today, every grade school child knows how to maintain ventilation by the cyclic inflation and spontaneous expiration of mouth to mouth resuscitation. Yet, this was not the path of thoracic surgery of the early 1900s. Comroe felt the delay was due to the discredit of one individual, Ernst Ferdinand Sauerbruch (1875–1951). Sauerbruch, while in the laboratory of Mikulicz, developed a negative chamber for thoracic surgery (1904). In this room, the patient, below his neck, and the entire operating team, were enclosed in a subatmospheric environment by means of vaccum pumps (Fig. 5a, b). Basically, Sauerbruch converted the entire room into the intrapleural space [8]. The practicality of such an operating suite was best described by Rudolf Nissen: "It was impossible to change the patient's position during operation without endangering the differential pressure; the surgeon and his assistants had very little room to

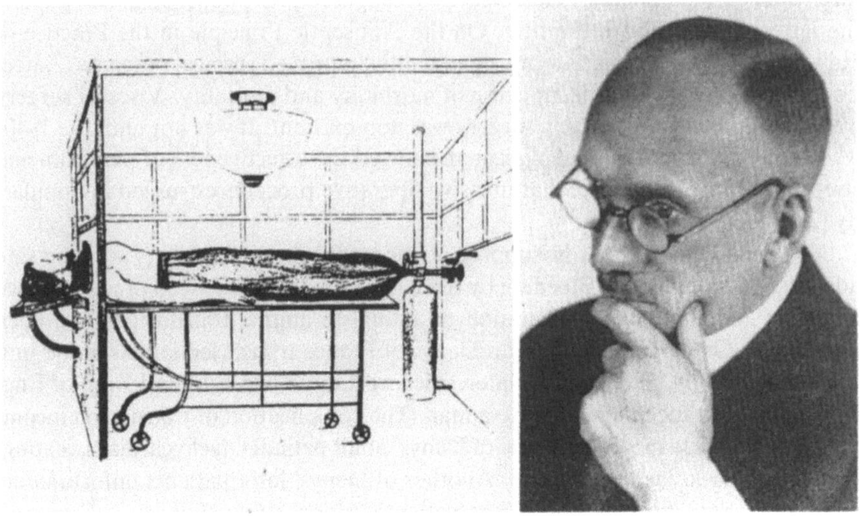

a b

Fig. 5. b Portrait of Ernst Ferdinand Sauerbruch (1875–1951); **a** the negative pressure operating chamber

move; the heat was almost unbearable; and, finally, it was extremely difficult to communicate satisfactorily with the anaesthetist outside the chamber" [26]. Today, it is still occasionally extremely difficult to communicate satisfactorily with the anaesthetist even in the same room. Bendixen opined that: "The dominant surgeons of that era chose to circumvent the need for endotracheal intubation, possibly because they did not wish to rely on any technique which they themselves had not mastered...They were not prepared to support the development of specialties or subspecialties" [4]. Sauerbruch's lack of flexibility and absolute authoritarian rule were seen in the reflections of Werner Forssmann, who had just published his paper on right heart catheterization:

> Every time I attempted to talk to the Old Man [about right heart catheterization] I got the feeling that independent thinking was regarded as a dangerous threat. This applied not only to scientific questions but also to problems with patients. An extraordinary inflexibility of thought reigned over the department, a rigid dogma based upon the teachings of Sauerbruch. Any divergent opinions were considered heresy...

After Forssmann mildly protested over Sauerbruch's statement, "You might lecture in a circus about your little tricks, but never in a respectable German university", Sauerbruch screamed, "Get out! Leave my department immediately" [11]. Forssmann did and in 1956 received the Nobel prize. Ironically, it was Forssmann's accomplishment which led to the flowering of cardiac surgery.

Unfortunately, Sauerbruch's reputation stimulated the chamber idea in America as well as in Europe. Willy Meyer's 1909 "Universal Negative Pressure Chamber", housed at the Rockefeller Institute in New York City reached near the pinnacle of absurdity. It was 1000 ft^3 in volume, containing 17 people including patient, surgeon, surgeon's assistants, visitors, an engineer and two anaesthetists, one of whom, along with the patient's head, were in a positive pressure chamber contained within the negative pressure room! [21]

Sauerbruch not only ignored his countrymen but also his colleagues from abroad. Rudolph Matas wrote in 1899 [20]:

> The procedure that promises the most benefit in preventing pulmonary collapse in operations on the chest is the artificial inflation of the lung and the rhythmical maintenance of artificial respiration by a tube in the glottis directly connected with a bellows. Like other discoveries, it is not only elemantary in its simplicity, but the fundamental ideas involved in this important suggestion have been lying idle before the eyes of the profession for years. It is curious that surgeons should have failed to apply for so long a time the suggestions of the physiological laboratory, where bellows and tracheal tubes have been in constant use from the days of Magendie (1783–1855) to the present, in practising artificial respiration on animals.

Although Sauerbruch significantly delayed thoracic surgery, the idea of the negative pressure chamber in support of respiration led to the development of the "iron lung" in the therapy of respiratory failure from poliomyelitis in the 1930s and 1940s [20].

World War I assisted the direction and development of positive pressure ventilation as it was cumbersome to set up negative pressure chambers at the front lines (except in Germany, where under Sauerbruch's influence they were still used in the 1930s). The early Meltzer-Auer technique involved a continuous positive pressure flow of compressed air via an endotracheal tube with air exiting between the tube and tracheal wall. Although neither CO_2 nor O_2 were ever measured, the authors claimed: "under these conditions the supply of oxygen and removal of carbon dioxide take place apparently in physiological fashion" [10, 27].

After 1930, anaesthesia and intermittent positive pressure controlled ventilation developed. One must appreciate the courage which our anaesthesiology colleagues embarked upon by controlling respiration. For nearly a century, anaesthesiologists had used spontaneous respiration as the indicator for the depth of anaesthesia. The present-day jocular response of "sign of life," upon complaint by the surgeon of patient movement, was indeed an accurate reflection of the near past. The use of muscle relaxants and narcotics led to the modern "balanced anaesthesia" [27]. Today, the paediatric anaesthesiologist is armed with an array of computerized gadgetry which monitors every conceivable parameter.

The final segment of this review will examine the development of a few specific techniques and equipment of the thoracic surgeon. As the seventeenth century was distinguished by advancements in static and dynamic anatomy, the eighteenth and nineteenth centuries were ones of pathological descriptions. Many perturbations of paediatric development discussed in this monograph were described; in chronological order:

1594 Bauhinus	– pectus excavatum
1670 Durston	– isolated oesophageal atresia
1687 Bartholinus	– pulmonary hamartoma
1696 Gibson	– esophageal atresia with tracheo-oesophageal fistula

1706 de Torres	– sternal cleft
1761 Morgagni	– substernal diaphragmatic hernia
	– congenital pulmonary agenesis
1810 Laennec	– pneumothorax; empyema
	– bronchiectasis
1828 Redenbacker	– cystic hygroma
1841 Poland	– deficient pectoralis major and minor and brachysyndactyly
1847 Morel-Lavallée	– congenital absence of ribs
1848 Bochdalek	– congenital diaphragmatic hernia
1854 Hess	– teratoma of neck

By the latter half of the nineteenth century, paediatrics, paediatric nursing and paediatric surgical care were on the ascent. Paediatrists, as they were then called, dedicated to the care of children were establishing specialty hospitals. The renowned Charles West established the Hospital for Sick Children (1852) in London and even appointed George Pollock as its inaugural paediatric surgeon. Unfortunately, this was a political appointment and Pollock left soon thereafter to pursue a more lucrative career. Other paediatrists, such as Rotch and Straus, were improving the nutritional and sanitary aspects of milk. Near the turn of the century, Tarnier had developed the incubator. Florence Nightingale was instituting standardized nurse training programmes and elevating nursing to a profession throughout England and abroad. In 1846, James Milman Coley wrote perhaps the first textbook of paediatric surgery entitled, Practical Treatise on the Diseases of Children. Finally, in 1895, Wilhelm Conrad Röentgen reported the discovery of the X-rays which within 1 year were used to diagnose foreign bodies and shortly thereafter in examining the gastrointestine and in the treatment of cancer [7, 34].

The treatment of the paediatric age group for various intrathoracic afflictions has been alluded to throughout this review. For example, W. S. Playfair's use of the underwater seal suction was in the treatment of empyema in children. He clearly showed that continuous underwater seal drainage not only obviated the risks of pneumothorax, but also eliminated the protracted illness and chest deformity of the older methods of repeated aspirations and of incision and open drainage [30].

Surgical treatment for pulmonary tuberculosis was attempted as early as 1822 by James Carson of Liverpool when he induced pneumothorax in order to collapse and "rest the lung". Thoracoplasty with rib resection was introduced by J. A. Estlander in 1879. This was followed by phrenic nerve cutting and later crushing in 1911 by C. A. E. Stuertz. After the development of lung resection in the 1940s, this mode of treatment became popular in adults and continued until the development of antituberculous drugs. DeForest Willard reported in his 1910 textbook on Surgery of Childhood of 75 surgical tuberculous cases: 61 pneumonotomies with 32 deaths; 6 pneumonectomies and 2 deaths; 8 rib resections with 3 deaths; overall mortality 49%. Prior to the discovery of streptomycin by Selman A. Waksman in 1943, paediatricians were far more likely to recommend fresh air, sunshine and generous doses of cod liver oil than a trip to the local surgeon.

The development of pulmonary resection played a central role in the overall development of thoracic surgery. Prior to the 1900s pulmonary resections were unusual (as in the case of Rolandus of 1499) and survival rare. Most reports were of chronic suppurations which, during incision and drainage, were debrided rather than resected. Any paediatric surgeon of today can appreciate the difficult predicament of pulmonary resection with isolation of hilar structures in the face of active inflammation and infection. Add to that the instability of airway control, the lack of antibiotics and the precariousness of blood products, this author doubts if modern paediatric surgeons could fare any better. The first purposeful pulmonary resection was reported in 1823 by Milton Anthony on a 17-year-old boy who developed a lung abscess 2 ½ years after falling off a horse. Surgery was performed without any drugs or whiskey and the encountered "grume, and old red coagula, intermixed with dense coagula of lymph, resembling fragments of membranes" were removed. The patient recovered from the surgery. In 1861, the renowned French surgeon, Péan, resected a lung tumor by first suturing the leaves of the pleura to the lung then excising it with galvanocautery. The wound was dressed with carbolic acid (4 years before Lister's report) and the patient recovered. The nature of the tumor was not revealed [21].

In the latter part of the 1800s, experimental pulmonary resections in rabbits and dogs were performed notably by Gluck, Marcus, Schmid, Bloch, Biondi and Zakharevitch. All had significant numbers of animal survivals and felt that their techniques could be applied to humans. Of the investigators, only Schmid suggested the individual ligation of the blood vessels and bronchus. Unfortunately, mass ligation of the hilum was to predominate for many years. Tragically, M.H. Bloch, a vocal advocate of this technique, attempted to perform this operation on a patient who did not fare as well as his animals. This was related in a letter by G.L. Walton in 1883 [15]:

> It seems that he operated on a young lady, I am told a relative, at her own request. The lungs are said to have been found healthy, but the patient died, according to one report, during the operation; according to another shortly after. Legal procedures were instituted, but the unfortunate operator took his own life by shooting himself through the head.

In 1891, Theodore Tuffier (1857–1929) performed the first successful lung resection for tuberculosis. The patient, a 25-year-old cook was placed under chloroform anaesthesia. Through an extrapleural approach, the hilum of the right upper lobe was ligated with a chain suture and resected. The chest was closed with catgut, the skin with Florentine horse hair and the wound dressed with iodoform. Eight days later, the patient climbed two flights of stairs to be presented at the meeting of the Society of Surgeons of Paris. Over the next 30 some odd years, successful reports of partial or total lung resections were generated by Krönlein, Macewen, Heidenhain and Riedinger. The first lobectomy according to modern standards was performed by Themistokles Gluck (1853–1943) in 1899. The successful left lower and partial left upper lobectomy was performed on a child with bronchiectasis. In 1912, Morriston Davies, of London, ligated the vessels and bronchus individually in a case of lung cancer diagnosed by X-ray. Even though the patient died, the autopsy showed the bronchus closure to be intact. Prior to 1933, the majority of pulmonary resections were staged affairs with initial mass ligation of the hilum and later excision of the necrotic tissue. The greatest fear was infection and bronchial disruption. The first successful lobectomy using the Davies technique of anatomical ligation was performed by Archibald Young of Glasgow in 1934. The year after, sulphonamide was introduced. In 1938, Clarence Crafoord demonstrated the use of positive pressure anesthesia in pneumonectomy. Pulmonary surgery then flowered under the care of Evarts Graham, Edward Churchill, Clarence Crafoord, Brian Blades, Rudolph Nissen and many others [15, 21].

Once anaesthesia, positive pressure ventilatory support and antibiotics became established, surgery of other thoracic organs flourished. While foreign bodies of the oesophagus were treated by the ancients, most were attempted extractions through the mouth by means of long clamps, hook-shaped wires attached to catheters or probangs which were usually made of horsehair attached to the ends of two telescoping tubes. The instrument was passed by the foreign body, then the inner tube was pulled up which caused the horsehairs to form a discoid shape. Extraction was successful if the foreign body was not sharp or lodged in the wall of the oesophagus. Operative removal was not performed until the latter part of the nineteenth century and those were limited to cervical oesophagostomies. Strictures of the oesophagus from lye ingestion were treated in similar fashion by the performance of a cervical oesophagostomy and gastrostomy. Various dilators were then passed guided by a string. The renowned Friedrich Trendelenburg (1844–1925) maintained the nutrition in a child by: "a long tube was attached to the gastrostomy tube and through the open end the boy directed the food he masticated straight from his mouth in the stomach, helping it descend by blowing the food along" [33]. Prior to the primary repair of oesophageal atresias, William Ladd would create skin tubes which connected the cervical oesophagostomy to the gastrostomy. The procedures which literally took years to complete are testimony of the patience and dedication of the founder of American paediatric surgery. Cameron Haight of Ann Arbor, Michigan, performed the first successful one-stage repair of an oesophageal atresia on 15 March 1941. It was of interest to note that Haight made an extrapleural approach, but from the left side. He attempted to perform the surgery using a local anaesthetic but had to resort to ether drip when the proximal oesophageal pouch would retract into the neck each time the child swallowed [25].

As mentioned previously tracheostomy was known from the time of Hippocrates and certainly used to advantage in cases of impacted foreign bodies or severe upper airway inflammation. The investigation of the airway (and the oesophagus), however, had to await the development of special instruments and lighting. In 1743, Levret, a French physician, invented a speculum which "reflected the luminous rays in the direction of the tumor" in the nostrils. Sixty-one years later, Bozzini utilized reflected light and mirrors to examine the larynx and upper oesophagus. His classic work was published in 1807 as Der Lichtleiter, The Light-Conductor, or Description of a Simple Apparatus for the Illumination of the Internal Cavities and Spaces in the Living Animal Body. Most medical historians are familiar with Manuel Garcia, a Spanish-French singing master, who in 1854

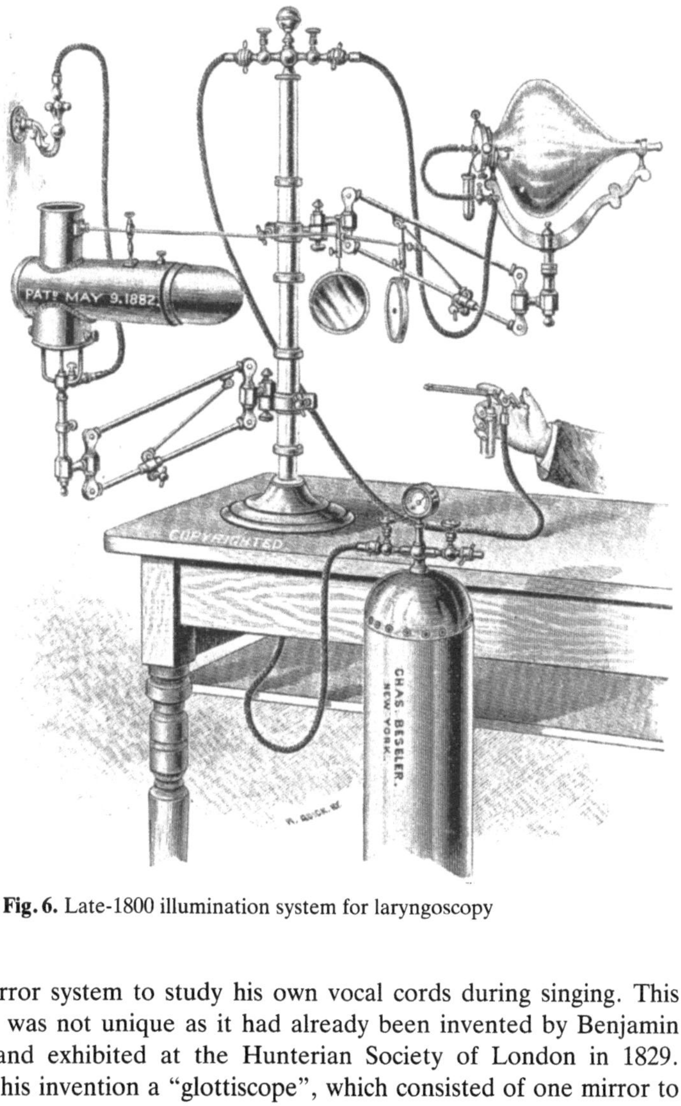

Fig. 6. Late-1800 illumination system for laryngoscopy

devised a two-mirror system to study his own vocal cords during singing. This autolaryngoscope was not unique as it had already been invented by Benjamin Guy Babington and exhibited at the Hunterian Society of London in 1829. Babington called his invention a "glottiscope", which consisted of one mirror to reflect light and another which was attached by a spring to a spatula tongue depressor. The equipment for illumination became elaborate to the point of being almost obstructive (Fig. 6). The first man to examine oesophageal mucosa via an endoscope was L. Walenburg. His initial instrument was a 14-cm-long tubular mirror. Later, he used a laryngeal mirror to examine through the tube. Walenburg even allowed the patient to hold the tube in order to use his free hand to pass sounds to dilate stenoses. The credit for the foundation of modern endoscopy was attributed to Johann von Mikulicz-Radecki (1850-1905) of Poland. His contribution, in 1881, was in showing that the curvature of the pharynx and the entire esophagus could be transformed into a straight line, thereby allowing direct examination through a rigid tube. His light source was a heated red-hot platinum wire attached to the distal part of the tube [15]. Endoscopic examination for diagnosis and treatment of both the esophagus and airway is a routine matter today. One wonders what Mikulicz's thoughts would be if he knew that one day we would have disposable 2-mm-diameter fibre optic endoscopes.

Space prohibits an examination of the development of the respirator, blood gas analysis and surgical instrumentation which added immeasurably to the effectiveness and safety of present-day paediatric thoracic surgery. Paediatric surgery, already a specialty in Great Britain and on the European Continent, started in America about the time pulmonary surgery had matured. The author has always been grateful that one of the founders of American paediatric surgery, Robert Gross, had an equally keen interest in thoracic and cardiovascular surgery. It is largely through his pioneering investigations and clinical successes on both sides of the diaphragm that present-day paediatric surgery has not been dismembered into organ specialties as has its parent field of general surgery.

This brief review is dedicated to the sage words of George Santayana: "Those who cannot remember the past are condemned to repeat it" and to Dr. David Sabiston, Jr., who too many years ago stimulated a young medical student into the field of paediatric surgery and the love of history.

References

1. Adams F (1846) The seven books of Paulus Ægineta. Adlard, London (Sydenham Society)
2. Adams F (1849) The genuine works of Hippocrates. Wood, New York (Sydenham Society)
3. Alexander B (1764) The seats and causes of diseases by John Baptist Morgagni, vol 3. Millar Cadell Johnson Payne, London, p 196
4. Bendixen HH (1982) Respirators and respiratory care. Acta Anaesth Scand 26:279–286
5. Breasted JH (1930) The Edwin Smith papyrus. University of Chicago Press, Chicago
6. Castiglioni A (1947) A history of medicine. Knopf, New York
7. Chang JHT (1986) Timelines in the history of pediatrics surgery. J Pediatr Surg 21:1068–1072
8. Comroe JH Jr (1975) Retroscope – inflation – 1904 model. Am Rev Resp Dis 112:713–716
9. Eloesser L (1970) Milestones in chest surgery. J Thorac Cardiovasc Surg 60:157–165
10. Fell GE (1910) Artificial respiration. Surg Gynecol Obstet 10:572–582
11. Forssmann W (1974) Experiments on myself. Memoirs of a surgeon in Germany (English edn). St Martin, New York
12. Garrison FH (1929) An introduction to the history of medicine, 4th edn. Saunders, Philadelphia
13. Goodall EW (1934) The story of tracheotomy. Br J Child Dis 31:167–176
14. Hamby WB (1960) The case reports and autopsy records of Ambroise Paré translation of JP Malgaigne's Oeuvres completes d'Ambroise Paré, Paris 1840. Thomas, Springfield
15. Hochberg LA (1960) Thoracic surgery before the 20th century. Vantage, New York
16. Keynes G (1653) The anatomical exercises of Dr. William Harvey De Motu Cordis 1628. Nonesuch, London
17. Killen DA, Gobbel Jr WG (1968) Spontaneous pneumothorax. Little Brown, Boston
18. Lister J (1909) Collected papers, vol 2. Clarendon, Oxford
19. Mason GA (1968) American and British thoracic surgery. J Thorac Cardiovasc Surg 55:1–5
20. Matas R (1899) On the management of acute traumatic pneumothorax. Ann Surg 29:409–434

21. Meade RH (1961) A history of thoracic surgery. Thomas, Springfield
22. Meade RH (1968) An introduction to the history of general surgery. Saunders, Philadelphia
23. Morse WR (1934) Chinese medicine. Hoeber, New York (Clio Medica Ser, vol 11)
24. Morton LT (1970) A medical bibliography: Garrison and Morton, 3rd edn. Trinity, London
25. Myers NA (1986) The history of oesophageal atresia and tracheo-oesophageal fistula – 1670–1984. In: Rickham PP (ed) Historical aspects of pediatric surgery. Springer, Berlin Heidelberg New York (Progress in pediatric surgery, vol 20)
26. Nissen R (1955) Historical development of pulmonary surgery. Am J Surg 89:9–15
27. Nuland SB (1983) The origins of anesthesia. Classics of Medicine Library, Birmingham
28. O'Dwyer J (1887) Fifty cases of croup in private practice treated by intubation of the larynx, with a description of the method and of the dangers incident thereto. Med Rec Ann 32:557–561
29. Perkins JF Jr (1964) Historical development of respiratory physiology. In: Fenn WO, Rahn H (eds) Respiration, vol 1. American Physiological Society, Washington DC (Handbook of Physiology, section 3)
30. Playfair WS (1872–1873) On the treatment of empyema in children. Obstet Trans 14:4–18
31. Potain (1869) Des difficultes que peut rencontrer l'evacuation complete du liquide dans l'operation de l'empyeme. Lyon Med 3:197–199
32. Smith RA (1982) Development of lung surgery in the United Kingdom. Thorax 37:161–168
33. Trendelenberg F (1878) Über einen Fall von Gastrotomie bei Oesophagusstrictur. Arch Klin Chir 22:227–234
34. White JW (1896) The use of skiagraphy for the detection and location of foreign bodies impacted in the esophagus. Ann Surg 24:238–242

Nursing Perspectives in the Management of Infants and Children Requiring Thoracic Surgery

H. Telfer and S. Willis

Summary

Nurses who care for infants and children undergoing thoracic surgery must function and make decisions which take into account a multiplicity of complex data. This necessitates a background of knowledge, skill and intuition which guides their nursing practice. The principles of holistic care in which the total needs of the infant and child are met within the context of the family are seen as an important approach to patient care. Selected perspectives in the care of infants with congenital and acquired thoracic anomalies are discussed, in particular infants with congenital diaphragmatic hernia and oesophageal atresia. The preparation of children for chest surgery and the postoperative nursing management are outlined and include aspects of pain management, physiotherapy and chest drain care.

Zusammenfassung

Krankenschwestern, die Kinder und Säuglinge mit throaxchirurgischen Eingriffen betreuen, sind vor Entscheidungen gestellt, die eine Vielzahl komplexer Daten implizieren. Dies erfordert einen soliden Wissensstand, Fertigkeit und Intuition für die tägliche Pflegepraxis. Die Prinzipien einer umfassenden Pflege, die alle Bedürfnisse der Säuglinge und Kinder auch im Kontext mit der Familie berücksichtigt, sind wichtig zur Bewältigung dieser Aufgabe. Ausgewählte Gesichtspunkte bei der Pflege von Säuglingen mit kongenitalen oder erworbenen Thoraxanomalien werden diskutiert, insbesondere bei Säuglingen mit angeborener Zwerchfellhernie und Ösophagusatresie. Die Vorbereitung der Kinder für einen thoraxchirurgischen Eingriff und die postoperative Pflege werden dargestellt; dabei werden Aspekte der Schmerzbekämpfung, der Physiotherapie und der Umgang mit Thoraxdrainagen erörtert.

Résumé

Les infirmières qui s'occupent des nourrissons et des enfants devant subir une intervention chirurgicale du thorax doivent agir et prendre des décisions en tenant compte d'une multiplicité de facteurs extrêmement complexes. Elles doivent donc disposer, , en plus de leur expérience, d'un important bagage de connaissances, d'adresse et d'intuition. Les principles de la théroie de la totalité (holistic care) prenant en considération l'ensemble des besoins d'un nourrisson et d'un enfants dans son contexte familial sont considérés comme un atout majeur.

Les auteurs traitent des soins à apporter aux nourrissons présentant des anomalies thoraciques congénitales et acquises et en particulier aux nourrissons avec hernie diaphragmatique congénitale ou atrésie oesophagienne.

Il est aussi question de la préparation des enfants à la chirurgie du thorax et de l'organisation des soins postopératoires, y compris la lutte contre la douleur, la physiothérapie et le drainage thoracique.

Department of Nursing, Royal Children's Hospital Melbourne, Flemington Road, Parkville 3052, Victoria, Australia.

Progress in Pediatric Surgery, Vol. 27
Myers and Angerpointner (Eds.)

Introduction

The modern history of thoracic surgery at the Royal Children's Hospital, Melbourne, began in the late 1940s. Prior to this surgery was limited to drainage of empyema and an occasional lobectomy. One of the first thoracic surgical procedures was a definitive repair of an oesophageal atresia in a neonate. Within the same year (1949) two more infants survived the same procedure. At that time cardiac surgery was beginning, the first operation being the closure of a patent ductus arteriosus in a child. This was courageous surgery at a time when anaesthetic techniques were limited and backup facilities minimal. Surgery within the chest created a challenge for nursing as there was little verbal and no written information to guide nursing practice for these patients.

Many changes have occurred since these early days. Paediatric anaesthesia is skilled and safe and affords the surgeon greater ease at surgery. Surgical techniques have been improved and refined, and surgery once deemed impossible is now performed regularly. Infants and children are assured of excellent results at an early age and our cardiac unit reports a fall in mortality from 62.5% to 4.2% in the past 7 years in babies under 6 months of age. The number of children helped by heart, and heart and lung transplants is increasing. We now rarely see patients requiring lung resection for bronchiectasis.

The development of intensive care with its highly specialized staff and modern technology has been a major factor in the advanced management and care of infants and children who are critically ill, resulting in improved results with a significant reduction in morbidity and mortality.

The purpose of this article is to discuss current perspectives in the nursing management of infants and children undergoing thoracic surgery, and to highlight aspects of the developing child which may influence the care provided. It is not intended to cover all conditions, but to discuss selected principles of care and to utilize a few more common conditions to illustrate these. Comments will be made on general aspects of the management of sick infants and then the specific care of infants with congenital diaphragmatic hernia and oesophageal atresia. This will be followed by a description of the principles of care as they relate to children with thoracic conditions.

Paediatric Nursing

Nurses who care for children must function and make decisions which take into account a multiplicity of complex data. Now, more than ever before, nurses are recognizing and valuing their nursing practice and the knowledge embedded in it [1] and also the unique contribution they make in the care of children and their families.

Expansion of education has resulted in a better knowledge of bioscience and pathophysiology, child development and family dynamics. This has provided an informed base for the development of skills of assessment, analysis and nursing actions. Critical thinking as well as the skills of doing are now the hallmark of paediatric nursing practice.

The fact that infants differ in many ways from adults is now more fully recognized. Physically they are not scaled-down adults, but have many anatomical and physiological differences. This is particularly so in the neonate. Psychosocially children must be considered according to their developmental age. They must also be considered within the context of their family. All these factors have important nursing implications.

The concept of a team approach with doctors, nurses, social workers, physiotherapists and technicians communicating and working together is one which is now well developed. This multidisciplinary approach means that all professionals are kept informed of the plan of care for the child and family.

The Infant with Congenital Thoracic Anomalies

When an infant is diagnosed with a condition which requires management at a specialized paediatric centre there are general principles of care which are relevant for all sick infants.

Transport

The development of neonatal transport has been a major factor in recent years in improving the clinical outcome of neonatal patients [2]. In Victoria the Newborn Emergency Transport Service (NETS) retrieves infants from all over the State and transfers them to neonatal intensive care units situated in Melbourne. The team consists of a neonatal nurse with specialized transport skills, and a neonatal paediatrician or registrar.

Initial management will be commenced at the referring hospital usually in consultation with the staff at the receiving hospital. It is important that the infant is stabilized before the journey is commenced. This may take some time to achieve [3]. Details of the perinatal history, the patient's condition and investigation results should be readily available for the team's information.

Of primary importance is adequate respiratory support. Endotracheal intubation may be required with or without assisted ventilation, according to clinical assessment and blood gas estimation. Intravenous fluids are commenced if necessary and volume expanders as required. Temperature control is of utmost importance.

The parents need to be considered and kept well informed. If at all possible they need to be given the opportunity to touch and hold their infant before the transfer is made [4]. A photograph of the baby given to the mother is a small way of helping to ease the temporary parting. We feel that it is best that the father travels independently to the receiving hospital so that he may have the opportunity to spend time with his infant and get to know the nursing staff. The surgeon will then have more time to spend with him to give explanations that are needed.

The father is an important link with the mother and the hospital until she is able to visit herself.

Admission

When the receiving unit is notified of an expected admission, preparations are made to ensure an orderly and coordinated admission procedure. This involves assembling equipment, making ready appropriate accommodation and assigning staff to receive the infant. When the patient arrives the principles of care already commenced are continued.

Nursing Assessment and Care

The initial nursing assessment of the infant on admission is an important aspect and gives a baseline for later comparison for improvement or deterioration. A statement of how infant appears generally is documented and is a valuable reference point. Nursing assessment is ongoing throughout hospitalization and guides nursing actions. Aspects appraised include assessment of respiratory and cardiovascular status, thermoregulation, fluids and nutrition and psychosocial needs.

Respiratory Aspects

There is a high incidence of respiratory distress and respiratory failure in neonates for a number of reasons. The ribcage is structurally immature and compliant, and the relatively soft sternum forms an unstable base [5]. The ribs are more horizontally placed than in adults, thus, eliminating the bucket-handle motion upon which thoracic respiration depends. The intercostal muscles are weak and underdeveloped and respiration is almost entirely dependent on the diaphragm [5]. Respirations may be readily embarrassed by anything that interferes with diaphragmatic movement such as abdominal distension.

The infant tires easily with increased respiratory effort and will preferentially quicken his rate of breathing to conserve energy [6]. In more severe situations there will be indrawing of the chest also in an effort to increase tidal volume.

The first signs of respiratory distress are restlessness, often a subtle cue, and tachypnoea. Other signs will be chest retraction, nasal flaring, and, when the condition is critical, pallor and cyanosis. Nursing assessment included respiratory rate, the degree of inspiratory effort and rib recession and the presence of grunting and colour changes. These are noted whilst the infant is undisturbed.

Early diagnosis of the cause is essential and respiratory support given as indicated by this and blood gas estimations until specific treatment is undertaken. The position of choice is prone with the head of the bed raised if ventilatory support is not immediately required. In this position the abdominal contents fall away from the diaphragm and allow an increase in lung volume [5]. The infant is usually more settled in this position. The introduction of pulse oximetry has been a welcome technical aid in the monitoring of respiratory function by enabling a constant oxygen saturation reading to be taken. This method is less complex to use than transcutaneous oxygen monitoring.

Cardiovascular Aspects

In the fetus only about 10% of the cardiac output goes to the lungs due to the very high pulmonary vascular resistance. This is the result of marked vasoconstriction of the muscular pulmonary arterioles. At birth, when the lungs expand, the pulmonary resistance falls, the foramen ovale closes and there is constriction followed by thrombosis and closure of the ductus arteriosus.

However, for a period the cardiovascular system and pulmonary vasculature remain reactive to episodes of hypoxia, hypercarbia, acidosis or hypothermia. In these situations the rise in pulmonary vascular resistance may cause a reversal to fetal circulation [7], which may occur with extreme rapidity. The neonate has a rapid heart rate and a small stroke volume; therefore bradycardia may cause a fall in cardiac output. The myocardium has less contractility than has an adult, and appears to respond more readily to an increased afterload with diminished cardiac output or heart failure [8].

Nursing assessment includes heart rate and rhythm. A slowing of heart rate may indicate hypoxia or vagal stimulation caused, for example, by the passing of a nasogastric tube. Increasing tachycardia may be a sign of a compromised circulation or perhaps overheating. Systolic, diastolic and mean blood pressures should be monitored in a very sick infant. It is well to realize that the normal parameters accepted for vital signs may not be appropriate signs for the critically ill infant [9]. Consistent trends or changes should be reported.

The implementation of medical instructions in the management of these aspects is a nursing responsibility. These may include directions regarding preload, contractility and afterload. Volume may be ordered to increase filling pressures and these need to be given carefully with an alert eye on the infant and monitor. Attention to acid base status and an inotrope infusion such as dopamine may be ordered to strengthen myocardial contractility. Reduction in ventricular afterload may be achieved by the use of a vasodilator drug.

Thermoregulation

For the surgical neonate the maintenance of temperature is a vital consideration. A neutral thermal environment is important to avoid the sequelae of cold stress, increased oxygen demands, metabolic acidosis, hypoglycaemia and pulmonary vasoconstriction [10]. A temperature which is too high will also increase oxygen requirements and may cause apnoea; therefore care needs to be taken to prevent inadvertent overheating. A labile temperature may indicate sepsis and further investigation is required.

Nurses have a responsibility to ensure that the infant's temperature is well controlled. Heat losses may occur through evaporation, conduction, radiation and convection.

Overhead heaters are a very useful way of providing radiant energy for body absorption to compensate for heat loss by radiation. Through a servo-controlled mechanism which utilizes a probe attached to the infant's trunk, the surrounding air is warmed according to the skin temperature sensor. The probe is covered with foil to reflect the heat, thus reducing the possibility of inaccurate sensing. It is important that the probe does not partially lift as it will result in overheating. Underheating may occur if the infant lies on the probe. Personnel need to be reminded of the possibility of their own bodies blocking warmth to the infant during procedures of any length. Bonnets and bootees help to conserve heat as well as providing a personalized effect.

Heat may be lost by convection through draughts. This may be caused by the fan in phototherapy lights, and a protective sheet needs to deflect the current of air from the infant. Conductive loss from cold surfaces such as X-ray plates is counteracted by warming them before use. Evaporative heat and water losses are high under a radiant heater and must be taken into account with fluid maintenance needs. Significant heat is lost from moist skin; therefore it is not appropriate for these infants to be bathed, nor is it necessary when they are very ill [11]. Inspired gases also need to be warmed and humidified.

Similar care needs to be taken when nursing an infant in an incubator. Radiant heat may be lost to a cooler environment such as a window. Convective and evaporative losses are not as great in incubators in comparison with radiant heaters. There has been a move to nurse more infants in cots in recent years [12].

Care to preserve heat must be taken when the infant is being transferred to the operating room. During surgery the operating room temperature will be increased and the table, lotions and inspired gas warmed [13]. It is thought provoking to consider that mortality can be cut by 25% in small babies by the provision of adequate warmth [12].

Fluid Balance

For any infant undergoing surgery the maintenance of fluid and electrolyte balance is essential. Fluids given must take into account the infant's weight, age and gestation. Requirements vary with the manner in which the infant is nursed. There will be increased fluid losses under a radiant heater or phototherapy lights. Patients on mechanical ventilation will require less fluid because of reduced respiratory loss with humidified gases, and the presence of raised levels of antidiuretic hormone [14].

All fluids used in therapy such as drugs, and saline which is used to flush intravenous lines, need to be taken into account. Hydration is assessed by skin turgor [15], urinary output, urine osmolality and serum sodium; also by the monitoring of central venous and arterial pressures in very ill infants. The accurate and safe delivery of fluids is a nursing responsibility and this has been made easier in recent years by the availability of infusion pumps.

Total Parenteral Nutrition

The increased knowledge and refinement of fluids and additives used in total parenteral nutrition has meant that infants unable to be given enteral feedings may be supported well intravenously. Sufficient nutrients, electrolytes and trace elements will make possible physiological stability, basal metabolism, healing and growth. However, complications of intravenous nutrition can still occur and some are preventable by good nursing practice.

The route may be by peripheral vein or, if a longer period is anticipated, by the central venous route. Sophisticated infusion pumps have enabled the delivery of nutrient solution and fat emulsion to be more accurrate and less time consuming for nurses. The inclusion of alarms has also made them safer.

Parenteral nutrition is always introduced and withdrawn slowly. If a cannula is dislodged it should be reinserted immediately to avoid rebound hypoglycaemia [14]. We use an infusion of similar dextrose concentration in water with sodium and potassium chloride if nutrient solution is not available when required. There is no place for "catching up" if delivery of fluid is behind schedule.

As nutrient solutions for neonatal use contain high concentrations of calcium, magnesium and phosphorus, it is important that they are delivered in a manner which prevents mixing with the fat emulsion. Either the fat emulsion is given through a separate line, or we use a cycle of 3 h nutrient and 1 h fat emulsion [16]. A separate closed system is used between each delivery to flush the line with saline. An awareness of the possibility of infection in a central line guides this aspect in meticulous aseptic techniques. Protocols vary in different hospitals. We have recently reviewed our nursing practice and central lines are now changed every 72 h and dressings once a week [17]. Previously all lines were changed each day. Monitoring for signs of infection locally or systemically needs astute and alert observation.

Measurements of electrolytes and serum lipaemia are performed each day. Blood glucose is monitored every 8 h until the dextrose intake is stable and urine is tested 8 hourly for the presence of glucose.

Care of the Family

It was not so long ago that the care of the family was considered mainly the role of the medical staff and medical social workers, and nurses concentrated their attention mostly on the infants in their care, giving support to the parents often only in a crisis situation.

These days nurses encompass the family as part of their holistic care, and place great emphasis on family welfare and the nurses' role in this. When an infant is critically ill after birth, the parents will usually have had little time to prepare for this crisis. Not only is there the adjustment to an infant quite different from the expected healthy baby, but an anticipatory grief response similar to that of parents whose infants die is experiences by most parents [18].

There may be a myriad of feelings of guilt, fear, anger and confusion compounded by tiredness. All will affect their ability to absorb information given to them. They need time, according to individual needs, and explanations given in a manner which they can understand. These may need to be repeated many times whilst they are in a state of stress. Many parents say that in these early contacts with the staff they remember vividly the way in which they were given information, the tone of voice and the caring and accepting attitude of them.

They also value early visits to see their infant, and speak of the reassurance felt when they observed nurses' proficient and caring handling of their child. The development of a trusting relationship between nurses and parents is one in which they feel comfortable to ask questions, to express their feelings [19] and to be able to relate to their infant. Many studies have been documented on the importance of the parent-infant bond [20–22]. This is a complex process and takes time to achieve. The parents' readiness is an important factor and needs to be sensitively assessed. We constantly have this in mind as we nurse these infants, always calling them by name and encouraging the parents to touch and caress. Toys and small items of clothing such as bonnets and bootees, and maybe cards drawn by siblings will help develop a feeling of family integration.

Congenital Diaphragmatic Hernia

Although a congenital diaphragmatic hernia may be diagnosed beyond the neonatal period and present in many different ways, it is in the early period after birth that it is most life threatening. The high mortality associated with this condition has been a concern for a number of years [23]. In spite of antenatal diagnosis, better transport and intensive care facilities there has been little improvement in the 50% survival rate of infants presenting in the first few hours after birth [24–27]. However, in recent years there have been changes in management of high-risk infants which appear promising. There are new techniques in the prevention and management of persistent fetal circulation and in many centres the surgery is being delayed [26].

Embryology

In the embryo the diaphragm develops from four structures, the septum transversum, the pleuroperitoneal membranes, the dorsal mesentery of the oesophagus and the body wall. The growth and fusion of these structures divide the thoracic and abdominal cavities by the closure of the pleuroperitoneal canal [28]. This occurs between the 8th and 10th week of life. If there is a failure of fusion or defective formation, an opening will persist. The most common site is the posterolateral segment, the foramen of Bochdalek. This occurs mainly on the left side and, less frequently, on the right side [29].

Pathophysiology

Lung growth will be affected if there is herniation of the intestines through the defect before the 16th week [30]. The degree of lung hypoplasia will vary depending on the stage of development and the severity of compression of the ipsilateral lung. Hypoplasia means that there is less capacity for gas exchange [25], the pulmonary arterial bed is decreased and the vessels are more muscular than normal [31]. Mediastinal shift displaces the heart to the contralateral side, and may result in bilateral pulmonary hypoplasia.

Clinical Presentation

Tachypnoea is the main sign in these infants and this may be noted by the nurse soon after delivery. The earlier the presentation after birth, the poorer the prognosis is likely to be. In some infants there may be rapidly developing cyanosis. Other infants may develop tachypnoea and a weak cry then, after several hours, chest retraction, nasal flaring and ultimately cyanosis. Heart sounds may be displaced depending on the amount of bowel in the chest, and the abdomen may be scaphoid [32]. In another group there may be only rapid breathing at rest, and tiring with feeds which alerts the nurse that further investigation may be needed, and medical staff should be notified.

An X-ray of the chest and abdomen confirms the diagnosis by the presence of a bowel gas pattern in the thorax. Biochemical investigation reveals hypoxaemia, hypercarbia and acidosis. A nasogastric tube when passed may enter an abnormally situated stomach [33].

Before Transfer

These infants are usually extremely ill and require intensive care management as soon as possible after diagnosis. With the expertise available through the specialist doctor and nurse transport team in Victoria, all measures are commenced in the referring hospital. When this is not practicable resuscitative measures according to the level of expertise available would be undertaken.

Gentle, minimal handling to avoid crying and gaseous bowel distension is important. A size 8–10 FG nasogastric tube is passed, aspirated frequently and left on open drainage. If intubation and ventilation are required this is performed as smoothly as possible. To minimize stress and the increase in pulmonary hypertension intravenous morphine may be given before this is performed. The intubation procedure can be greatly facilitated by the nurse's assistance in positioning the infant, making ready the tape for tube fixation and placing connections at hand for suction and mechanical ventilation.

Blood gas measurements are taken and metabolic acidosis corrected. These results will guide ventilation in the attempt to provide adequate oxygenation and a reduction of $PaCO_2$ to 35 mm Hg. This is done with the aid of muscle relaxants. Intravenous volume expanders are given as necessary.

Management Following Admission

All previous management is continued on arrival at the intensive care unit of the receiving hospital. The infant is nursed with the head of the cot elevated. Sedation is established using a continuous infusion of fentanyl or morphine to minimize stress.

Until recently repair of the diaphragm and replacement of the intestines into the abdominal cavity was considered to be a surgical emergency, and was performed after a short period of stabilization. Many centres are now questioning this and are delaying surgery until the infant's labile respiratory and haemodynamic status have been stabilized [26, 34, 35]. In one study the mean time of delay was 24.4 h [26]; another has waited up to 7 days [35]. There are suggestions that surgery itself may be partly responsible for the delayed onset of persistent fetal circulation [26]. The timing of surgery is the subject of much debate and further evaluation is being undertaken.

Because these infants have small, hypoplastic lungs and exquisitely sensitive pulmonary vasculature, the pattern of ventilation aims to achieve optimal oxagen and carbon dioxide exchange with minimal barotrauma. The use of muscle relaxants will assist this. A rapid ventilation rate with moderate peak inspiratory pressure and a short inspiratory time is usual, but each infant will have differing needs and responses. Frequent arterial sampling enables the measurement of blood gases.

There must be constant surveillance for the complication of air leaks such as pneumothorax. Nursing anticipation of this possibility will need prior preparation of the equipment needed to evacuate the air. The care of chest drains will be discussed later in the chapter.

Persistent pulmonary hypertension leads to intractable right-to-left shunting through the foramen ovale and the ductus arteriosus. This is known as persistent fetal circulation and is the main cause of mortality [34]. Measures to counteract this are taken before as well as following surgery. The many factors which increase shunting are those which cause pulmonary vasoconstriction and include hypoxia, hypercarbia, acidosis, pain, noise, cold stress and stress from handling. The aims of nursing care are directed towards preventing or ameliorating these, providing the delivery of fluids, drugs and nutrition, and the support of the parents.

Ventilatory parameters are constantly checked and suction of the endotracheal tube performed quickly and gently to minimize any drop in PaO_2. Oxygen is increased before and after suction and a close watch is kept on the infant and heart rate during the procedure. Oximetry enables continual surveillance of haemoglobin saturation.

We minimize stress and pain by handling the infant as little as possible, and group the necessary activities together to allow rest periods. A continuous opiate infusion is maintained to keep the infant well sedated and pain free. The lights and noise level are kept as low as it is safe and practical to avoid unwanted sensory stimulation.

Pulmonary hypertension may respond to vasoactive drugs such as tolazoline; however, these also dilate the systemic circulation and may cause hypotension. A cautious delivery is therefore necessary, taking note of circulatory pressures. Intravenous volume expanders should be on hand.

Cardiac output may be impaired by the high pulmonary vascular resistance. Right ventricular dilation may lead of left ventricular failure by impairing left ventricular filling needing the use of an inotrope such as dopamine to increase left ventricular function. The delivery of dopamine is by continuous infusion and its effect on the infant and monitor pressures noted by the nurse. We label all drug lines close to the patient and do not flush the lines. No bolus injections of other drugs are made into these lines.

A careful account is kept of fluids given. Urinary output is measured and charted, and urine osmolality noted and recorded. If a catheter is not in situ we find small paper drinking cups useful in urine collection. Monitoring includes heart rate and rhythm, central venous and arterial pressures and ventilatory pressures. These are displayed in digital and wave form on the monitor. Assessment of cardiac output, using indicators such as right atrial pressure, arterial systemic pressure, peripheral pulses and the temperature and capillary refill of the extremities, is important. The onset of pulmonary hypertension and consequent right to left shunting can be monitored by the comparison of arterial oxygenation in the distribution of pre- and postductal perfusion areas. At our hospital we use preductal samples from a right radial line and samples from an arterial line in a leg (postductal). The most important monitor is the nurse who is in constant attendance observing with all senses, interpreting according to her knowledge, experience, and intuition [36] and recording data. The information is communicated to the medical staff and care is coordinated to an optimal degree. Weaning from the ventilator will be slow and cautious [29] and during this time the nurse is particularly alert for signs of returning persistent fetal circulation.

Skin integrity in these sedated and paralyzed infants needs to be watched carefully. We nurse the infant on a sheep skin with alternate lateral tilting, and use a soft doughnut under the head to prevent pressure injury.

Extracorporeal Membrane Oxygenation

Extracorporeal membrane oxygenation (ECMO) has been used in the past decade in infants with intractable post-operative persistent fetal circulation. Numerous centres in the United States have reported success with infants who would otherwise have died [24, 37, 38]. However, recent evidence is suggesting that ECMO in the postoperative phase has not appreciably affected the high mortality in the high-risk group [35].

In addition to the strategies of hyperventilation, paralysis, sedation and minimal stress now in use, attention is now being directed to the preoperative use of ECMO in those infants with continued poor gas exchange. As mentioned previously, this leads to a considerably longer period before surgery, sometimes up to 1 week, and the results are very promising [35].

Extracorporeal membrane oxygenation is an expensive procedure in terms of resources, and there are complications which have caused concern. However, with improved technology and equipment design the complications associated with heparinization, carotid ligation and blood membrane interaction should be eliminated. The system, and infant care, will be able to be managed by one nurse instead of the two staff currently needed, thus conserving resources [39].

Parents

Throughout this difficult time of hospitalization, nursing interaction with the parents is vital. We hold the infant in trust for the parents and our relationship with them must reflect this. Even at busy times there are small ways of letting them know that they and their feelings are respected. They also need times for our undivided attention for explanations and verbalization of their feelings.

Outcome

The time in hospital for those infants who do survive is sometimes prolonged with many setbacks. As lung development will continue up to the age of 8 years [30], the lung function will eventually be near normal [34].

Oesophageal Atresia

Over the past decade there have been major advances in the management of infants born with oesophageal atresia. This has been attributed to refinements in surgery, anaesthesia and intensive care facilities. There has been a considerable reduction in mortality and morbidity particularly in low birth weight infants. The contribution of nursing has been a significant one.

Diagnosis

It has sometimes been suggested that all newborn infants should have a nasogastric tube passed into the stomach after birth to exclude oesophageal atresia. This does seem to be an unnecessary intrusion. We rarely admit an infant these days following a delay in diagnosis. Nurses in delivery rooms are very aware of the signs of oesophageal obstruction, and are especially alert if the mother has had polyhydramnios [40]. Infants with excessive bubbly secretions should certainly have a firm size-10 FG catheter passed to check for patency. An X-ray will confirm the diagnosis. It is most important that the diagnosis is made before the first feeding is given to prevent aspiration pneumonitis.

Embryology and Pathophysiology

In the embryo the gut and respiratory tract begin as a single tube. This tube becomes longer and separates into two separate tubes during the 4th and 5th week of gestation [41]. Both tubes are joined at the pharynx. Defective growth of endodermal cells results in atresia. A fistula is present when there is incomplete separation of the tubes. The most common form of anomaly (86%) is a blind upper pouch with a distal tracheo-oesophageal fistula. Oesophageal atresia with a long gap and no fistula accounts for 8% of oesophageal anomalies [42].

Transport

The most important nursing goals before and during transport are to prevent aspiration of secretions accumulating in the blind oesophageal pouch, and the reflux of acid gastric juice through the fistula (if present) into the lungs. Frequent suctioning of the oesophageal pouch is mandatory, at at least every 10–15 min, but we find it is needed more frequently when the infant is crying. We endeavour to prevent crying by comfort measures and gentle handling. It is important to do this as air forced through the fistula may distend the stomach, and increase the possibility of gastric juice with air reflux. We place the infant in a prone position with the head of the cot raised, to minimize reflux. The infant's face must always be in full view of the nurse for observation and assessment. All these measures are continued on admission to the referral centre. As there is an incidence of associated anomalies [43], ultrasound of the heart and kidneys will be performed to detect these. The severity of anomalies will affect the clinical outcome.

Oesophageal Atresia with Tracheo-oesophageal Fistula

Infants with this anomaly have surgical correction within 12 h of birth. Gestational age no longer is a reason for delay [44].

Postoperative Management

Following surgery there will be an initial need for suctioning until adequate swallowing can clear secretions. Care is taken to protect the anastomotic site, and the suction catheters are carefully measured to avoid this.

Extubation is usually performed in the operating room or soon after return to the neonatal unit. Pain in the neonate is difficult to assess and treat as opiates are not well tolerated in non-ventilated patients. Local anaesthetic nerve block at surgery may be effective for some hours. We try and relieve any strain on the thoracotomy wound by supporting the infant's back and arm with a soft towelling roll and being gentle with changes of position. Stroking the infant with quiet talking may help to ameliorate the pain sensation; however, there needs to be sensitivity not to overstimulate and thus increase discomfort.

Intravenous nutrition is commenced on the 2nd day, and oral feedings introduced after 3–5 days. We encourage mothers to breast feed, and infants are able to be put to the breast very soon after commencing oral feeds. The incidence of gastro-oesophageal reflux is high [45], and the raising of the head of the cot will assist in minimizing this.

As chest drains and gastrostomy tubes are now not used in our institution convalescence is usually straightforward and the infant is discharged in about 10 days.

Long-Gap Oesophageal Atresia

This type of anomaly means that the infant will be hospitalized for several months until the oesophagus has grown sufficiently for a delayed primary repair to be achieved [46]. The philosophy for surgery at the Royal Children's Hospital has always been "the best oesophagus is the patient's own oesophagus", and much effort has gone into achieving this [40].

Management of Secretions

The care of an infant with an unrepaired oesophagus is a challenge for the nursing staff. Cervical oesophagostomy is now rarely used; therefore the infant relies completely on the nurse to remove secretions by suctioning at frequent intervals. There is a constant risk of pulmonary aspiration if these secretions are not meticulously removed. This is an intrusive procedure and must be done effectively; however, it also needs to be performed without trauma and with an attitude of caring.

Nutritional Needs

Feedings are given by gastrostomy, taking care that the infant receives optimal nutrients and calories for growth. Losses from aspiration of saliva are replaced. We find that sodium replacement is needed for satisfactory weight gains. During this time we encourage the parents to participate in the care of their baby as much as possible. This involves gastrostomy feeding and care as well as all nurturing tasks and pleasures. Following delayed primary anastomosis at the age of 8–10 weeks the parents play a major role in the establishment of oral feedings.

Care at Home

One of the goals of nursing is to help parents gain confidence in parenting. Specific to the care of infants following oesophageal repair is the knowledge of what to expect, and when to seek medical advice. A "brassy" cough is common due to a degree of tracheomalacia, and many infants need positioning to minimize gastro-oesophageal reflux. Stricture at the site of anastomosis can be a problem and any signs of difficulty with feeding or swallowing of saliva need to be notified.

The Child with Thoracic Surgical Problems

There are a variety of thoracic problems which require surgery in childhood. These may be congenital or acquired. Some of the more common conditions seen are listed as follows:

1. Congenital diaphragmatic hernia with delayed presentation
2. Chest wall deformities
3. Cystic fibrosis with pneumothorax
4. Mediastinal tumours
5. Localized lobar infection
6. Unusual infections such as *Pneumocystis carinii,* or conditions such as broncho-pulmonary dysplasia
7. Spontaneous pneumothorax

In the following section selected principles of nursing care which illustrate changes in nursing practice for these children will be discussed.

Before Admission

Many children who are to undergo thoracic surgery are admitted to hospital on an elective basis. Any hospitalization is a stressful time for both child and family, and preparation beforehand is one way in which this stress may be reduced. Nurses are able to do this more effectively these days with the increase of literature and knowledge available to them and their own experience. It is an area in which there has been a number of nursing research studies, and there is a need for ongoing evaluation [47].

A number of strategies are in use, often for groups of children. These include a hospital and ward tour with a question and answer session, play therapy and videos or films. Difficulties exist with children in groups because of the age differences and levels of understanding. Each child in their parents need individual preparation as well.

Some factors to be considered during preparation, in addition to the child's age, are previous hospital experiences, the anxiety level of the parents and the child's developmental age. The latter is very important as children of like age vary considerably in cognitive development. Young children will understand best if able to use play materials. Older children benefit from diagrams, discussions and videos [47].

Children are able to cope better subsequently in hospital when they have previous knowledge of what they will see, hear and feel as well as know what will be happening [48]. For example, a child who is to have a chest drain will benefit from seeing the catheter, hearing the suction (or a description) and what the drain will feel like.

Honesty, and language at their level of understanding, without ambiguity, is important. For instance words like "cut" are best avoided in the 2–7 age group as it implies pain, and they will not understand the meaning of a "test". To a school-age child "test" means something that results in a pass or fail [49].

Preoperative Preparation

The child may be admitted several days before operation depending on the surgery. Preparation includes an X-ray of the chest, blood for grouping and cross-matching and physiotherapy. Sputum or a throat swab may also be cultured. Chest physiotherapy sessions are conducted by a physiotherapist and aim to clear the chest as much as possible. According to the child's age, ability to cooperate and the surgery being undertaken, breathing exercises to increase lung expansion and exercises to increase arm and spine mobility are also taught.

Postoperative Care

Following surgery respiratory function is assessed constantly, noting respiratory rate and effort, colour and pulse rate. Babies are monitored in addition by the use of oximetry. Oxygen may be given for an initial period, then as indicated subsequently.

The child is nursed flat in bed until all vital signs are stable. Gradually pillows are used for a sitting position. An "armchair" arrangement of the pillows is avoided as patients will favour the operative side, thus increasing a tendency to stiffness. A baby will be more comfortable nursed without pillows and the head of the bed raised. It is important to "cradle lift" the child under the thighs and back when changing position, as a "shoulder lift" will cause pain and discomfort from tension on the thoracotomy wound.

A careful watch is kept for signs of bleeding from the wound or chest drain. Early ambulation in 24–48 h is now usual and can be achieved safely even when a chest drain is in place.

Pain Management

Children of all ages require individual assessment in relation to pain. This enables titration of amounts of analgesia and safe delivery to the child.

It is not long since pain was thought to be a negligible consideration in the management of the postoperative child. Yet in the 1980s, in spite of ever-increasing knowledge and information in the literature, much remains to be applied in practice [50]. Many myths were common in the past and some still persist: "children don't feel pain", a "child's pain is different to that experienced by an adult", or "narcotics are dangerous in children and always cause respiratory depression". The fear of addiction was uppermost in the minds of medical and nursing staff, and often only one or two doses of analgesia were given postoperatively. A reluctance is still seen on the part of the medical staff adequately to prescribe and the nursing staff to administer analgesia to patients [51], especially young children.

Determination and assessment of pain in very young children may be difficult. Infants may respond by crying, facial expression, body movements and autonomic responses [52]. Children generally are able accurately to describe the pain they are experiencing, even those as young as 4 years [52]. Many children will not complain as the fear of a "needle" is worse than the pain itself, and some choose to remain silent. Frequent regular doses of intramuscular analgesia, besides causing the distress of injections, give only intermittent pain relief. The child swings from states of euphoria and stupor to uncooperative rigidity and pain.

Pain management in the postoperative paediatric patient has improved markedly with the introduction of opiate infusions. Once used selectively and exclusively in an intensive care setting under controlled conditions, opiates have now proved safe and effective for routine pain management in the ward situation. An opiate infusion permits a lower total daily dose of drug to be administered whilst providing a serum level which allows the patient to stay awake, responsive and cooperative during physiotherapy and other procedures. Pain-free activities may be undertaken earlier such as sitting out of bed, playing, school work or occupational therapy. Infusion rates may be adjusted or a bolus given during times of added stress, such as procedures.

At the Royal Children's Hospital, Melbourne, our early experience with opiate infusions was with morphine. This has been effective and we have chosen to continue to use this in preference to other drugs. Pethidine and papaveretum are occasionally prescribed for those children for whom morphine is contraindicated.

In a recent study at the hospital morphine infusions were found to be safe as well as effective, easy to manage and well accepted by staff, patients and parents [53]. As with any innovation in care, a protocol is needed for the use of opiate infusions in the ward setting.

It is recommended that:

1. Opiate infusions must be regulated by an infusion pump.
2. All orders for opiate infusions automatically expire after 48 h. Review and reordering of infusion is necessary.
3. Naloxone is available in the ward.
4. Trained staff should prepare and supervise the infusion.

Our management of infants under the age of 6 months still warrants greater thought and research. It has been suggested that a reduction in the dose, rather than total deprivation, should be considered. However, the response of infants to opiates is variable. Comfort measures such as supporting limbs, position changes, cuddling and stroking are some of the ways which can be helpful.

The aim of postoperative pain control should be to maintain the patient in a comfortable, humane and cooperative state at all times for as long as it is necessary after surgery.

Physiotherapy

If a child is pain free he or she is able to cooperate with physiotherapy with minimal discomfort. The physiotherapist and nurse work closely together in this aspect of care. Often a great deal of ingenuity is needed with a small child to achieve deep breathing and coughing. A child will breathe in more deeply if he or she first "blows out". Small tissue "rabbits" and puffs of cotton wool are two devices to encourage this. Firm, even pressure over the wound whilst the child coughs may help. Sometimes sips of warm fluid or external tracheal pressure will stimulate coughing. Coughing and deep breathing should be encouraged hourly during the early postoperative phase.

We tell a story, for example, "The Three Little Pigs", to make arm and body exercises more fun when the child is able to begin these. Physiotherapy will be continued at home following discharge.

Chest Drain Care

This aspect of care is often not well understood. Bringing to mind knowledge of the mechanics of breathing makes intelligent management of chest drains much easier.

The lungs are surrounded by two layers of pleura. A thin layer, the visceral pleura, is attached to the lungs. Continuous with this is a thicker layer which lines the chest wall and covers the diaphragm, the parietal pleura. Both membranes are in close apposition, and between them exists a subatmospheric or negative pressure. This occurs because of the elastic tendency of the chest wall to expand and the lungs to collapse, and is vital for normal breathing. On inspiration the diaphragm descends and the chest wall lifts up and out, taking the pleura with it, thus expanding the chest. Air is drawn in due to a pressure gradient. Expiration follows as the diaphragm relaxes.

Any air or fluid in the pleural space will interfere with the negative pressure, and cause partial lung collapse. If air collects under tension there may be complete lung collapse with a mediastinal shift, an urgent situation. The negative pressure will be restored when the air of fluid are removed. An underwater seal allows drainage and prevents air being "sucked in" from the higher atmospheric pressure.

To avoid discomfort and tension on the chest drain we strap the catheter tubing on to the chest, and support the drainage tubing by pinning it to the bed with an elastic band. All connections are reinforced by a plastic tie on longitudinal strapping for safety. We try and avoid dependent loops by coiling some of the tubing flat on the bed, securing it and allowing the rest to fall in as straight a line as possible to the collection bottle.

Fluctuations of the underwater seal tube are observed and will become less as the lung expands. They will also lessen as the level of fluid in the collection bottle rises. Swinging will cease when suction is applied, and if the child is on artificial ventilation it will be reversed. The amount of drainage, air or fluid, is noted and recorded.

Whether to "milk" the tube or not is controversial. Some consider that tissue damage may result from this. Research points out that when as little as 10 cm of the tube is stripped as much as −100 cm water negative pressure can be generated [54]. Those who recommend regularly "milking" of tubing are positive about its effect of dislodging clots and debris to achieve patency, and believe it is a necessary procedure. We recommend that each patient be individually asessed.

The practice of clamping chest drains before moving the patient, far from being a safety manoeuvre, is now being looked at critically. In fact it can be a dangerous practice, particularly in a child with pneumothorax. There is no need to clamp the tubing if the bottle or unit is kept below the child's chest. It is well to remember too to disconnect suction tubing when suction is ceased as tension pneumothorax may develop in a child who has an air leak, because the system will have no exit for the escape of air. After the chest drain has been removed observation of respiratory function is continued and any breathing difficulty notified.

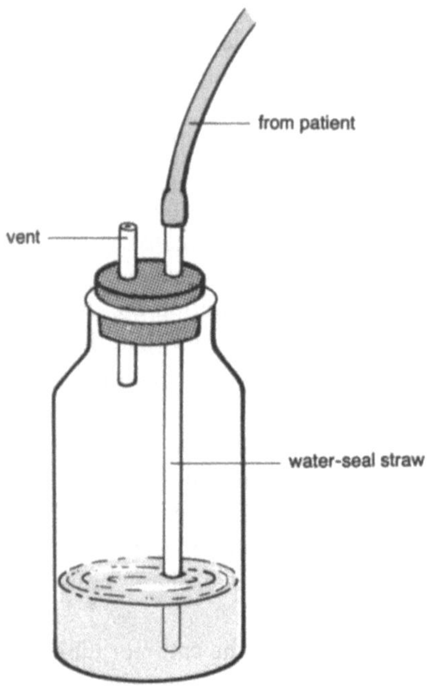

Fig. 1. Pleural drainage: single-bottle system

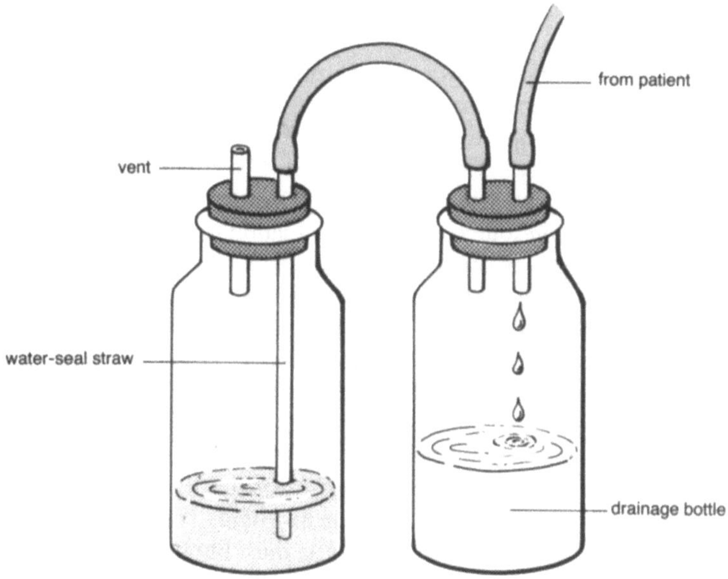

Fig. 2. Pleural drainage: double-bottle system

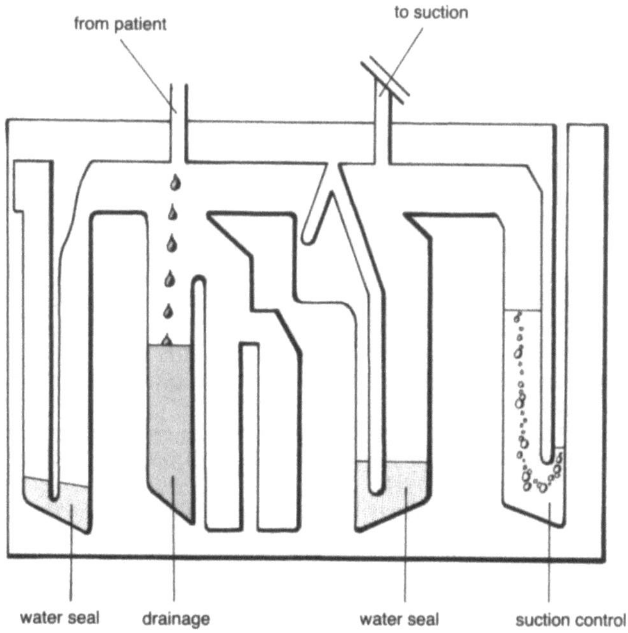

Fig. 3. Pleural drainage: Argyle "double-seal" unit

Drainage Systems

Although a number of systems exist, the principles of all remain the same. The simplest and least expensive is a single bottle with a glass tube submerged 1–2 cm under water (Fig. 1). This must be sufficiently under water to be safe, but not too deep to cause an increase in respiratory effort. If suction is applied we add a suction control bottle to the system; also a "trap" bottle to prevent accidental suction of fluid into the suction source (Fig. 2). The suction control bottle is a safety measure to prevent surges of negative pressure, thus allowing constancy of suction. The length of the tube under water determines the suction pressure applied. Bubbling in this tube will increase if the suction source is turned higher thus drawing in atmospheric air, but will not affect suction to the chest drain. Commercially produced chest drainage systems have been in use now for some years. These are expensive but have the advantage of convenience and ease of use. The Pleur-evac system has an infant and adult unit (Fig. 3). The necessity for applying suction is debated, as is the amount of suction pressure needed. In a child usually 20 cm water suction is applied and 10 cm water in an infant. To be sure that this amount of suction is being applied, the control bottle must bubble constantly.

References

1. Benner P (1982) From novice to expert. Am J Nurs 82:402–407
2. Roy N (1977) Neonatal transport. Med J Aust 2:862–864
3. Roy N, Brown M (1983) Stabilization and treatment. Newborn Emergency Transport Service, Melbourne, Victoria
4. Kennell JH, Klaus MH (1988) Care of the parents. In: Carlo WA, Chatburn RL (eds) Neonatal respiratory care, 2nd edn. Yearbook Medical, Chicago, pp 213–234
5. Muller NL, Bryan AC (1979) Chest wall mechanics and respiratory muscles in infants. Pediatr Clin North Am 26:503–515
6. McMahon RA (ed) (1984) Physiological differences between adults and children. In: An aid to paediatric surgery. Churchill Livingstone, Edinburgh, pp 4–7
7. Liebman J, Borkat G, Hirschfeld S (1979) The heart. In: Klaus MH, Fanaroff AA (eds) Care of the high-risk neonate. 2nd edn. Saunders, Philadelphia, pp 294–323
8. Friedman WF (1973) The intrinsic physiologic properties of the developing heart. In: Friedman WF et al (eds) Neonatal heart disease. Grune and Stratton, New York
9. Hazinski MF (1984) Children are different. In: Hazinski MF (ed) Nursing care of the critically ill child, Mosby, St Louis, p 2
10. Rushton CH (1988) The surgical neonate: principles of nursing management. Pediatr Nurs 14:141–150
11. Hazinski MF, Pacetti ASP (1988) Nursing care of the infant with respiratory disease. In: Carlo WA, Chatburn RL (eds) Neonatal respiratory care, 2nd edn. Yearbook Medical, Chicago, pp 154–211
12. Hey E, Scopes JW (1987) Thermoregulation in the newborn. In: Avery GB (ed) Neonatology: pathophysiology and management of the newborn, 3rd edn. Lippincott, Philadelphia, p 209
13. Dienno ME (1987) Esophageal atresia, corrective procedures and nursing care. AORN J 45: 1364
14. Shann F (1985) Paedriatric fluid and electrolyte therapy. In: Oh TE (ed) Intensive care manual, 2nd edn. Butterworths, Sydney, pp 425–429

15. Dorrington KL (1981) Skin turgor, do we understand the clinical sign? Lancet I:264–266
16. Smith LJ (ed) (1989) Intravenous nutrition. In: Paedriatric handbook, Roxal Children's Hospital, Melbourne. Endata Pty Ltd, Australia, pp 224–225
17. Central venous lines: descriptions, protocols and procedures (1988) Royal Children's Hospital, Melbourne
18. Benfield DG, Leib SA, Reuter J (1976) Grief response of parents following referral of the critically ill newborn. N Engl J Med 294:975
19. Mercer RT (1974) Mother's responses to their infants with defects. Nurs Res 23:133
20. Klaus MH, Kennell JN (1982) Parent-infant bonding. Mosby, St Louis
21. MacFarlane JA, Smith DM, Garrow DH (1978) The relationship between mother and neonate. In: Kitzinger S, Davis JA (eds) The place of birth, Oxford University Press, New York
22. Anisfeld E, Lipper E (1983) Early contact, social support and mother, infant bonding. Pediatrics 72:79
23. Berman L, Stringer D, Ein S, Shandling B (1988) The late-presenting pediatric Bochdalek hernia. J Pediatr Surg 23:735–739
24. Johnston PW et al (1988) Clinical use of extracorporeal membrane oxygenation in the treatment of persistent pulmonary hypertension following surgical repair of congenital diaphragmatic hernia. J Pediatr Surg 23:908–912
25. Bohn D et al (1987) Ventilatory predictors of pulmonary hypoplasia in congenital diaphragmatic hernia, confirmed by morphologic assessment. J Pediatr Surg 111:423–430
26. Langer JC et al (1988) Timing of surgery for congenital diaphragmatic hernia: is emergency operation necessary? J Pediatr Surg 23:731–734
27. Reynolds M, Luck SR, Lapper R (1984) The 'critical' neonate with congenital diaphragmatic hernia: a 21-year perspective. J Pediatr Surg 19:364–369
28. Moore KL (1982) The developing human, 3rd edn. Saunders, Philadelphia, pp 172–174
29. Anderson KD (1986) Congenital diaphragmatic hernia. In: Welsh KJ et al (eds) Pediatric surgery, 4th edn. Yearbook Medical, Chicago, pp 590–600
30. Phelan PD, Landau LI, Olinsky A (eds) (1982) Lung growth and development. In: Respiratory illness in children, 2nd edn. Blackwell, Oxford 5
31. Geggel RL et al (1988) Congenital diaphragmatic hernia: arterial structural changes and persistent pulmonary hypertension after surgical repair. J Pediatr 107:457–463
32. Moynihan P, Gerraughty A (1985) Diaphragmatic hernia, low stress = higher survival. Am J Nurs June:662–665
33. Filston HC, Izant RJ (1985) Congenital anomalies that present with respiratory distress. In: Filston HC, Izant RJ (eds) The surgical neonate. Appleton Century Crofts, Norwalk, Connecticut, p 94
34. Burge D (1989) Diaphragmatic hernia. Matern Child Health, January:21–25
35. Lillehei CW et al (1989) Preoperative ECMO in high-risk CDH. Fifth Annual Children's Hospital National Medical Center ECMO Symposium, p 68
36. Schraeder BD, Fischer DK (1986) Using intuitive knowledge to make clinical decisions. MCN 11:161–162
37. Stolar C, Dillon P, Reyes C (1988) Selective use of extracorporeal membrane oxygenation in the management of congenital diaphragmatic hernia. J Pediatr Surg 23:207–211
38. Gerraughty AB, Younie PLJ (1987) ECMO, the artificial lung for gravely ill newborns. Am J Nurs May:655–658
39. Nicks JJ, Bartlett RH (1988) Extracorporeal membrane oxygenation and other new modes of gas exchange. In: Carlo WA, Chatburn RL (eds) Neonatal respiratory care, 2nd edn. Yearbook Medical, Chicago, pp 405–407
40. Myers NA (1974) Oesophageal atresia: the epitome of modern surgery. Ann R Coll Surg Eng 54:277–287
41. Hopkins WA (1972) The esophagus. In: Gray SW, Skandalakis KE (eds) Embryology for surgeons. Saunders, Philadelphia, p 63
42. Guzetta PC et al (1987) Surgery of the neonate. In: Avery GB (ed) Neonatology: pathophysiology and management of the newborn, 3rd edn. Lippincott, Philadelphia, pp 952–953

43. Barry JE, Auldist AW (1984) The VATER association, one end of the spectrum of anomalies. Arch Dis Child 128:769
44. Connolly B, Guiney EJ (1987) Trends in tracheoesophageal fistula. Surg Gynecol Obstet 164:308–312
45. Spitz L, Kiely E, Bereton RJ (1987) Esophageal atresia: five-year experience with 148 cases. J Pediatr Surg 22:105–106
46. Puri P, Blake N, O'Donnell B, Guiney EJ (1981) Delayed primary anastomosis following spontaneous growth of esophageal segments in esophageal atresia. J Pediatr Surg 16:180–183
47. Bates TA, Broome M (1986) Preparation of children for hospitalization and surgery: a review of the literature. J Pediatr Nurs 1:230–238
48. Piaget J, Inhelder B (1969) Psychology of the child. Basic, New York
49. Pontious SL (1982) Practical Piaget: helping children understand. Am J Nurs, January:115
50. Bradshaw C, Zeanah PD (1986) Pediatric nurses' assessments of pain in children. J Pediatr Nurs 1:314
51. Cousins MJ, Mather LE (1989) Relief of post operative pain: advances awaiting application. Med J Aust 150:355
52. Dale JC (1986) A multidimensional study of infants' responses to painful stimuli. Pediatr Nurs 12:27
53. Beasley S, Tibballs J (1987) Efficacy and safety of continuous morphine infusion for post operative analgesia in the paediatric surgical ward. Aust NZJ Surg 57:233–237
54. Erickson R (1981) Chest tubes, they're really not that complicated. Nurs 11:41

Influence of Anatomy and Physiology on the Management of Oesophageal Atresia

S. W. Beasley

Summary

Anatomical and physiological considerations specific to newborn infants with congenital thoracic abnormalities directly affect the timing and nature of surgical intervention during the neonatal period. This paper uses oesophageal atresia as an example of a common neonatal thoracic condition to highlight the way in which these considerations have influenced the approach to their surgical management. The type of surgical approach employed during thoracotomy determines the likelihood of subsequent chest wall deformity: an intercostal approach is preferable to rib resection. Multiple thoracotomies adversely affect the chest wall appearance and lung function. In premature infants with respiratory distress syndrome early surgical closure of the tracheo-oesophageal fistula is advantageous, and gastrostomy alone often prolongs the ventilatory difficulties. The upper oesophagus can be extensively mobilized with little danger to its blood supply, whereas the lower oesophagus, because it receives a segmental supply, is more vulnerable to ischaemia. The severity and distribution of tracheomalacia is reflected in its symptomatology. Tracheomalacia often coexists with gastro-oesophageal reflux, which should be corrected by a fundoplication if respiratory symptoms persist or an oesophageal stricture develops. The numerous factors producing heat loss in the newborn during thoracotomy are discussed.

It is clear that an understanding of the anatomy and physiological changes which occur in the neonate is required if these infants are to be treated effectively and safely.

Zusammenfassung

Anatomische und physiologische Gesichtspunkte, die spezifisch für Neugeborene mit angeborenen Anomalien der Brustorgane sind, beeinflussen direkt die zeitliche Folge und die Art der Operation während der Neugeborenenperiode. Die vorliegende Arbeit zeigt anhand der Ösophagusatresie als Beispiel einer häufigen thoraxchirurgisch zu behandelnden Erkrankung im Neugeborenenalter, wie diese Gesichtspunkte das chirurgische Management beeinflußt haben. Die Art des chirurgischen Zugangs während der Thorakotomie bestimmt das Auftreten einer späteren Thoraxwanddeformität: der interkostale Zugang ist der Rippenresektion vorzuziehen. Multiple Thorakotomien beeinflussen die Form der Thoraxwand und die Lungenfunktion negativ. Bei Frühgeborenen mit Atemnotsyndrom hat sich der frühe Verschluß der tracheoösophagealen Fistel als vorteilhaft erwiesen, wohingegen die alleinige Gastrostomie häufig Beatmungsprobleme verlängert. Der obere Ösphagusstumpf kann ohne Gefährdung der Blutversorgung ausgiebig mobilisiert werden. Der untere Ösophagusstumpf hingegen ist wegen seiner segmentalen Blutversorgung empfindlicher gegenüber einer Ischämie. Ausprägung und Art der Ösophagusatresie sind häufig mit einem gastroösophagealen Reflux assoziiert, der durch eine Fundoplicatio korrigiert werden sollte, wenn respiratorische Symptome persistieren oder wenn eine Ösophagusstriktur entsteht. Die vielfältigen Faktoren, die beim Neugeborenen während der Thorakotomie zum Wärmeverlust führen, werden beschrieben. Logischerweise ist ein profundes Ver-

Department of General Surgery, Royal Children's Hospital Melbourne, Flemington Road, Parkville 3052, Victoria, Australia.

Progress in Pediatric Surgery, Vol. 27
Myers and Angerpointner (Eds.)

ständnis der anatomischen und physiologischen Veränderungen bei diesen Neugeborenen notwendig, um eine effektive und sichere Behandlung zu erreichen.

Résumé

Les données anatomiques et physiologiques spécifiques des nouveaux-nés présentant des anomalies thoraciques congénitales déterminent le moment choisi et la nature d'une intervention chirurgical durant la période néo-natale. Pour ce communiqué, nous avons pris comme exemple l'atrésie oesophagienne que l'on rencontre fréquemment durant la période néo-natale pour mettre en lumière l'influence des aspects indiqués ci-dessus sur la conception du traitement chirurgical. La technique utilisée pour la thoracotomie va déterminer l'ampleur de la déformation subséquente de la cage thoracique: la technique intercostale est préférable à la résection costale. Des thoracotomies répétées endommagent la cage thoracique et lèsent la fonction pulmonaire. Chez les prématurés présentant une insuffisance respiratoire grave, une intervention chirugicale pratiquée très tôt pour fermer la fistule trachéo-oesophagienne présente de grands avantages alors que la gastrotomie risque souvent de prolonger les difficultés respiratoires. La partie supérieure de l'oesophage peut être mobilisée sans risquer d'interrompre l'afflux sanguin alors que pour la partie inférieure de l'oesophage qui est alimentée par un segment, le risque d'ischémie est plus important. Dans les cas graves, il y a aussi souvent reflux gastro-oesophagien. Il faudra alors pratiquer une fondoplication si les symptômes persistaient ou s'il survenait une sténose (stricture) oesophagienne. Les auteurs traitent aussi des différents facteurs pouvant provoquer une perte de chaleur chez le nouveau-né durant la thoracotomie.

Introduction

Anatomical and physiological considerations specific to the newborn infant affect the surgical management of many neonatal thoracic conditions. While the basic anatomical structure of the thorax and its contents is established at birth, further development and growth continues throughout childhood. For example, while the number of airways proximal to the alveolar ducts (the basic anatomical structure of the airways) increases little from birth to adult life, there is a major increase in the number of alveolar ducts and sacs [1].

The physiological changes which occur in the newborn are rapid and complex as the infant quickly adapts to the different requirements of extrauterine life. Changes in lung compliance, airways resistance and the transition to postnatal circulation take several days before they are complete. These alterations in physiology, together with the pathophysiology of thoracic disease in the neonate, often influence the timing and extent of surgical intervention.

In this paper, oesophageal atresia and tracheo-oesophageal fistula is used as an example to highlight the ways in which anatomical and physiological considerations in the newborn influence the management of neonatal thoracic conditions.

Surgical Approach

The approach employed in thoracotomy in neonatal surgery is determined by consideration of the exposure required and the effect the incision will have on subsequent function and growth of the chest wall. In past years a variety of incisions have been popular in surgery for oesophageal atresia, but, recently, the postero-lateral thoracotomy with rib resection or through an intercostal approach have been the most popular. In our institution, both these approaches have been used. Recently, we conducted a review of adults with repaired oesophageal atresia to determine the effect of surgical approach on the development of subsequent chest wall deformity in patients who had no congenital vertebral anomaly [2]. It was found that the rib bed approach with rib resection was associated with a higher incidence of chest wall deformity than the intercostal approach (Fig. 1). This

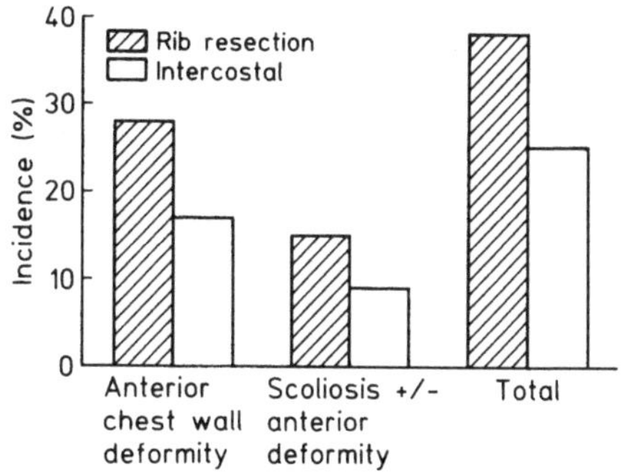

Fig. 1. Effect of surgical approach on chest deformity

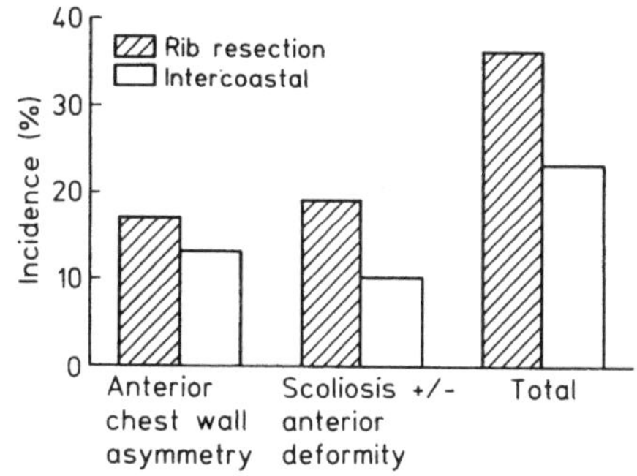

Fig. 2. Effect of surgical approach in children less than 15 years of age

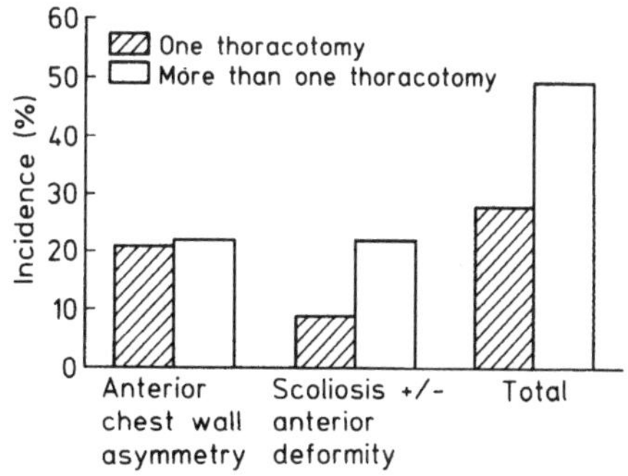

Fig. 3. Effect of thoracotomy number on chest deformity

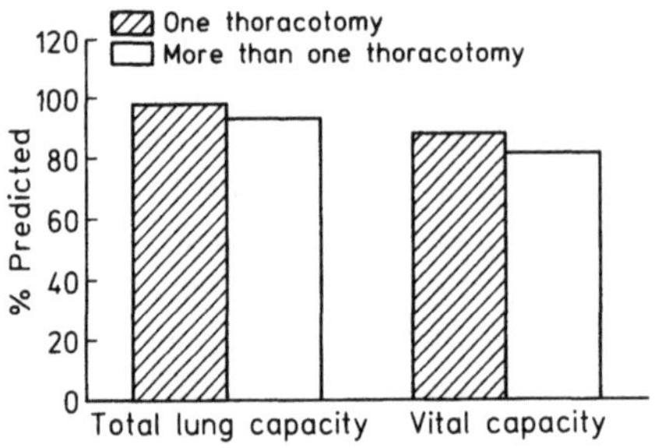

Fig. 4. Effect of thoracotomy number on lung function

effect on the chest wall first appeared during childhood (Fig. 2) and was maintained throughout life.

Likewise, thoracotomy number was found to have an effect on later chest wall deformity in that multiple thoracotomies increased the incidence of both anterior chest wall asymmetry and scoliosis (Fig. 3). Multiple thoracotomies had been performed deliberately in staged repairs, or in the management of complications of a previous thoracotomy. Total lung capacity and vital capacity were reduced after multiple thoracotomies (Fig. 4), in part because of the repeated thoracotomies in themselves, and in part due to the reasons for which the thoracotomies were performed, e.g. anastomotic dehiscence or empyema.

What are the factors which contribute to chest wall deformity? Interference with a rib and its periosteum might be expected to affect subsequent growth. Denervation of muscles, in particular the lower fibres of serratus anterior which are supplied by the long thoracic nerve from above, and the latissimus dorsi, may be further factors. Retraction of the edge of the wound inferiorly following division of the latissimus dorsi allows mobilization of the serratus anterior off its origin, and preserves its innervation. The muscle can be resutured to its origin low on the chest wall during closure. An intercostal approach is quick and easy in the neonate, does not disrupt the periosteum, requires no resection of ribs and would appear to result in less deformity than an approach which involved rib resection.

The Tracheo-oesophageal Fistula

Many infants with oesophageal atresia and a distal tracheo-oesophageal fistula are premature. The escape of air down a tracheo-oesophageal fistula through the stomach and beyond may result in gaseous distension of the abdomen, elevation of the diaphragm and restriction of ventilation. The neonate depends almost entirely on diaphragmatic movement for effective ventilation as the transverse rather than oblique configuration of the ribs means that intrathoracic volume increases little with intercostal contraction. In premature infants the combination of respiratory distress syndrome and splinting of the diaphragm may cause respiratory embarrassment and necessitate ventilatory support. In order to minimize respiratory compromise the lowest ventilatory pressures required to achieve adequate oxygenation must be used, and the tracheo-oesophageal fistula should be divided early [3]. These infants do best if operated on before the respiratory distress of prematurity becomes fully established and the complications of inadequate ventilation against an elevated diaphragm or ruptured stomach occur. The earlier practice of performing emergency gastrostomy in infants with major escape of air through a distal tracheo-oesophageal fistula causing gastric dilatation has been abandoned. This is because the massive leak often continued after gastrostomy and made ventilation ineffective as the air preferentially passed through the fistula [3]. As hyaline membrane disease takes 24–48 h to develop, the tracheo-oesophageal fistula should be divided on the 1st day, before the respiratory distress is fully established. Closure of the fistula improves the ease of subsequent ventilation because: there is no escape of air down the fistula; there is no diaphragmatic splinting; and soiling of the lungs with gastric secretions is less likely. In virtually all infants oesophageal continuity can be achieved at the time of thoracotomy to close the fistula.

Influence of the Vascular Supply of the Oesophagus on Oesophageal Mobilization

The cervical portion of the oesophagus is supplied by the inferior thyroid artery, a branch of the thyrocervical trunk [4]. The inferior thyroid artery gives off oesophageal and tracheal branches which run vertically downwards on their respective structures as far as the arch of the aorta in the superior mediastinum where they anastomose with oesophageal branches from the aorta and bronchial arteries. The remainder of the thoracic portion of the oesophagus, i.e. below the tracheal bifurcation, is supplied entirely by segmental oesophageal branches from the aorta, which are of relatively small calibre [5]. These form a rich anastomosis with adjacent vessels as well as with branches from intercostal and bronchial arteries. The distal oesophagus is supplied by the left gastric artery with some support from the inferior phrenic artery. In oesophageal atresia the blood supply to the oesophagus usually follows the same pattern [6].

The surgical significance of this supply is that the cervical and abdominal portions of the oesophagus are supplied richly by vessels which run along the oesophagus, whereas the thoracic portion is supplied segmentally, and has the most tenuous connections [6]. Mobilization of the thoracic oesophagus, therefore, is more liable to render it ischaemic. In oesophageal atresia without a tracheo-oesophageal fistula or where there is a long gap between the two oesophageal segments following division of a tracheo-oesophageal fistula, an oesophageal anastomosis may only be achievable after mobilization of both oesophageal segments. Knowledge of the vascular anatomy of the oesophagus enables us to be confident in dealing with mobilization of the upper pouch: the mobilization can be extensive and continued well up into the neck with little risk of devascularization because the arterial supply from the inferior thyroid artery remains intact. On the other hand, excessive mobilization of the lower oesophagus, by disrupting its segmental supply, may devascularize it and should be discouraged. In short, where the gap between the oesophageal ends necessitates oesophageal mobilization, full mobilization of the upper segment should be performed first, and the lower segment mobilized only as much as is required to achieve an end-to-end anastomosis. Procedures such as circular myotomy may compromise the blood supply, which may account for their high complication rate [7].

Tracheomalacia

In most infants and children with repaired oesophageal atresia and distal tracheo-oesophageal fistula there is some degree of structural and functional weakness of the tracheal wall which may result in intermittent respiratory obstruction. There is an absolute deficiency in cartilage and an increase in the length of the transverse muscle of the posterior tracheal wall [8]. The cartilage is shorter than normal and fails to give adequate support to the tracheal wall which has a perimeter greater than normal. The abnormality primarily affects the area around the site of the tracheo-oesophageal fistula, but may extend to involve the lower half of the trachea and, occasionally, the whole trachea. When the abnormality is confined to the intrathoracic trachea the signs are those of expiratory obstruction. Situations which increase the intrathoracic pressure, e.g. lower respiratory infection and inhalation of fine material, exacerbate the degree of tracheal collapse. Once expiration ceases to be forced, and the positive intrathoracic pressure is reduced, normal respiration is usually regained. Consequently, the signs of tracheomalacia are those of intermittent expiratory obstruction with normal inspiration. Infants with tracheomalacia often have a history of feeding difficulty and vomiting. An oesophageal stricture predisposes to inhalation of saliva and food and distension of the proximal oesophagus compressing the trachea and worsening the obstruction of the tracheomalacia. In turn, the expiratory obstruction facilitates gastro-oesophageal reflux by increasing the intra-abdominal pressure. Gastro-oesophageal reflux, therefore, may be both a cause and result of tracheomalacia.

When the symptoms of tracheomalacia are mild no active intervention is necessary, and as childhood progresses they tend to become less significant, although the so-called TOF cough may persist into adult life [9]. The management of severe tracheomalacia is less clear cut. Careful attention must be paid to feeding and the infant is given small amounts of soft foods until late in the 1st year. If there is associated gastro-oesophageal reflux this should be managed by posturing and thickened feeds in the first instance and by Nissen fundoplication if the respiratory symptoms persist or an oesophageal stricture develops. In the absence of gastro-oesophageal reflux, any oesophageal stricture should be dilated. Aortopexy should be considered in the child with recurrent cyanotic episodes due to expiratory obstruction in whom these measures have not been successful. The rationale for aortopexy relies on the observation that there are fibrous connections between the posterior surface of the aorta and the anterior wall of the trachea. By drawing the ascending arch of the aorta forward and suturing it to the body of the sternum the fibrous connections to the trachea pull the anterior wall of the trachea forward and hold open its lumen [10]. In the absence of gastro-oesophageal reflux, any oesophageal stricture should be dilated. Although the success of this procedure has varied from institution to institution, it would seem an appropriate procedure to be performed if life-threatening episodes continue despite the conservative measures mentioned above. External splinting operations of the trachea have not been shown to be effective in this condition.

Gastro-oesophageal Reflux

Gastro-oesophageal reflux is extremely common in infants but becomes less so during the 1st year of life. In part, this decrease in incidence of gastro-oesophageal reflux relates to the development of an intrinsic high pressure zone at the gastro-oesophageal junction. The normal neonate has a low oesophageal sphincter (LES) pressure but by 6 weeks has attained normal LES pressures [11]. Other factors which may contribute to the decrease in incidence with age include the increase in the length of the intra-abdominal portion of the oesophagus with growth, and the assumption of an erect posture.

The exact mechanism of competence of the gastro-oesophageal junction is argued but there is increasing evidence that the intrinsic muscular tone of the lower end of the oesophagus is the most important factor [12]. Although the macroscopic and histological appearance of the lower end of the oesophagus is not distinctive, manometric studies have shown active relaxation and contraction in this region in response to a variety of physical, chemical and hormonal stimuli. The angle at which the oesophagus enters the stomach at the cardia, and the length of the intra-abdominal portion of the oesophagus have also been suggested as factors contributing to competence of the gastro-oesophageal junction. In addition to these, infants with oesophageal atresia may have inherent dysfunction of the vagus nerve, trauma to vagal fibres during division of the fistula and mobilization of the oesophagus, and upward traction of the lower end of the oesophagus to achieve oesophageal anastomosis. It is suspected that these all may contribute to the high incidence of gastro-oesophageal reflux seen in oesophageal atresia patients following repair.

The sequelae of gastric acid reflux into the oesophagus is oesophagitis and, in severe cases, oesophageal stricture. In oesophageal atresia patients an oesophageal stricture may occur at the site of the oesophageal anastomosis or at the lower end of the oesophagus. Oesophageal dilatation for an oesophageal stricture secondary to gastro-oesophageal reflux is not effective as definitive treatment because the stricture tends to recur rapidly, often within weeks. The correct treatment for such strictures is fundoplication to prevent further reflux and to enable the stricture to resolve.

The abnormal motility with discoordinated peristalsis of the distal oesophagus from the level of the fistula [13] suggests that abnormal oesophageal motility is a feature of the anomaly itself and not purely secondary to operative manipulation.

Temperature Homeostasis

Heat loss in the newborn may be critical on account of the high surface area to body volume ratio. When the infant is born, unless dried promptly, considerable heat loss occurs from evaporation. In the premature infant, the smaller size, thinner skin and immaturity of the temperature-regulating centre in the hypothalamus compound the problem. The infant with recognized congenital abnormalities is subjected to repeated examination and frequent manipulation to attach or insert various monitoring devices and intravascular lines. This may delay the infant's placement in the controlled temperature of an incubator.

Upset in the control of temperature may occur as a result of the administration of anaesthetic drugs which depress those reflexes which maintain body temperature [14]. Muscle relaxants prevent shivering, and some anaesthetics, e.g. halothane, produce peripheral vasodilatation which increases heat loss.

The period of greatest risk is at induction of anaesthesia prior to draping of the infant. Measures which the anaesthetist can take to minimize temperature loss during thoracotomy include the use of a heating blanket, placement of a heat lamp over the operating table until the infant is draped, use of a rectal probe to monitor temperature, control of the temperature of warmed humidified inspired gases, warming of the operating theatre, keeping the infant covered as much as possible and infusion of warmed intravenous solutions. If blood loss leads to circulatory impairment, maintenance of body temperature will be further compromised [14]. Therefore the anaesthetist should ensure that there is an adequate circulatory blood volume at all times.

Where the surgical procedure involves thoracotomy, the moist exposed surfaces lose heat rapidly. The surgeon is obliged to ensure that the temperature is being monitored and controlled adequately, and that the duration of open thoracotomy is no longer than necessary.

References

1. Thurlbeck WM (1975) Postnatal growth and development of the lung. Am Rev Resp Dis 111:803–845
2. Chetcuti P, Myers NA, Phelan PD, Beasley SW, Dickens DRV (1989) Chest wall deformity in patients with repaired esophageal atresia. J Pediatr Surg 24:244–247
3. Holmes SJK, Liely EM, Spitz L (1987) Tracheooesophageal fistula and the respiratory distress syndrome. Pediatr Surg Int 2:16–18
4. Last RJ (1978) The posterior mediastinum. In: Last RJ (ed) Anatomy – regional and applied, 6th edn. Churchill Livingstone, Edinburgh, pp 238–240
5. Amoury RA (1986) Structure and function of the esophagus in infancy and early childhood. In: Ashcraft KW, Holder TM (eds) Pediatric esophageal surgery. Grune and Stratton, Orlando, pp 1–29
6. Lister J (1964) The blood supply to the oesophagus in relation to oesophageal atresia. Arch Dis Child 39:131–137
7. Taylor RG, Myers NA (1989) The management of a post-Livaditis procedure oesophageal diverticulum. Pediatr Surg Int 4:238–240

8. Wailoo MP, Emery JL (1979) The trachea in children with tracheo-oesophageal fistula. Histopathology 3:329–338
9. Checuti P, Myers NA, Phelan PD, Beasley SW (1988) Adults who survived repair of congenital oesophageal atresia and tracheo-oesophageal fistula. Br Med J 297:344–346
10. Benjamin B, Cohen D, Glasson M (1976) Tracheomalacia in association with congenital tracheo-oesophageal fistula. Surgery 79:504–508
11. Boix-Ochoa J, Cannals J (1976) Maturation of the lower oesophagus. J Pediatr Surg 11:749–756
12. Mann CV, Greenwood RK, Ellis FH (1964) The oesophago-gastric junction. Surg Gynecol Obstet 118:853–862
13. Sieber WK, Sieber AM (1974) Oesophageal manometry in postoperative oesophageal atresia with tracheo-oesophageal fistula. Z Kinderchir (suppl) 17:109
14. Brown TCK, Fisk GC (1979) Anaesthesia for children. Blackwell, Oxford, pp 14–18

Cervical, Cervicomediastinal and Intrathoracic Lymphangioma

M. J. Glasson and S. F. Taylor

Summary

Lymphangiomas result from abnormal development of the lymphatic system, with obstruction to lymph drainage from the affected area. The neck is the most common site (25%). In this study, we review the literature of lymphangioma in the neck and thorax and have undertaken detailed analysis of 52 children with cervical lymphangioma treated during the 20 years 1969–1988. Cervicomediastinal lymphangioma is uncommon (4%) and lesions confined to the thorax are rare, with none in our series. Neck lymphangiomas occur in early childhood with half being diagnosed at birth and almost 90% before school age. All have a mass. Two-thirds are asymptomatic; sudden enlargement, inflammation, infection, feeding difficulties and respiratory symptoms occur in the remainder. Pharyngeal and laryngeal involvement, usually associated with large infiltrating lesions, results in acute airways obstruction. The respiratory symptoms caused by mediastinal extensions are usually less dramatic. Lymphangiomas have a characteristic appearance on ultrasound examination and CT scan. These investigations are mandatory for an undiagnosed intrathoracic mass and when there is clinical suspicion of mediastinal extension of cervical lymphangioma but should be obtained for neck swellings only when the clinical diagnosis is in doubt. The recommended treatment is surgical excision which can be achieved with no mortality and little morbidity. An initial period of observation is justified for asymptomatic cervical lesions because there is a small incidence (6%) of spontaneous regression. Cervicomediastinal lymphangiomas can be removed at one operation using a neck incision combined with median sternotomy. The surgeon must preserve vital structures (especially vagus, recurrent laryngeal and phrenic nerves) and should not necessarily attempt total removal of all lymphangiomatous tissue. Massive infiltrating cervical lesions pose a particular challenge and may require multiple operations over many years before a satisfactory result with good-quality survival is attained.

Zusammenfassung

Lymphangiome resultieren aus einer abnormen Entwicklung des lymphatischen Systems mit Obstruktion der Lymphdrainage aus dem betroffenen Gebiet. Die Halsregion ist die häufigste Lokalisation (25%). In der vorliegenden Arbeit haben wir die Literatur zum Hals- und Thoraxlymphangiom durchgesehen und eine Analyse von 52 Kindern mit zervikalen Lymphangiomen während der letzten 20 Jahre (1969–1988) durchgeführt. Das zervikomediastinale Lymphangiom ist selten (4%). Ungewöhnlich sind Läsionen, die allein auf den Thorax beschränkt sind; wir hatten keinen derartigen Fall in unserer Serie. Halslymphangiome treten in der frühen Kindheit auf, wobei etwa 50% schon bei Geburt bestehen und fast 90% vor dem Schulalter diagnostiziert werden; dabei ist immer ein Tumor vorhanden; ⅔ sind asymptomatisch. Plötzliches Wachstum, Entzündung, Infektion, Ernährungsschwierigkeiten und respiratorische Symptome treten beim restlichen Drittel auf. Ein Befall von Pharynx und Larynx, gewöhnlich im Zusammenhang mit ausgedehnten Infiltrationen, führt zur akuten Atemwegsobstruktion. Die respiratorischen Sym-

Department of Paediatric Surgery, Royal Alexandra Hospital for Children, PO Box 34, Camperdown 2050, New South Wales, Australia.

Progress in Pediatric Surgery, Vol. 27
Myers and Angerpointner (Eds.)

ptome bei Befall des Mediastinums sind hingegen gewöhnlich weniger dramatisch. Lymphangiome zeigen eine charakteristische Struktur bei der Ultraschall- und CT-Untersuchung. Diese Untersuchungen sind unverzichtbar bei einem noch undiagnostizierten intrathorakalen Tumor oder wenn klinisch der Verdacht auf mediastinalen Befall eines zervikalen Lymphangioms besteht. Bei anderen Schwellungen im Halsbereich sollten sie aber nur durchgeführt werden, wenn Zweifel an der klinischen Diagnose bestehen. Die Behandlung der Wahl ist die chirurgische Exstirpation, die ohne Letalität und mit nur geringer Morbidität durchgeführt werden kann. Bei asymptomatischen zervikalen Läsionen kann man sich zunächst auf die Beobachtung beschränken, da in einigen Fällen (6%) die spontane Rückbildung erfolgen kann. Zervikomediastinale Lymphangiome können in einer Sitzung mit einer kombinierten Halsinzision und medianen Sternotomie exstirpiert werden. Der Chirurg muß die wichtigsten Strukturen schonen (besonders N. vagus, N. recurrens und N. phrenicus) und sollte nicht unbedingt versuchen, das gesamte lymphatische Gewebe in toto zu entfernen. Ausgedehnte infiltrierende Zervikalläsionen stellen eine besondere Herausforderung dar und können multiple Operationen über viele Jahre erforderlich machen, bis ein befriedigendes Ergebnis mit guter Lebensqualität erreicht ist.

Résumé

Les lymphangiomes sont dus à un développement anormal du système lymphatique avec obstruction du drainage lymphatique de la région touchée. Le siège d'élection est le cou (25%). Dans cet article, nous avons passé en revue la littérature sur le lymphangiome du cou et du thorax et nous avons analysé en détail les 52 cas d'enfants traités pour lymphangiome cervical en l'escape de 20 ans, entre 1969 et 1988. Le lymphangione cervico-médiastinal est peu fréquent (4%) et les lésions, limitées exclusivement au thorax, sont rares. Nous n'en présentons pas dans notre série. Les lymphangiomes du cou apparaissent chez les enfants en bas âge, la moitié des diagnostics étant possible dès la naissance, et près de 90% avant l'âge scolaire. Tous ont une masse. Les deux tiers sont asymptomatiques: dans les autres cas, on observe des augmentations de volume brusques, des inflammations, des infections, des problèmes lors de l'alimentation et des symptômes respiratoires. Une participation du pharynge et du larynge, accompagnée le plus souvent de grandes lésions infiltrantes, provoque une obstruction aigue des voies respiratoires. Les symptômes respiratoires causés par les extensions médiastinales sont en général moins dramatiques. Les lymphangiomes ont un aspect caractéristique qui permet des les discerner nettement à l'échographie et à la tomodensitométrie. Ces examens sont indispensables en présence d'une masse intrathoracique non diagnostiquée et quand il y a lieu de soupçonner une extension médiastinale d'un lymphagiome cervical. Dans les cas de gonflements cervicaux, on ne devra les pratiquer que si le diagnostic clinique est douteux. Le traitement de choix est l'excision chirurgicale qui peut se pratiquer sans mortalité et avec un très faible pourcentage de morbidité. Il est recommandé de prévoir une période d'observation du début dans les cas de lésions cervicales asymptomatiques car il arrive qu'il se produise (dans 6% des cas environ) une régression spontanée. Un lymphangiome cervico-médiastinal peut être excisé en une seule opération, en pratiquant une incision cervicale associée à une résection médiane du sternum. Le chirurgien se doit de préserver les structures vitales (en particulier le nerf pneumogastrique, les nerfs recurrents laryngé et phrénique et ne doit pas essayer obligatoirement de supprimer tout le tissu lymphangiomateux. Les infiltrations cervicales majeures posent un problème considérable et peuvent exiger des interventions répétées sur plusieurs années avant de pouvoir obtenir un résultat satisfaisant et une survie dans de bonnes conditions.

Introduction

A lymphangioma is a benign abnormal collection of lymphatic vessels which forms a mass. Most are present at birth but some do not become clinically evident for many months or years. The first descriptions of lymphangioma were in the European literature during the nineteenth century. Although relatively rare, lymphangioma now has a vast bibliography and should be well understood by paediatricians and paediatric surgeons alike.

Lymphangiomas have been described in almost every part of the body; the neck is the most common site. Mediastinal lymphangioma is most uncommon but is known as the most dangerous form of lymphangioma [16]. Mediastinal lymphangiomas usually exist as a downward extension of a cervical lymphangioma but may be confined to the thoracic cavity.

This article details the experience of lymphangioma at a large paediatric institution with emphasis upon lesions in the neck and thorax and attempts to review all aspects of the disorder occurring in these sites.

Clinical Experience

At the Royal Alexandra Hospital for Children, Sydney, Australia, 200 children were treated for lymphangioma during the 20-year period 1969–1988. The lesions occurred all over the body (Table 1) with the neck being the most common site. The lower limb (13%) and chest wall (12.5%) were next most frequent. Lymphangiomas at sites other than the neck are excluded from the following analysis.

Amongst the 52 cases of cervical lymphangioma, there were 30 boys and 20 girls. Some examples are illustrated in Fig. 1–5. Seven children (5 boys, 2 girls) had additional involvement of tongue, floor of mouth, pharynx or larynx. Two boys had a mediastinal extension and there were no examples of lymphangioma

Table 1. Site of lymphangioma, RAHC, 1969–1988

Site		No.	%	Site		No.	%
Neck		52	26	Upper limb		16	8
Neck only	50			Shoulder	3		
Cervicomediastinal	2			Arm	2		
Intrathoracic		0	0	Forearm	6		
				Hand/finger	5		
Head		20	10	Chest wall		25	12.5
Face	12						
Postauricular	5			Abdominal wall		3	1.5
Occiput	1			Inguinoscrotal		12	6
Postauricular	1						
Submental	1			Intra-abdominal		11	5.5
Intra-oral		19	9.5	Lower limb		26	13
Tongue	12			Thigh	13		
Buccal	3			Leg	10		
Pharynx/larynx	4			Foot	3		
Axilla		16	8		Total	200	

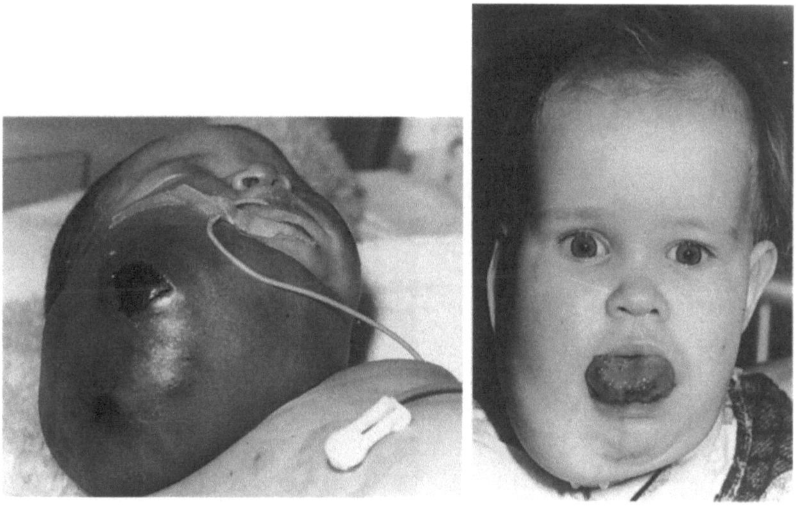

a b

Fig. 1. **a** Massive infiltrating lymphangioma of neck at birth. Note skin ulceration. **b** Same patient age 2 years with tracheostomy prior to subtotal glossectomy

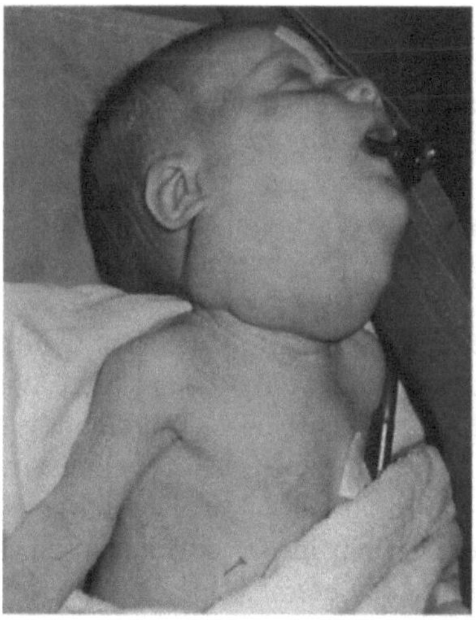

2

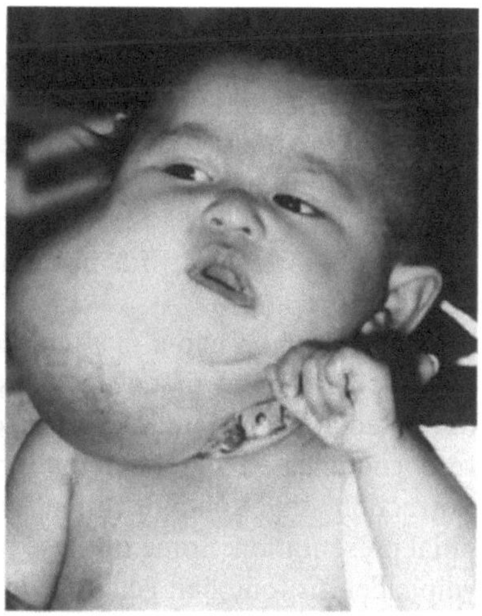

3

Fig. 2. Neonate with very large cervical lymphangioma and respiratory distress. (Reproduced from *An Aid to Paediatric Surgery*. Edited by R. A. McMahon. By kind permission of Churchill Livingstone, Edinburgh)

Fig. 3. This patient required tracheostomy at age 3 months

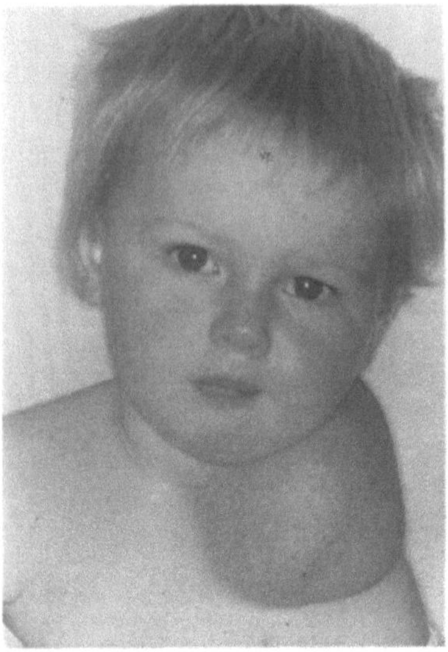

4

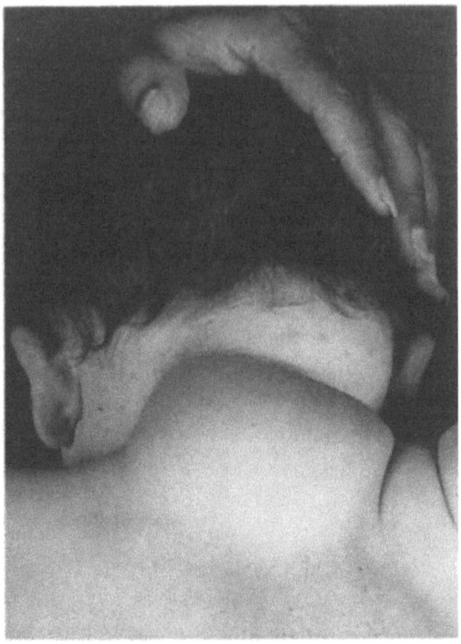

5

Fig. 4. Infant with large lymphangioma low in left neck. Mediastinal extension possible

Fig. 5. Lymphangioma in the midline of the posterior neck

confined to the thorax. The neck swelling was on the left side in 28 patients; 1 of these had an extension across the midline. Twenty-three were on the right and one was in the midline posteriorly (see Fig. 5).

Table 2 outlines the ages of the 52 children at time of presentation. Almost half were noted at birth. Sixty-five percent had been diagnosed by age 12 months and 88% before their fifth birthday. Three lymphangiomas were not detected until age 10 years.

All 52 children had a mass in the neck (Table 3). More than two-thirds were asymptomatic when first seen. Most remained well although three lymphangiomas noted at birth increased in size during the early weeks and months of life and were complicated by inflammation; one of these also developed respiratory obstruction. Eight patients (15.5%) had inflammatory change in the mass at the initial presentation. Some of these were initially incorrectly diagnosed as infective lymphadenitis; one had generalized infantile eczema. One child presented in the newborn period with feeding difficulties caused by a sublingual extension of the cervical lymphangioma. Eight patients (15.5%) had respiratory difficulty in addition to their mass when first seen. Three with extensive infiltrative lymphangioma involving neck, tongue, floor of mouth, pharynx, epiglottis and supraglottic larynx presented as a neonatal emergency (see Figs. 1, 2). The other five presented at ages 4 months to 2 years usually with noisy breathing and minor respiratory difficulty; one progressed to marked respiratory obstruction with stridor and cyanosis. Overall, 11 patients had respiratory symptoms directly associated with the lymphangioma either at the time of presentation or subsequently. The two

Table 2. Cervical lymphangioma RAHC, 1969–1988 – age at presentation

	No.	%
Birth	25	48
Birth – 6 months	6	11
6–12 months	3	6
1 year	2	4
2–4 years	10	19
5–9 years	3	6
10 years	3	6
	52	

Table 3. Cervical lymphangioma RAHC, 1969–1988 – mode of presentation

	No.	%
Asymptomatic mass	35	67
Mass plus inflammation	8	15.5
Mass plus feeding difficulty	1	2
Mass plus airways obstruction	8	15.5
	52	

Table 4. Cervical lymphangioma, RAHC, 1969–1988: investigations

	No.	%
Nil	26	50
Chest X-ray	22	42
Ultrasound	13	25
CAT scan	8	15
Endoscopy	7	13

children with mediastinal extension had respiratory difficulties and chest infections but did not have airways obstruction (see below).

No associated developmental anomalies were identified.

The radiological and other investigative procedures obtained in the 52 children are outlined in Table 4. A confident clinical diagnosis of lymphangioma could usually be made on the basis of the physical characteristics of the neck swelling. As a result, half of the children had no investigations. Chest X-ray was obtained most frequently (42%). Ultrasound examination of the swelling (Fig. 6) was undertaken in one-fourth of the children. The lymphangioma of one infant was suspected from antenatal ultrasound appearance. Eight children underwent computerized tomographic scanning (Fig. 7); this sometimes required general anaesthesia. Seven of the eight children with clinical evidence of airways obstruction underwent endoscopic examination of the larynx, pharynx, trachea and bronchi and oesophagus under general anaesthesia, usually as a preoperative manoeuvre. Three of these infants subsequently required repeated endoscopic evaluation during the course of their treatment.

The neck masses of three children who presented at birth, 3 months and 10 months respectively, disappeared spontaneously and no active treatment was required (Table 5). All three had a multilobulated appearance on ultrasound con-

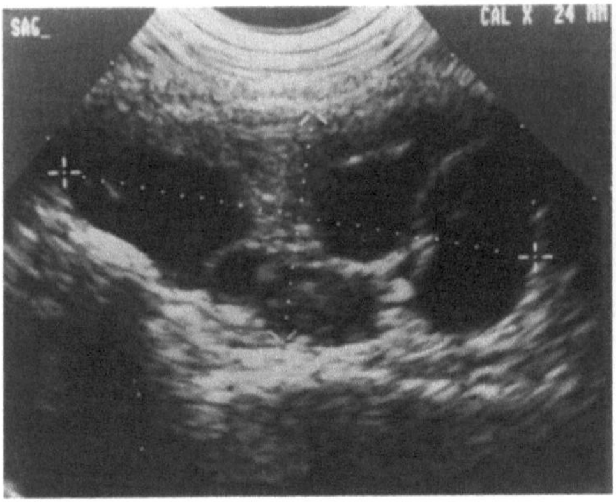

6

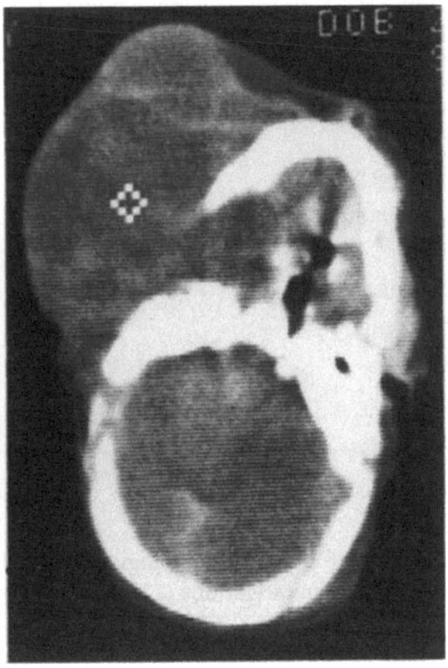

7

Fig. 6. Ultrasound of neck lymphangioma. Note cystic spaces of variable size and multiple septae

Fig. 7. Computed tomographic scan at birth of the patient illustrated in Fig. 1. Large infiltrating homogeneous mass

Table 5. Cervical lymphangioma, RAHC, 1969–1988: surgical treatment

	No.
No operation	3
One excision	38
Two excisions	7
More excisions	4
Tracheostomy	4
Gastrostomy	2

Table 6. Lymphangioma present at birth, RAHC, 1969–1988

Age at first operation	No.
Neonate	8
1–5 months	7
6–11 months	2
1 year	6
2 years	1
3 years	1
	25

sistent with lymphangioma; one also had a suggestive CT scan. With two of these children, the cystic mass resolved over intervals of 6 and 12 months whilst the third varied in size but when admitted for operation at age 4 years there was no palpable abnormality.

Forty-nine children underwent surgical excision of lymphangioma. Of the 25 diagnosed at birth, 8 with severe symptoms required treatment during the neonatal period but some waited for many months or years (Table 6). Table 7 outlines

Table 7. Lymphangioma not present at birth, RAHC, 1969–1988

Interval between diagnosis and operation	No.
1 month	6
2–5 months	8
6–11 months	6
1 year	3
2 years	1
	24

Table 8. Cervical lymphangioma, RAHC, 1969–1988: postoperative morbidity

	No.
Abnormal fluid accumulation	13
Haematoma	1
Wound infection	5
Damage to cervical branch facial nerve	7
Horner's syndrome	2
Phrenic nerve paralysis	2

the interval between diagnosis and operation with the 24 lymphangiomas which were not present at birth. Six were treated within a month whereas four waited for more than a year.

Thirty-eight patients (77%) had one procedure only (see Table 5). Three of these have documented residual or recurrent lymphangioma but have not required further surgery. Seven children required two excisional operations. The four who had more than two excisions included three with massive infiltrating lesions involving neck, tongue, pharynx, supraglottis or chest wall. Feeding gastrostomy was necessary for two of these children because of deglutition problems and all three had debulking operations in the neck or tongue and a number of microlaryngoscopic procedures which included laser destruction of lymphangioma with two. These three children underwent tracheostomy for respiratory obstruction in the neonatal period; another child had tracheostomy at age 3 months (see Fig. 3).

The diagnosis of lymphangioma was confirmed histologically in all 49 patients. Forty-seven were reported as having cystic lymphangioma and there was one example each of cavernous and capillary lymphangioma. All except two were multilocular. Sixteen showed pathological evidence of recent or old haemorrhage.

There was no mortality. Persistent fluid accumulation beneath the wound was the most common postoperative complication (Table 8). Suction wound drainage was usually utilized in the immediate postoperative period. Following removal of the wound drain, ten patients subsequently required intermittent needle aspiration and a further formal drainage procedure was necessary with three. The operation notes record involvement of or damage to the great auricular and supraclavicular nerves in eight patients and accessory nerve in five but none of these had documented postoperative nerve deficits. Seven patients with lymphangioma in the submandibular region experienced weakness of the lower lip postoperatively from damage to the cervical branch of the facial nerve; all resolved spontaneously. Two patients developed Horner's syndrome and diaphragmatic paralysis from phrenic nerve injury. One of these was an 18-month-old boy whose lymphangioma infiltrated the right neck widely and was closely associated with sympathetic chain, phrenic nerve, vagus nerve and carotid sheath. Both the Horner's syndrome and the diaphragmatic paralysis resolved. The other patient was one of the two with cervicomediastinal lymphangioma whose case histories are now detailed.

Case 1

Admitted in 1973 at age 2 weeks with a large soft mass in the right infraclavicular region. Needle aspiration produced 38 ml clear fluid. Operation at age 3 weeks revealed an appearance consistent with multiloculated lymphangioma infiltrating the clavicular head of pectoralis major muscle and extending into the right neck between the heads of the sternomastoid muscle. The lesion was excised incompletely and the microscopic report was resolving, partly calcified old haematoma. Postoperatively, good progress was made but fluid accumulation beneath the wound necessitated aspiration on two occasions. Chest X-ray was normal. The child remained well but returned at age 2 years with a history of persistent dry cough, intermittent bronchitis and the reappearance of right infraclavicular swelling. A further biopsy demonstrated fibrous and fibrocellular tissue with bundles of smooth muscle suggestive of lymphangioma. Mild dyspnoea developed and chest X-ray revealed a sharply demarcated opacity in the medial portion of the right upper lung field with slight indentation of the trachea. The child's symptoms did not progress over the following 3 months but repeat chest X-ray showed increased widening of the superior mediastinum. Utilizing median sternotomy, the lymphangioma was found to be adherent to the lower pole of the thyroid gland and intimately associated with major blood vessels, vagus and phrenic nerves and pericardium. The mass was dissected away from these structures with great difficulty; complete removal was not possible. Histologically, the lesion was a lymphangioma with cysts of varying size up to 4 cm in diameter.

Postoperatively, chest drainage continued for several days and there were no problems apart from minor cellulitis around the wound. There was no evidence of nerve damage. Further operation was required at age 7 years for a recurrent lymphangioma involving the right anterior chest wall.

Case 2

This boy was noted to have a very large cystic swelling in the left axilla at birth in 1977. Incomplete excision was undertaken at age 3 weeks; the histological diagnosis was lymphangioma. At age 8 months, noisy breathing developed in association with an enlarging mass in the left lower neck which augmented with crying. On chest X-ray soft tissue swelling was noted in the cervical region and in the superior mediastinum, mainly on the left. There was narrowing of the trachea with displacement of its mid portion to the right. Dyspnoea developed and progressed to stridor. Through a left neck incision and median sternotomy, a very extensive lymphangioma was encountered in the superior mediastinum extending into the left paravertebral space, neck and axilla. The innominate vein and left phrenic nerve were stretched over the lesion and the left vagus nerve and the great vessels passed through it. The lymphangioma was multiloculated and contained dark fluid. Almost complete removal of the mediastinal mass in continuity with the cervical mass was achieved. Microscopically, the diagnosis of lymphangioma was confirmed. Postoperatively, there was significant drainage of fluid from the intercostal catheter for several days. The patient developed left Horner's syndrome and over the following few months had frequent chest infections due predominantly to left diaphragmatic paralysis from left phrenic nerve palsy. There was good response to antibiotics and physiotherapy. Unfortunately, the patient has been lost to further follow-up.

Discussion

Embryology

The development of the lymphatic system is poorly understood. It is known that two paired (jugular and sciatic) and two unpaired (retroperitoneal) endothelial sacs appear during the 3rd and 4th month and constitute the primitive lymphatic system. Sabin [41] stated that these sacs develop from the venous system. Outgrowth of epithelium from the primitve sacs results in lymphatic channels which make new connections with the parent veins. According to this "centrifugal" theory, lymphangiomas would arise from growth of portions of the sacs which become sequested during embryonic life. Goetsch supported this idea, believing that active growth of epithelium is the explanation for the lymphangioma mass [14]. Godart rejected the centrifugal theory because it was based upon experiments using retrograde injections [13].

The alternative "centripetal" theory of Huntington is that mesenchymal slits appear in the reticulum of a rich venous plexus and coalesce to form lymphatic vessels; definitive lymph channels establish their own connections with veins and the parent veins degenerate [21]. Lymphangioma results from failure of mesenchymal clefts (primary lymphatic spaces) to establish connection with the developing main venous channels. Lymph sacs therefore enlarge and lymph accumulates in tissues.

Godart believed that lymphangioma growth occurs through accumulation of peripheral lymph secondary to atresia of main collectors [13]. The studies of Touloukian et al. injecting radioactive-labelled xenon gas into lymphangiomas gave support to this proposal by demonstrating that a functional lymphaticovenous block contributes to the size of lymphangiomas [49].

It is understandable that lymphangiomas most commonly occur in the neck close to the position of a primitive lymph sac. It is not surprising that some cervical lymphangiomas descend along vessels into the superior, anterior and posterior mediastinum. The embryological explanation for lymphangioma confined to the mediastinum is less clear and may be the result of abnormal development of the thoracic duct. The thoracic lymph channels are originally paired and have numerous cross-anastomoses. Usually the right embryonic trunk persists in the lower thorax and the definitive trunk crosses at the fourth to sixth thoracic vertebral level from where the left embryonic trunk persists to ascend and enter the left subclavian vein. There are many variations in the final course of the duct. It is reasonable to postulate that mediastinal lymphangioma could arise from sequestration or failure of connection of lymphatic vessels during thoracic duct development.

Pathology

Whether lymphangiomas are neoplasms or hamartomas is controversial. A neoplasm is an aberrant new growth of abnormal cells or tissues. A hamartoma is a developmental anomaly which produces a mass composed of tissues normally present in that locality but of improper proportion and distribution with dominance of one type of tissue. Goetsch observed that lymphangiomatous cysts enlarged by endothelial sprouting with extension along tissue planes between and around structures such as vessels or nerves and argued that it is an infiltrating neoplasm [14]. Willis believed that lymphangiomas are vascular hamartomas and that enlargement is due to the opening up of new channels in dormant lymphangioma and to fluid accumulation and not proliferative new growth [50]. This view is probably correct; malignant transformation of lymphangioma has not been reported [39].

Macroscopically, lymphangiomas are lobulated, multicystic lesions which usually infiltrate surrounding tissues but occasionally are encapsulated. Microscopically, the cyst walls are lined with a single layer of flattened endothelium and often contain smooth muscle. Lymphoid tissue is an integral part of the lesion and large irregular blood vessels are sometimes seen. Landing and Farber classified lymphangiomas into three varieties (simplex or capillary, cavernous, cystic) according to the size of the cystic spaces within the lesion [27]. Harkins and Sabiston showed that combinations of the three varieties occur in one patient [20]. Bill and Sumner suggested that the size of cystic areas is determined by the nature of surrounding structures. In areas of loose areolar tissue such as neck, axilla and mediastinum, large cysts develop (cystic lymphangioma) [3]. In areas such as the tongue or cheek where muscle and fibrous tissue intermingle with areolar tissue, the spaces are small (capillary/cavernous lymphangioma).

Lymphangiomas in the neck may be very large containing a network of intercommunicating cystic cavities of great complexity. The term "cystic hygroma" was first used to describe a neck lymphangioma and corresponds with the cystic variety of Landing and Farber [27]. With long usage lymphangiomas at any site are often called cystic hygroma. Although the pathologist reported almost all of our cases as cystic lymphangioma we believe that elements of all three varieties are almost always present. The Landing and Farber classification is not very helpful and the term "cystic hygroma" should be abandoned.

Associated Anomalies

Lymphangiomas usually occur in isolation. Associated malformations are mentioned by few authors other than Galofre et al. [11], who found disparate disorders such as thyroglossal duct cyst, cleft lip, congenital heart disease, hypertrophic pyloric stenosis and spina bifida sporadically amongst their patients. None of our patients had other abnormalities.

Chervenak et al. observed fetuses with lymphangiomas in the neck and other tissues associated with Turner's syndrome or other chromosomal anomalies [8]. None survived postnatally. Another extremely rare disease is Gorham's syndrome in which there is generalized lymphangiomatosis and osteolysis (disappearing bone disease) [6, 33]. The diagnosis is not usually made until adult life and the mediastinal lymphangioma is often complicated by chylothorax. We have had no experience with this syndrome.

Incidence

No data are available concerning the number of live births for each one with lymphangioma. Whilst uncommon, lymphangioma does occur with sufficient frequency for clinicians who work with children to need to be familiar with its various manifestations. All authors agree the neck is the most common site for lymphangioma. Of the patients reported by Galofre et al., 81.5% had lymphangioma predominantly in the neck but many of the diagnoses were not confirmed histologically [11]. Ravitch and Rush believed that three-fourths of lymphangiomas are in the neck [39]. Almost half of the patients reported by Ninh and Ninh [31] had their lesion in the neck. Other series had incidences in the neck of 41% [3] and 36% [2]. Although the neck is the most common site in our series (26%), we clearly have a lower incidence there than other authors and a higher incidence in other parts of the body, especially lower limb and chest wall.

In our series, 2 of 52 neck lymphangiomas had a mediastinal extension (3.8%). Ravitch and Rush [39] believed the incidence is lower (2%–3%). Other series have a higher incidence of mediastinal extension varying from 5% [2] to 9.5 [11].

Lymphangioma confined to the thorax is rare. There were no examples at our hospital during the period of review but we did find the medical records of two children with this variety of lymphangioma treated in the early 1960s. Intrathoracic lymphangioma is more common in adults than children. Childress et al. [9] reported 1 adult and reviewed 18 other cases in the literature of which only 4 were children. Bratu et al. [4] found 52 cases and reported 1 more. Rasaretnam et al. [37] stated that 1.3% of all primary mediastinal tumours are lymphangiomas. Sumner et al. [47] found 24 cases of isolated mediastinal lymphangioma in children in the literature. Ravitch [38] collected 320 cases of cysts and primary neoplasms of the mediastinum in infancy and childhood; 9 (2.8%) were lymphangiomas.

Clinical Aspects

Age at Presentation

Lymphangiomas in the neck are usually detected in very early life. Twenty-five of our cases (48%) were noted at birth (Table 2); many of these were very large (Figs. 1–3) and there were four with widespread infiltration of the neck. Bill and Sumner found that 59% of their total cases were noted at birth [3]. Ninh and Ninh believed that more than two-thirds of their cases (neck and other sites) were present at birth but in Vietnam medical attention was frequently delayed for weeks or months [31]. Ravitch and Rush stated that 50%–60% of lymphangiomas appear before the end of the 1st year of life and 80%–90% by the end of the 2nd year. Only 69% of our cases were diagnosed before their 2nd birthday [39]. Late presentation does occur presumably because of disruption of a tenuous balance between production and drainage of lymph in the affected area. Two of our patients had no abnormality in the neck until age 10 years; Galofre et al. had 8 patients aged more than 15 years [11].

Cervicomediastinal lymphangioma is also usually diagnosed in early infancy. Our two cases had obvious lymphangioma in the neck in the neonatal period; the mediastinal components were not recognized initially and required treatment at age 8 months and 2 years respectively. Gross and Hurwitt had one patient at age 7 months and another at age 14 months [18]. The patients of Camishion and Templeton presented at age 2 years and 4 years [7]. Other authors have reported cervicomediastinal lymphangioma in children aged 4 years or less [1, 3, 17, 29, 30, 45, 46]. Late diagnosis does occur. Rasaretnam et al. reported two patients diagnosed in adult life and not treated until their 4th decade [37].

Although lymphangiomas confined to a thoracic cavity occur mostly in adults, children have been reported at age 2 months [4], 14 months [47] and 11 years [23]. Bratu et al. found six children in the literature diagnosed during the first 2 years of life and eight over the age of 2 years [4]. Both cases treated at our hospital before the period of review were diagnosed at age 2 years.

Sex

Ravitch and Rush stated that lymphangiomas occur with equal frequency in males and females [39]. In our series of 52 lymphangiomas in the neck, there was a slight but not significant preponderance of boys. Bill and Sumner [3] and Ninh and Ninh [31] also found more boys than girls. Both our cases of cervicomediastinal lymphangioma were boys as were those of Camishion and Templeton [7]. Grosfeld et al. had six boys and four girls [17]. On the other hand, the two cases reported by Khoury and Demong were girls [24]. There appears to be an equal distribution of boys and girls amongst the examples of lymphangioma confined to the thoracic cavity which have been reported. The two treated at our hospital were girls.

Symptoms and Signs

Lymphangiomas in the neck cause a soft swelling which may have a multilobular appearance and which to palpation may appear cystic (see Figs. 1–5). The mass may be circumscribed but very often its infiltrative nature is obvious clinically. The physical sign of transillumination is not always present. The submandibular region and posterior triangle are affected most commonly. Two-thirds of neck lymphangiomas are asymptomatic (see Table 3).

Symptoms which occur in the neonatal period are usually related to breathing, feeding or both. Massive infiltrating lymphangioma (see Figs. 1, 2) may create an urgent clinical situation in the perinatal period. Urgent assisted delivery was necessary for one of our patients (see Fig. 1) because of obstructed labour. This patient and two others developed stridor and progressive respiratory difficulty soon after birth. Broomhead [5] and Barrand and Freeman [1] reported similar experience. The airways obstruction in these patients is due partly to the soft tissue mass in the neck and partly to lymphangioma in the glottis and supraglottic region.

One of our patients with a small mass in the left neck at birth could not be established on oral feeding because of a fairly large sublingual component. Macroglossia (see Fig. 1B) and pharyngeal coordination can also contribute to feeding and swallowing difficulties.

Older children develop acute symptoms such as pain and discomfort when there is sudden enlargement of the lymphangioma. This can be caused by haemorrhage into the lesion, fluid accumulation or secondary infection. With some of our patients, inflammatory changes were present when the neck swelling first appeared and the clinical features mimicked acute bacterial lymphadenitis. None progressed to abscess formation but this did occur in one of the patients reported by Camishion and Templeton [7]. There were patients in our series who experienced sudden enlargement of the lymphangioma at the time of an acute upper respiratory tract infection. This phenomenon has been noted by other authors [11, 17, 18] and presumably results from tissue fluid disturbance.

A mediastinal extension should be suspected when the lymphangioma is in the lower neck (see Fig. 4) especially if its size fluctuates with straining and respiration [29]. The respiratory symptoms in our two patients with cervicomediastinal lymphangioma were less alarming than the airways obstruction in the patients with massive lesions involving the supraglottic region as well as the surrounding neck. Nevertheless, cervicomediastinal lymphangioma can produce a dramatic clinical picture with acute respiratory distress, cyanosis and poor feeding [25]. Eight of ten cases reported by Grosfeld et al. required urgent treatment [17].

Lymphangiomas confined to the thorax can cause dramatic respiratory symptoms in early infancy [10]. The neonate with respiratory failure reported by Man et al. [28] had obstruction to the left main stem bronchus and a mediastinal lymphatic cyst of uncertain significance. Bratu et al. [4] described a child with anterior mediastinal lymphangioma causing severe respiratory distress at age 2 months. Our patients both presented with cough, fever and physical signs of bronchitis at age 2 years. Other authors reported patients with similar mild to moderate respiratory symptoms [26, 34, 47]. Recent haemorrhage into the pre-existing lymphangioma probably explained the short duration of symptoms before diagnosis. Prominent veins over the chest wall [24] and unresolved pneumonia [35] have also provided clues to the diagnosis of intrathoracic lymphangioma. Other associations include superior vena caval obstruction [22], primary chylopericardium [19] and chylothorax [4, 23, 46].

Investigation

With many lymphangiomas in the neck, management can be planned without the aid of investigations. Alternative diagnoses such as teratoma, haemangioma, thyroglossal duct cyst, lipoma, branchial cyst or lymphadenopathy may often be excluded on the basis of physical signs alone. Investigations are helpful if the diagnosis is in doubt or if there is a possibility of a mediastinal extension.

Some authors recommend that all patients with a lymphangioma in the neck have a chest X-ray [9, 17, 45]. With the low incidence (4%) of mediastinal extension, the validity of this recommendation is doubtful. Chest X-ray is mandatory for all patients with respiratory symptoms and is wise for those whose swelling is in the lower neck (see Fig. 4). Chest X-ray was obtained in 42% of our patients.

Ultrasound examination is an extremely useful investigation for selected patients and was obtained in one-fourth of those reported here. On ultrasound, there is a characteristic appearance (see Fig. 6); the lymphangioma mass is randomly divided by incomplete septa of variable thickness. Groves and Sumner [19] reported the value of ultrasound in preoperative diagnosis of an intra-abdominal lymphangioma. Grosfeld et al. [17] found ultrasound of use in the diagnosis of cervicomediastinal lymphangioma. Chervenak et al. [8] used ultrasound antenatally accurately to diagnose lymphangioma. Rueda et al. [40] studied an infant with a posterior mediastinal mass with an ultrasound appearance considered typical of lymphangioma; the diagnosis was subsequently confirmed histologically. Sheth et al. [42] correlated sonographic findings with histological appearance in eight children and demonstrated that the echogenic component of the lymphangioma corresponds to clusters of abnormal lymphatic channels. Ultrasound examination is non-invasive and is easily obtained at all ages.

Silverman et al. [44] used computed tomographic (CT) scan to confirm the diagnosis of lymphangioma in a 5-year-old girl with a swelling in the neck and demonstrated no mediastinal extension. Pilla et al. [36] used this modality to investigate two patients with a mediastinal mass; the findings were sufficiently characteristic to suggest the diagnosis of lymphangioma. The lesions were well-circumscribed, enveloped normal mediastinal structures, and had low attenuation. Other authors have also found CT scan useful for the diagnosis of lymphangiomas in the anterior and superior mediastinum [6, 26, 43]. The display of the precise extent of the lesion in relation to surrounding structures helps plan treatment. CT scan was obtained in 15% of our patients (see Fig. 7). This method of investigation was not available during the first 10 years of the review.

Endoscopic examination of the pharynx, larynx, trachea and oesophagus is a necessary investigation for patients who have clinical evidence of respiratory obstruction with stridor. It was undertaken with seven of our patients but was not considered necessary in the two children with cervicomediastinal lymphangioma. Endoscopy affords the opportunity accurately to assess the distribution of lymphangioma and determine whether airways compromise is caused by mucosal or extramural disease.

Fluroscopy may help diagnose mediastinal lymphangioma by visualizing wavy motion of the outline of the mass [29].

Investigations which are not helpful include barium swallow, mediastinoscopy, diagnostic pneumothorax and diagnostic aspiration of a neck mass with or without injection of radiopaque contrast material [39].

Management

Surgical excision is the treatment of choice. Alternative treatments which have been described for lymphangioma include simple aspiration, incision and drainage, irradiation and injection of sclerosants. None were used with our patients.

Irradiation using standard radiotherapy or the implantation of radon seeds is ineffective [3, 11] and may provoke lymphangitis [31] or increased swelling and the need for urgent intervention [1]. Irradiation is irrational treatment for a benign process such as lymphangioma and in the neck or mediastinum unacceptably exposes the patient to the risks of thyroid cancer and damage to cervical and thoracic vertebral epiphyses. Irradiation caused some of the deaths in the series of Galofre et al. [11].

The injection of sclerosing agents has appeal as a therapeutic manoeuvre for lymphangioma but there are no reports of good results. Sclerosants which have been tried include sodium morrhuate, glucose, boiling water, quinine, ethanolamine, saturated saline, lipidol, tincture of iodine and bleomycin. Broomhead found subsequent excision was made more difficult by resulting fibrosis [5]. Tanigawa [48] used bleomycin as an oil emulsion which is retained within the lesion. There was some benefit but most patients developed fever and increased swelling immediately following the injection. One patient with cervico-mediastinal lymphangioma became dyspnoeic and required urgent operation. This technique may prove to be a valuable adjunct to surgery for selected patients who do not have a mediastinal component.

Spontaneous regression has been reported [5, 31, 32]. Infection in a lymphangioma may provoke fibrosis and disappearance [7]. Three of our patients had neck swellings which disappeared without active treatment. None had documented infections. Two had sonographic features suggestive of lymphangioma with haemorrhage. In these patients, resolution of the haemorrhage may have stimulated improved lymphatic drainage and hence regression of the lymphangioma. Despite this, prolonged watchful expectancy is justified for only a small number of patients. Without operation, the neck swelling creates anxiety and there is the risk of sudden enlargement.

When there are no symptoms, operation can be planned as an elective procedure. For children diagnosed in the early weeks or months of life, it is sensible to wait until a later age, when general anaesthesia is better tolerated. Forty per cent of our neck lymphangiomas diagnosed at birth had no treatment until after the age of 6 months (see Table 6); one waited until age 3 years. Similarly, 42% of those diagnosed at an older age waited for more than 6 months before operation (see Table 7). The possibility of spontaneous regression justifies a period of observation before advising surgical treatment. Operation should be postponed for 3 months following an episode of infection [31]. Prompt intervention is mandatory when there are acute respiratory symptoms. Eleven of our patients had respiratory symptoms; six required urgent operation.

In the neck, an incision placed over the site of maximum swelling provides good access. For cervicomediastinal lesions, a two-stage approach can be used with initial operation in the thorax [7] or in the neck [18, 30]. The latter has appeal because adequate removal of the mediastinal extension might be achieved from above, thus avoiding thoracotomy. We have preferred the one-stage combined approach advocated by Kirschner [25] and Mills and Grosfeld [29]. A hockey stick incision from the neck onto the midline anterior chest is utilized and with median sternotomy excellent exposure is obtained.

At operation, a plane of dissection is carefully developed on the surface of the lymphangioma mass, preferably with its capsule intact. Cystic spaces which are entered can be sutured; alternatively a gloved finger inside the cyst provides traction to facilitate further dissection [17]. Sometimes complete removal may be achieved especially with encapsulated lymphangiomas in the neck. More often, excision is incomplete because there is no plane of cleavage between the mass and surrounding tissues which may include carotid sheath, subclavian vessels, superior vena cava, thymus, sympathetic chain, vagus, recurrent laryngeal, phrenic and accessory nerves and pericardium. There is agreement in the literature that total excision must not be attempted when vital structures are at risk, especially nerves.

The surgical task is particularly difficult when there is massive infiltration of the neck. Barrand and Freeman [1] were sufficiently discouraged with their results in this group to recommend against excision. This recommendation cannot be sustained especially when there is danger of mediastinal compression [2]. To become asymptomatic and socially acceptable, these unfortunate infants may require a large number of operations. Tracheostomy and/or gastrostomy relieve respiratory and feeding difficulties caused by lymphangiomatous involvement of tongue, floor or mouth, epiglottis and supraglottic structures and are required until much of the lymphangioma has been eliminated. One of our patients (see Fig. 1) over a 6-year period had a total of six debulking procedures in the neck and tongue and seven endoscopic procedures in the pharyngeal and laryngeal areas before removal of tracheostomy could be considered. We have found the carbon dioxide laser very effective for endoscopic destruction of lymphangioma in the airway and as an adjunct to operation on the tongue.

Lymphangiomas confined to the thoracic cavity should be excised at thoracotomy; the diagnosis may not be appreciated preoperatively. Both intrathoracic lymphangiomas treated at our hospital before the period of review were in the anterior and superior mediastinum predominantly on the left and were completely removed. Similar success in children has been reported by other authors [4, 34]. Bratu et al. [4] noted from the literature that all children offered surgical treatment for mediastinal lymphangioma had survived. Sumner et al. [47] thought their case was a mediastinal teratoma and therefore sacrificed the left phrenic and recurrent laryngeal nerves. Increasingly sophisticated preoperative non-invasive imaging techniques might prevent this error in the future. Subtotal removal of the lymphangioma relieved symptoms of superior vena caval obstruction in the patient reported by Issa et al. [22]. The 6-year-old boy with persistent pneumonia reported by Pike et al. [35] responded well to excision of lymphangioma from his left lower pleural cavity. Groves and Effler [19] successfully treated an adult with primary chylopericardium by excision of the associated mediastinal lymphangioma and ligation of thoracic duct. Pedicelli et al. undertook excision of anterior mediastinal lymphangioma and parietal pleurectomy to create adhesion between the lung and the chest wall in a patient with chylothorax associated with Gorham's syndrome [33].

As with other reported series, the most common postoperative complication experienced by our patients was excessive fluid accumulation (see Table 8). The cause is exudation either from lymphatics transected at the periphery of the mass or from the lining of incompletely removed cysts. Despite meticulous search it may not be possible at operation to identify and ligate all major lymphatics which have been divided. An effort should be made to destroy the endothelium of portions of lymphangioma which cannot be removed completely. Gross and Hurwitt used chemical sclerosis by swabbing the interior of residual cysts with iodine. We have not employed this method but have found diathermy coagulation useful [18]. The fluid accumulation in our patients responded to intermittent needle aspiration or a period of formal drainage; most other authors report similar experience. Fibrin glue can be used for lymph leaks which persist despite prolonged drainage [12]. The two patients in our series with cervicomediastinal lymphangioma had persistent serosanguinous intercostal catheter drainage for 7 or more days following thoracotomy. Chylothorax can occur following operation for intrathoracic lymphangioma [7, 23, 32].

Operation for cervical and mediastinal lymphangiomas carries significant risk of damage to important nerves. In particular danger are the cervical branch of the facial nerve, accessory nerve, sympathetic chain and the vagus, recurrent laryngeal and phrenic nerves. Barrand and Freeman [1] were sufficiently dismayed by their high incidence of vocal cord paralysis and facial nerve palsy following operation for massive infiltrating lymphangioma to contemplate non-intervention. Rasaretnam et al. [37] and Grosfeld et al. [17] reported Horner's syndrome, sometimes transient, after operation for cervicomediastinal lymphangioma. The two examples of Horner's syndrome in our series were permanent whereas those with damage to the cervical branch of the facial nerve all recovered. One of our two cases of phrenic nerve injury followed a neck dissection; the other was one of the children with cervicomediastinal lymphangioma (case 2). Increased intraoperative use of nerve stimulators may mean fewer damaged nerves in the future.

Prognosis

There were no deaths in our series but we are aware of an infant born in our city who died very soon after birth from respiratory failure associated with infiltrating lymphangioma of much of the upper body (Fig. 8). No treatment could be offered. Singh et al. [45] mentioned a similar neonate with massive lymphangioma of the chest wall extending into the mediastinum who died at age 2 days. The distribution of lymphangioma in these cases was incompatible with survival. Chervenak et al. [8] reported 16 cases of lymphangioma diagnosed by antenatal ultrasound examination with no postnatal survivors. Most were in the neck, some had fetal hydrops and all had chromosomal anomalies. Chromosome studies could not be obtained in the patient illustrated in Fig. 8.

All other forms of lymphangioma should have an excellent prognosis. Very large lesions in the neck do threaten life. These patients can succumb from acute asphyxiation whilst awaiting operation [2, 3, 45]; early intervention is therefore essential to provide a secure airway. One of our four patients with massive neck lesions underwent tracheostomy at age 3 days. Another patient had a period of nasotracheal intubation prior to tracheostomy at age 4 weeks. The other two had no respiratory distress initially but symptoms developed as the lymphangioma enlarged and tracheostomy was performed at age 1 months (see Fig. 2) and 3 months (see Fig. 3).

There have been reports of death from haemorrhage or anaesthetic difficulties during operation for excision of enormous lymphangiomas [2, 3, 31]. With skilled paediatric anaesthesia and the avoidance of radical aggressive surgery, operative death should not occur. The surgical aim must be to debulk tissue and relieve symptoms rather than achieve complete removal.

Broomhead [5] and Barrand and Freeman [1] experienced postoperative respiratory deaths in patients who had tracheostomy, nerve damage or residual lymphangioma in the larynx or superior mediastinum. Such deaths are avoidable. Tracheostomy is necessary when the lymphangioma is causing upper airways

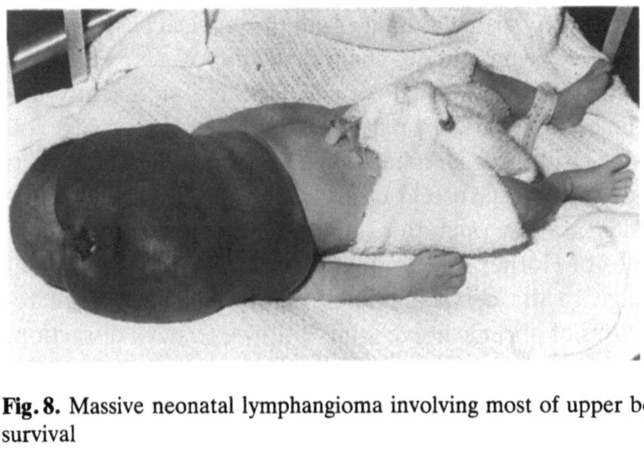

Fig. 8. Massive neonatal lymphangioma involving most of upper body and not compatible with survival

obstruction and must be retained until all abnormal tissue in the airway has been destroyed. The carbon dioxide laser delivered with microlaryngoscopic technique facilitates this process. Meticulous tracheostomy care is essential at all times and discharge from hospital should not be considered if there is need for frequent aspiration of secretions. One of our patients (see Fig. 1) remained in hospital continuously from birth until age 3 years, 2 months. His tracheostomy was removed at age 5 years.

Our two patients with cervicomediastinal lymphangioma both survived surgical treatment. Without operation these patients can die from mediastinal compression [2]. With operation, the outlook should be good. Bill and Sumner [3] lost a patient during operation. Stratton and Grant [46] reported a complex patient whose lymphangioma affected both sides of the neck, both axillae and mediastinum with a chylopericardium. The child died at age 10 months despite a number of operations. Early ligation of the thoracic duct may have helped.

Satisfactory quality of life can be anticipated following surgical treatment of lymphangioma. Galofre et al. [11] attempted to follow up their patients and classify the late result as good, fair or poor. More than half had a good result with no symptoms referrable to lymphangioma. One-fourth had a poor result with adverse sequelae due to treatment or the need for further surgery. We have not been able to study our patients in this manner but believe that current standards of anaesthesia and surgery should produce a good result for almost all patients. Those with massive lesions in the neck may have cosmetic deformity from residual or recurrent lymphangioma, Horner's syndrome, lower lip palsy or accessory nerve injury. When the recurrent laryngeal or phrenic nerve is damaged, the patient will have ongoing adverse symptoms and the late result may be poor.

Acknowledgments. We wish to thank our various surgical colleagues for permission to review their patients. The assistance of Dr. Patricia Bale, who reviewed the pathology specimens, is gratefully acknowledged. This work would not have been possible without the support and secretarial services of Mrs. Maryellen Sgro.

References

1. Barrand KG, Freeman NV (1973) Massive infiltrating cystic hygroma of the neck in infancy. Arch Dis Child 48:523–531
2. Bhattacharyya NC, Yadav K, Mitra SK, Pathak IC (1981) Lymphangiomas in children. Aust NZJ Surg 51:296–300
3. Bill AH, Sumner DS (1965) A unified concept of lymphangioma and cystic hygroma. Surg Gynecol Obstet 120:79–86
4. Bratu M, Brown M, Carter M, Lawson JP (1970) Cystic hygroma of the mediastinum in children. 119:348–351
5. Broomhead, IW (1965) Cystic hygroma of the neck. Br J Plast Surg 17:225–244
6. Brown LR, Reiman HM, Rosenow EC, Gloviczki PM, Divertie MB (1986) Intrathoracic lymphangioma. Mayo Clin Proc 61:882–892
7. Camishion RC, Templeton JY (1962) Cervicomediastinal cystic hygroma. Paediatrics 29:831–834

8. Chervenak FA, Issacson G, Blakemore KJ, Breg WR, Hobbins JC, Berkowitz RL, Tortora M, Mayden K, Mahoney MJ (1983) Fetal cystic hygroma. N Engl J Med 309:822–825
9. Childress ME, Baker CP, Samson PC (1956) Lymphangioma of the mediastinum. J Thorac Surg 31:338–348
10. Feutz EP, Yune HY, Mandelbaum I, Brashear R (1973) Intrathoracic cystic hygroma. Radiology 108:61–66
11. Galofré M, Judd ES, Pérez PE, Harrison EG (1962) Results of surgical treatment of cystic hygroma. Surg Gynecol Obstet. 115:319–326
12. Giberson W, McCarthy PM, Kaufman BH (1988) Fibrin glue for the treatment of persistent lymphatic drainage. J Pediatr Surg 23:1188–1189
13. Godart S (1966) Embryological significance of lymphangioma. Arch Dis Child 41:204–206
14. Goetsch E (1938) Hygroma colli cysticum and hygroma axillare; pathologic and clinical study and report of 12 cases. Arch Surg 36:394–479
15. Gordon MJ, Sumner TE (1975) Abdominal ultrasonography in a mesenteric cyst presenting as ascites. Gastroenterology 69:761–764
16. Gray SW, Skandalakis JE (1972) Embryology for surgeons: the embryological basis for the treatment of congenital defects. Saunders, Philadelphia
17. Grosfeld JL, Weber TR (1982) One-stage resection for massive cervicomediastinal hygroma. Surgery 92:693–699
18. Gross RE, Hurwitt ES (1948) Cervicomediastinal and mediastinal cystic hygromas. Surg Gynecol Obstet 87:559–610
19. Groves LK, Effler DB (1954) Primary chylopericardium. N Engl J Med 250:520–523
20. Harkins GA, Sabiston DC (1959) Lymphangioma in infancy and childhood. Surgery 47:811–822
21. Huntington GS (1911) The anatomy and development of the systemic lymphatic vessels in the domestic cat. Wistar Institute of Anatomy and Biology, Philadelphia
22. Issa PY, Brihi ER, Janin Y, Slim MS (1983) Superior vena cava syndrome in childhood: report of ten cases and review of the literature. Pediatrics 71:337–341
23. Johnson DW, Klazynski T, Gordon WH, Russell DA (1986) Mediastinal lymphangioma and chylothorax: the role of radiotherapy. Ann Thorac Surg 41:325–328
24. Khoury GH, Demong GV (1963) Mediastinal cystic hygroma in childhood. J Pediatr 62:432–434
25. Kirschner PA (1966) Cervicomediastinal cystic hygroma: one-stage excision in an eight-week-old infant. Surgery. 60:1104–1107
26. Korman MJ, Steiner R, Fish JE (1986) Dyspnoea and stridor in a young woman. Chest 89:579–581
27. Landing BH, Farber S (1956) Tumours of the cardiovascular system. Atlas of tumour pathology, Sect 3, vol 7. Armed Forces Institute of Pathology, Washington DC
28. Man, DWK, Donell ST, Raafai F, Eckstein, HB (1984) Congenital obstructive emphysema of the left lung associated with a mediastinal lymphatic cyst. Thorax 39:211–212
29. Mills NL, Grosfeld JL (1973) One-stage operation for cervicomediastinal cystic hygroma in infancy. J Thorac Cardiovasc Surg 65:608–611
30. Nanson EM (1968) Lymphangioma (cystic hygroma) of the mediastinum. J Cardiovasc Surg 9:447–452
31. Ninh TN, Ninh TX (1974) Cystic hygroma in children: a report of 126 cases. J Pediatr Surg 9:191–195
32. Pachter MR, Lattes R (1963) Mesenchymal tumours of the mediastinum. III. Tumours of lymphatic vascular origin. Cancer 16:108–117
33. Pedicelli G, Mattia P, Zorzoli A, Sorrone A, De Martino F, Sciotto V (1984) Gorham syndrome. Jama 252:1449–1451
34. Perkes EA, Haller JO, Kassner, EG, Wolf E, Velcek FT (1979) Mediastinal cystic hygroma in infants. Clin Pediatr 18:168–170
35. Pike MG, Wood AJ, Corrin B, Warner JO (1984) Intrathoracic extramediastinal cystic hygroma. Arch Dis Child 59:75–76
36. Pilla TJ, Wolverson MK, Sundaram M, Heiberg E, Shields JB (1982) CT evaluation of cystic lymphangiomas of the mediastinum. Radiology 144:841–842

37. Rasaretnam R, Chanmugam D, Sabanathan, Paul AT (1976) Cervicomediastinal lymphangioma. Aust NZJ Surg 46:378–381
38. Ravitch MM (1986) In: Paediatric surgery, 4th edn. Welch KJ, Randolph JG, Ravitch MM, O'Neill JA, Rowe MI (eds) Mediastinal cysts and tumours. Yearbook medical, Chicago
39. Ravitch MM, Rush BF (1986) In: Paediatric surgery, 4th edn. Welch KJ, Randolph JG, Ravitch MM, O'Neill JA, Rowe MI (eds) Cystic hygroma. Yearbook Medical, Chicago
40. Rueda A de O, Arellano CP, Rojas FD de, Mateo A (1984) Ultrasound diagnosis of mediastinal cystic hygroma. J Clin Ultrasound 12:180–182
41. Sabin FR (1912) The development of the lymphatic system. In: Manual of human embryology, vol 2. Keibel F, Mall FP (eds) Lippincott, Philadelphia
42. Sheth S, Nussbaum AR, Hutchins GM, Sanders RC (1981) Cystic hygromas in children: sonographic-pathologic correlation. Radiology 162:821–823
43. Sanders R (1987) Cystic hygromas in children: sonographic-pathologic correlation. Radiology 162:821–823
44. Shin MS, Berland LL, Ho KJ (1985) Mediastinal cystic hygromas: CT characteristics and pathogenetic consideration. J Comput Assist Tomogr 9:297–301
45. Silverman PM, Korobkin M, Moore AV (1983) CT diagnosis of cystic hygromas of the neck. J Comput Assist Tomogr 7:519–520
46. Singh S, Baboo MZ, Pathak IC (1971) Cystic lymphangioma in children: report of 32 cases including lesions at rare sites. Surgery 69:947–951
47. Stratton VC, Grant RN (1958) Cervicomediastinal cystic hygroma associated with chylopericardium. Arch Surg 77:887–891
48. Sumner TE, Volberg FM, Kiser PE, Shaffner L de S (1981) Mediastinal cystic hygroma in children. Pediatr Radiol 11:160–162
49. Tanigawa N, Shimomatsuya T, Takahashi K, Inomata Y, Tanaka K, Satomura K, Hikasa Y, Hashida M, Muranishi S, Sezaki H (1987) Treatment of cystic hygroma and lymphangioma with the use of bleomycin fat emulsion. Cancer 60:741–749
50. Touloukian RJ, Rickert R, Lange RC, Spencer RP (1971) The microvascular circulation of lymphangiomas: a study of Xe^{133} clearance and pathology. Pediatrics 48:36–40
51. Willis RA (1956) The borderland of embryology and pathology. Butterworth, London

Intralobar Pulmonary Sequestration

M. Kent

Summary

Intralobar pulmonary sequestration is a rare congenital anomaly, comprising a mass of non-functioning lung tissue, without normal bronchial and vascular connections. The condition has two distinct clinical presentations:

1. In the 1st year of life, it may present as the site of a significant arterio-venous shunt, and then is usually associated with other cardiac anomalies, becoming defined in the course of appropriate cardiovascular investigations.
2. In older children, the condition becomes manifest because of persistent radiological changes and inadequate response to treatment, following one or more bouts of respiratory infection.

Occlusion of the shunt or removal of the sequestration is the definitive management; the importance of the condition relates to the need to consider the diagnosis in evaluating the clinical presentations indicated above.

Zusammenfassung

Die intralobäre Lungensequestration ist eine seltene angeborene Anomalie, bestehend aus nicht funktionierendem Lungengewebe ohne normale bronchiale und vaskuläre Verbindungen. Diese Erkrankung zeigt 2 ausgeprägte klinische Bilder:

1. Im 1. Lebensjahr kann sie der Sitz eines signifikanten arteriovenösen Shunts sein und ist gewöhnlich mit anderen Herzfehlbildungen kombiniert. Sie wird im Verlauf geeigneter kardiovasculärer Untersuchungen diagnostiziert.
2. Bei älteren Kindern manifestiert sie sich im Rahmen persistierender radiologischer Veränderungen und Therapieresistenz nach einer oder mehreren Atemwegsinfektionen.

Verschluß des AV-Shunts oder chirurgische Entfernung sind die definitiven Behandlungen. Die Schwere der Erkrankung macht differentialdiagnostische Überlegungen in dieser Richtung erforderlch, wenn klinische Symptome auftreten, wie sie oben beschrieben sind.

Résumé

La séquestration intralobaire pulmonaire est une anomalie congénitale rare, caractérisée par une masse de tissu pulmonaire ne fonctionnant pas, sans jonctions bronchiales ou vasculaires normales. Cette affection se présente sous deux formes cliniques bien distinctes:

1. Chez un enfant de moins d'un an, elle peut se présenter comme le siège d'un shunt artéroveineux significatif et va le plus souvent de pair avec d'autres anomalies cardiaques qui se révèlent au fur et à mesure de l'investigation cardio-vasculaire.

Department of Surgery, Royal Children's Hospital Melbourne, Flemington Road, Parkville 3052, Victoria, Australia.

Progress in Pediatric Surgery, Vol. 27
Myers and Angerpointner (Eds.)

2. Chez les enfants plus agés, l'affection devient manifeste et est révélée par des modifications radiologiques persistantes et l'absence de réaction au traitement entrepris après une ou plusieurs infections respiratoires.

Le traitement définitif consistera en une occlusion de la dérivation ou suppression de la séquestration.

Definition

The term "pulmonary sequestration" refers to lung tissue which is separated from its usual connections. By common usage, it has come to be applied to a congenital malformation comprising a mass of non-functioning lung tissue, with no normal bronchial communication, receiving its blood supply from anomalous systemic arteries instead of from pulmonary arteries. In most instances, the abnormal lung tissue is incorporated within the normal lung, and is additional to the normal pulmonary lung segments; this anomaly is called intralobar sequestration. (When the abnormal pulmonary tissue is separate from the normal lung, with its own pleural covering, it is called extralobar sequestration.)

The sequestration may be of bronchial elements alone, of pulmonary artery supply alone, or, most commonly, of both elements. The disconnections imply that pulmonary structures (bronchial and alveolar elements, with mucus-secreting epithelium), without normal communications, develop static accumulations of secretions, which are prone to infection, and that vascular structures may have abnormal communications with significant arteriovenous shunts. These two abnormal features, in varying degree, determine the pathological progression and the various clinical presentations.

Pathology

Location

Intralobar pulmonary sequestration is almost always situated within the posteromedial basal segments of the lower lobe, adjacent to the mediastinum (Fig. 1); it is commoner on the left side than the right; occasionally, both lower lobes have contained sequestrations. Rarely, sequestrations have been reported in the middle lobe, usually in association with a sequestration in the lower lobe. Lesions in the upper lobe are very rare.

Blood Supply

Large systemic arteries (usually more than one) enter the sequestration by way of the pulmonary ligament in most cases. The arteries most commonly arise from the descending aorta (Fig. 2), but can arise from the abdominal aorta (Fig. 3), reach-

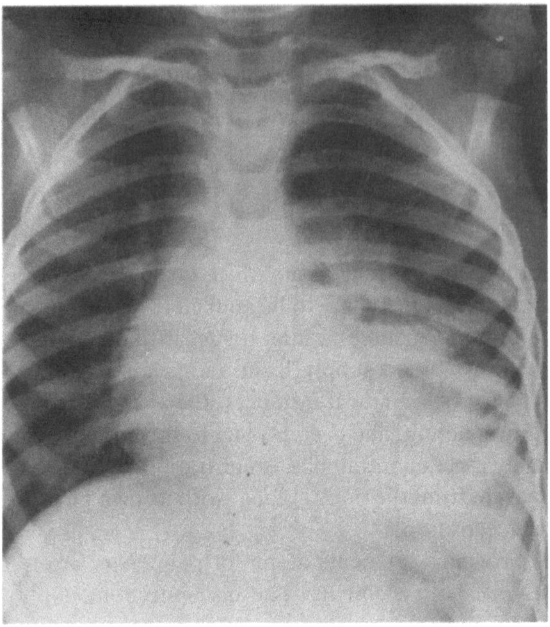

Fig. 1. Intralobar sequestration of left lower lobe. Presented with pneumonic-like illness; clinical improvement was unassociated with radiological change

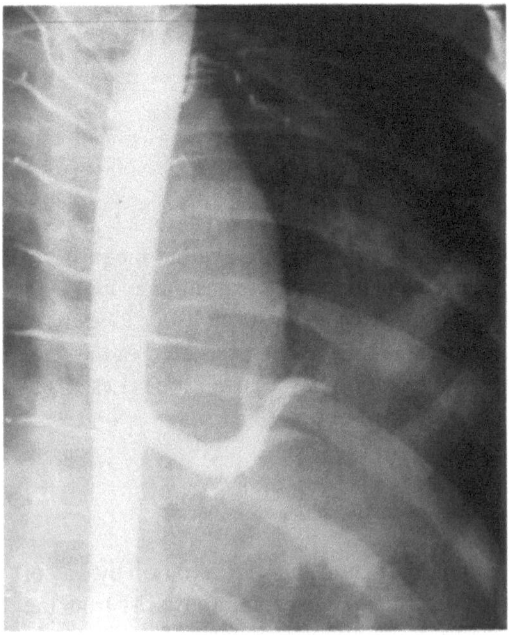

Fig. 2. Aortogram revealing aberrant blood supply from descending aorta (same patient as Fig. 1)

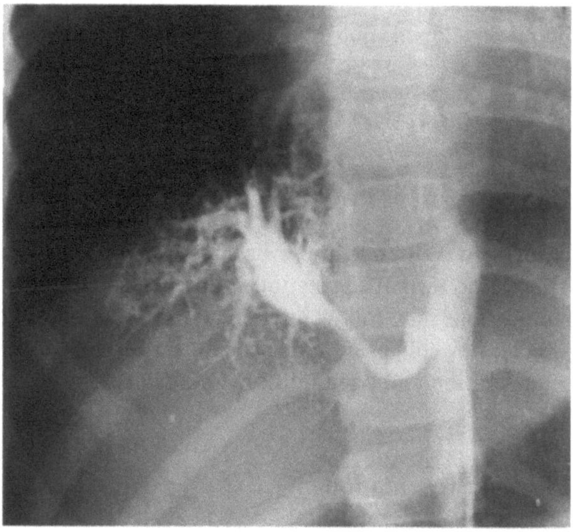

Fig. 3. Aortogram revealing aberrant artery arising from abdominal aorta and supplying intralobar sequestration of right lower lobe

ing the sequestration through the diaphragm. A single trunk may divide into several branches before entering the sequestration. The aberrant artery has, on rare occasions, been described as arising from the aortic arch, or from other major arteries in the mediastinum. Frequently, the abnormal artery shows atherosclerotic changes, and may be abnormally fragile.

The venous drainage from the sequestration is usually by way of the inferior pulmonary veins, thus creating a left-to-right shunt, which may be large enough to give rise to a murmur, and to cause cardiac failure.

Associated Anomalies

In its typical form, intralobar pulmonary sequestration is an isolated phenomenon. However, there have been many descriptions of associated cardiac anomalies: septal defects, coarctation, patent ductus arteriosus and anomalous pulmonary venous drainage have been described. The disturbed haemodynamics of these lesions may be further complicated by the presence of a large shunt; the presence of the shunt leads to recognition of the sequestration.

Communication between the alimentary tract and the pulmonary sequestration has been described, and diaphragmatic defects have also been recorded in association with sequestration.

Pathogenesis

The most widely accepted theory of aetiology is that sequestrations develop from an accessory lung bud, on the ventral aspect of the primitive foregut, distal to the normal lung bud. During caudal migration of the normal lung bud, the accessory bud is enveloped, but retains its systemic blood supply.

Natural History

Before the supervention of infection or other secondary changes, the lung tissue is not aerated, the lung spaces being filled with mucus. Cysts of various size may be present, either multiple or single. With infection, the cysts may contain air. There is no formal connection with the tracheobronchial tree, but secondary communications may follow infection. Compression of surrounding lung may lead to infection or collapse in adjacent lung. Rarely, tension cysts may arise within the sequestration and pneumothorax may develop.

Clinical Presentation

Most cases present in infancy or in childhood, but occasional reports of presentation in later life have been made.

Infancy

The presentation in the first few months of life may take several forms:

1. Incidental finding on chest X-ray. A basal paramediastinal density may be apparent on chest X-ray taken for other reasons.
2. As an incidental finding during investigation or treatment of associated cardiac anomalies.
3. Cardiac failure because of the presence of a large shunt within the sequestration. There may be a murmur associated with the shunt.
4. Repeated chest infection, associated with persistent X-ray findings in spite of resolution of associated infection.
5. Respiratory distress, either due to cardiac failure or to tension within the sequestration.

Older Children

1. As an incidental finding on chest X-ray.
2. Repeated chest infection and persisting X-ray changes. The infection is not usually associated with a productive cough, because of absence of a formal communication with the tracheobronchial tree.
3. Haemoptysis is an unusual presentation.
4. Alimentary symptoms have occasionally been reported, e.g. haematemesis and dysphagia.

Diagnosis

Chest X-ray

The typical appearance is of an abnormal dense shadow in the posteromedial basal portion of the lower lobe, adjacent to the mediastinum. There may be associated diffuse infiltration of the lower lobe. The dense mass may show cavitation, sometimes with fluid levels. Persistence of X-ray changes after there has been symptomatic improvement is typical. Chest films taken before the first clinical episode of infection may show changes, but normal X-rays do not exclude sequestration.

Aortography

Aortography defines the presence and position of the abnormal systemic vessels, and is an appropriate investigation when there is strong suspicion of the diagnosis. The descending aorta and abdominal aorta are the important areas to be examined.

Other Investigations

Occasionally, barium studies may be indicated if there are alimentary symptoms. Bronchoscopy and bronchography have now largely been superseded by aortography. The role of computed tomography, and ultrasound, has not been clearly defined.

When the clinical and plain radiology features provide a strong suspicion of sequestration, angiography is mandatory, providing clear definition of abnormal blood supply, and a "road map" for planning treatment. If the clinical and plain radiography features are less demanding, then further clinical observation must be contemplated as an alternative to invasive investigation.

Treatment

Untreated sequestration has a morbidity related to infection, or to vascular shunting; the natural history of "symptomless" sequestration is not clear, however, because experience relates almost entirely to those cases with clinical manifestations.

1. Resection of the sequestration, by segmental resection, has been regarded as the ideal form of treatment. It is necessary to identify the arterial supply, often situated within dense scar tissue on the inferior or medial aspect of the lower lobe. Separation of the sequestration from the surrounding lower lobe may be possible, if there is a clear line of demarcation between the normal and abnormal lung [1].

2. Lobectomy, removing the lower lobe and the included sequestration, has been the accepted operation, particularly if repeated infection has rendered separation of the abnormal segement from the lower lobe hazardous, or indeed impossible.
3. Ligation of the abnormal systemic arteries has been undertaken as an isolated procedure, and may be appropriate if there is a very large shunt through the sequestration, in the absence of infection.
4. Arterial embolization [2] may be an appropriate means of occluding circulation through the sequestration, and is particularly applicable if the shunt is causing cardiac failure, or is aggravating an associated congenital cardiac problem. The presence of infection in the sequestration, however, would render embolization a hazardous venture.
5. Evacuation of abscesses or of cystic spaces within the sequestration may be a necessary preliminary procedure, prior to definitive resection of the sequestration.
6. Observation, rather than operation or embolization, may be appropriate for asymptomatic intralobar sequestration. There is insufficient information concerning the natural history of intralobar sequestration to permit a definitive answer to this question, but the likelihood of infection occurring in the sequestration leads to a recommendation for intervention in most cases, particularly those recognized in early life.

Significance of Intralobar Pulmonary Sequestration

This anomaly is a rare condition, 34 cases being identified over a 24-year period from 1963 to 1987 at the Royal Children's Hospital, Melbourne. The condition shows a wide variety of clinical presentations, and thus the diagnosis should be entertained under the following situations.

1. Infants and children showing persistent chest X-ray findings in the medial portion of the lower lobe of the lung.
2. Infants with congenital cardiac anomalies, especially heart failure due to a large shunt.
3. Infants with respiratory distress in the 1st year of life.
4. Healthy patients with suggestive findings on chest X-ray.

The condition has surgical significance, because of the importance of identification of the large abnormally fragile systemic arteries entering the pathological lung, frequently within dense scar tissue. Without prior knowledge of the presence of these large vessels, surgery may be hazardous or fatal.

Incidence

The data of the Royal Children's Hospital, Melbourne, series has recently been reviewed by John, Beasley and Mayne [3]. Of 20 cases identified in the 1st year of life, only 6 showed symptoms directly related to the sequestration; presentation in the remaining 14 was most commonly related to associated cardiac anomalies, a vascular shunt often contributing to the cardiac problem. Beyond the 1st year of life, 12 of 14 cases presented with symptoms related to infection in the sequestration. In this latter group, an average of 19 months was the time between presentation and treatment; this delay is explained by the need to allow observation of the response of pulmonary infection to standard treatment: when this response is incomplete or inadequate, then the diagnosis of sequestration should be entertained.

Conclusions

The congenital anomaly of intralobar pulmonary sequestration is an uncommon condition, with a variety of clinical manifestations. Its two commonest clinical forms are as part of a complex congenital cardiovascular complex in the 1st year of life, and as persistent chest infection in older children. The diagnosis should be entertained in both of these clinical situations. Full definition of the cardiovascular status in the infant leads to recognition of the anomaly in the first group. Incomplete or inadequate response to treatment of pulmonary infection in the lower lobe of a child should point to the possibility of intralobar pulmonary sequestration, and further investigation should be contemplated. There are other causes of such inappropriate response to treatment, however, and invasive investigation should only proceed if the suspicion of sequestration is strong.

Once recognized, there are various treatment options. Observation may be appropriate. If the vascular shunt is the dominant feature, management of the shunt may be by vessel embolization, by vessel ligation, or by surgical excision of the sequestration; management should proceed in concert with management of the coexisting cardiovascular anomalies. When infection in the sequestration is the mechanism of presentation, then surgical resection is the definitive management, with preservation of normal lung tissue, if technically possible.

References

1. Howard R (1963) Conservative excision in intralobar sequestration of the lung. Lancet II: 1295
2. Wensley DF, Goh TH, Menahem S, et al (1989) Management of pulmonary sequestration and scimitar syndrome presenting in infancy. Pediatr Surg Int 4(6):381–385
3. John PR, Beasley SW, Mayne V (1989) Pulmonary sequestration and related congenital disorders. Pediatr Radiol 20:4–9

Mediastinal Masses in Childhood: A Review from a Paediatric Pathologist's Point of View

I. Simpson and P. E. Campbell

Summary

From 1970 to 1989, 121 children with mediastinal masses of various sorts were seen in the Department of Pathology, Royal Children's Hospital, Melbourne. The series is considered representative of the true incidence of these conditions in the state of Victoria, which had an average paediatric population during the time of this series of 900000 children.

The commonest cause of a mediastinal mass was NHL (36 cases). This was followed by HD (24 cases), then neuroblastoma and ganglioneuroma (16 and 9 cases respectively), duplication cysts (10 cases), teratomas (7 cases), neurofibroma (4 cases) and lymphangioma (3 cases). A great variety of rare conditions made up the remainder of the series and included mediastinal abscess, thymic cyst, pericardial cyst, accessory lobe of lung, plasma cell granuloma, fibromatosis, paravertebral Ewing's tumour, carcinoid tumour and neurofibrosarcoma. Presentation of the children with NHL was often acute with respiratory distress, while the child with HD was usually older and symptoms were more often systemic than local. The surgeon's role in diagnosis of these most frequently encountered mediastinal masses can be crucial and biopsy when indicated must be carried out with great care to produce material that is adequate for diagnosis and for the performance of cell marker studies and chromosome analysis.

Neuroblastoma (NBL) and ganglioneuroma (GN) together were the third largest group. Children with neuroblastoma were usually young; 15 of the 18 cases were less than 2 years old. One-third of the infants with neuroblastoma presented with paraplegia and one-third with respiratory symptoms including wheeze, stridor and respiratory difficulty. Three children had Horner's syndrome. Prognosis of children with thoracic neuroblastoma is very good and contrasts with the poor outlook for those with abdominal neuroblastoma. Stage at presentation is probably the most important single prognostic variable. Ganglioneuroma presents at a later age than neuroblastoma and symptoms may be present for a long time or may be completely absent. Catecholamines, usually raised in neuroblastoma, are mostly normal in ganglioneuroma. Duplication cysts were the next most frequent group. Symptoms can often be acute and life threatening, although in three of our ten cases the cyst was an incidental finding on chest X-ray. However, only three of our patients had a normal respiratory examination. Teratomas were usually large and more often benign than malignant. Excision is the mandatory treatment and is usually curative. Although teratomas in young infants are often cellular and composed of many immature tissue types, their behaviour is benign. Nevertheless careful search for yolk sac tumour elements should be made since these are malignant and their presence completely alters the prognosis.

The role of the surgeon in the management of mediastinal masses in children is usually a key one, being either that of surgical excision or in some instances the obtaining of tumour tissue for histological diagnosis on which further definitive treatment is based.

Zusammenfassung

Von 1970 bis 1989 wurden Mediastinaltumoren verschiedener Art von 121 Kindern an der pathologischen Abteilung des Royal Children's Hospital, Melbourne, untersucht. Diese Serie kann als

Department of Anatomical Pathology, Royal Children's Hospital Melbourne, Flemington Road, Parkville 3052, Victoria, Australia.

Progress in Pediatric Surgery, Vol. 27
Myers and Angerpointner (Eds.)

repräsentativ gelten für die Häufigkeit bei den 900000 Kindern, die im Untersuchungszeitraum im Staat Victoria gelebt haben.

Der häufigste Mediastinaltumor war das Non-Hodgkin-Lymphom (36 Fälle), gefolgt vom M. Hodgkin (24), Neuroblastom und Ganglioneurom (16 bzw. 9), zystischen Duplikaturen (10), Teratomen (7), Neurofibromen (4) und Lymphangiomen (3). Eine Vielzahl seltener Erkrankungen stellte den Rest der Serie und umfaßte Mediastinalabszesse, Thymuszysten, Perikardzysten, akzessorische Lungenlappen, Plasmazellgranulome, Fibromatosen, paravertebrale Ewing-Sarkome, Karzinoidtumoren und Neurofibrosarkome.

Kinder mit NHL wiesen häufig ein akutes Atemnotsyndrom auf, wogegen Kinder mit M. Hodgkin gewöhnlich älter waren und häufiger systemische als lokale Symptome hatten. Die Rolle des Chirurgen bei der Diagnosestellung der häufigsten Mediastinaltumoren kann schwierig sein, da die Biopsie, wenn indiziert, mit großer Sorgfalt erfolgen muß, um Material zu gewinnen, das für die Diagnosesicherung ausreicht und Zellmarkeruntersuchungen und Chromosomenanalysen erlaubt.

Neuroblastome und Ganglioneurome zusammengenommen, stellten die dritthäufigste Gruppe. Kinder mit Neuroblastom waren normalerweise sehr jung: in 15 der 18 Fälle waren sie jünger als 2 Jahre. Ein Drittel der Kinder mit Neuroblastom wies eine Paraplegie auf, ein Drittel hatte respiratorische Symptome mit Keuchen, Stridor und Atemnot; 3 Kinder litten unter einem Horner-Syndrom. Im Gegensatz zu Kindern mit abdominellen Neuroblastomen haben Kinder mit thorakalen Neuroblastomen eine sehr gute Prognose. Das Studium bei Diagnosestellung ist wahrscheinlich der wichtigste prognostische Einzelfaktor.

Ganglioneurome treten später auf als Neuroblastome; die Symptome bestehen oft über lange Zeit oder fehlen völlig. Die Katecholamine, beim Neuroblastom gewöhnlich erhöht, sind beim Ganglioneurom meist normal.

Zystische Duplikaturen stellten die nächsthäufigste Gruppe. Symptome können oft akut und lebensbedrohlich auftreten, obwohl bei 3 unserer 10 Fälle die Zysten zufällig bei einer Thoraxaufnahme gefunden wurden. Bei nur 3 unserer Patienten war jedoch die Lungenfunktion normal.

Teratome waren gewöhnlich sehr groß und häufiger benigne als maligne. Die chirurgische Exstirpation ist die Behandlung der Wahl und normalerweise kurativ. Obwohl die Teratome bei Säuglingen oft aus zellulären und vielen unreifen Gewebetypen bestehen, ist ihr Verhalten benigne. Trotzdem muß immer sorgfältig nach Dottersacktumorelementen gefahndet werden, da diese maligne sind und die Prognose völlig verändern.

Der Chirurg hat bei der Behandlung von Mediastinaltumoren eine Schlüsselrolle inne, sei es durch die chirurgische Exstirpation oder durch die Gewinnung von Gewebeproben zur histologischen Diagnose, die die weitere Behandlung bestimmt.

Résumé

Entre 1970 et 1989, 121 enfants présentant différentes sortes de masses médiastinales ont été traités au Department of Pathology, Royal Children's Hospital, Melbourne. Cette étude peut être considérée comme représentative en ce qui concerne la fréquence véritable de ces affections dans l'état de Victoria, la population infantile à l'époque de cette étude étant de 900000 sujets.

La cuase la plus fréquente d'une masse médiastinale était un lymphome non hodgkinien (36 cas), suivie par la maladie de Hodgkin (24 cas), les neuroblastomes et les glangioneuromes (16 et 9 cas), les formations kystiques de duplication (10 cas), les tératomes (7 cas), les neurofibromes (4 cas) et les lymphangiomes (3 cas). Le reste était composé d'affections rares telles qu'abcès médiastinal, kyste du thymus, kyste du péricarde (péricardique), lobe accessoire du poumon, granulome des cellules plasmatiques, fibromatose, sarcome d'Ewing paravertébral, tumeur carcinoïde et neurofibrosarcome.

Les enfants hospitalisés pour lymphone non hodgkinien présentaient souvent une détresse respiratoire aigue tandis que les enfants avec maladie de Hodgkin étaient souvent plus âgés et les symtômes plutôt systémiques que localisés. Le rôle du chirurgien du point de vue diagnostique dans ces cas les plus fréquents de masses médiastinales est d'une importance capitale et, si la biopsie est indiquée, elle doit être pratiquée avec le plus grand soin afin d'obtenir un tissu permettant le diagnostic, l'étude avec des marqueurs cellulaires et l'analyse chromosomique.

Les neuroblastomes et les ganglioneuromes constituent ensemble le troisième groupe dans l'ordre de fréquence. Les enfants atteints de neuroblastome sont en général jeunes; dans 15 des 18 cas, les enfants avaient moins de deux ans. Un tiers des enfants atteints de neuroblastome présentaient une paraplégie et un tiers des symptômes respiratoires y compris un bruit respiratoire (signe de Jackson), stridor (laryngé) et troubles respiratoires. Trois des enfants présentaient le syndrome de Claude Bernard-Horner. Le prognostic pour les enfants présentant un neuroblastome thoracique est très bon, contrairement à celni du neuroblastome abdominal. Le stade lors de la première consultation est probablement la variable la plus importante du point de vue prognostique.

Le ganglioneurome se révèlent comme neuroblastome et les symptômes peuvent exister depuis assez longtemps ou être complètement absents. Les catécholamines qui sont normalement plus élevées dans le cas du neuroblastome, sont le plus souvent normales dans le cas du ganglioneurome.

Viennent ensuite dans l'ordre de fréquence les kystes de duplication. Les symptômes peuvent être aigus et mettre en danger le pronostic vital, bien que dans trois de nos dix cas, le kyste ait été découvert per hasard sur une radiographie du thorax. Trois de nos patients avaient obtenu des résultats normaux à l'examen respiratoire.

Les tératomes étaient en règle générale étendus et plus souvent bénins que malins. L'excision est le traitement qui s'impose et elle garantit généralement la guérison. Bien que les tératomes des enfants en bas âge soient souvent cellulaires et composés de nombreux types de tissus embryonnaires (non adultes), ils se comportent comme un tératome bénin. Toutefois, il faut s'assurer avec minutie qu'il n'y a pas de signes de tumeur de la vésicule ombilicale car ces tumeurs sont malignes et leur présence bouleverse complètement le prognostic.

Le rôle du chirurgien lors du traitement des masses médiastinales chez les enfants est en général d'une importance capitale qu'il s'agisse de pratiquer une excision ou d'obtenir des tissus tumoraux pour le diagnostic histologique devant servir de base au traitement ultérieur définitif.

Introduction

The role of the surgeon in the diagnosis and treatment of mediastinal lesions in childhood can vary from nil to total management, depending on the nature of the mass. For example, a child with a large anterior mediastinal mass and stridor may have the diagnosis of lymphoma/leukaemia established by bone marrow aspiration so that no surgical management is indicated; on the other hand the nature of a posterior mediastinal mass discovered incidentally on chest X-ray will only be diagnosed after surgical excision, which may be the only therapy required.

In considering the different types of masses that may be encountered in the *mediastinum* of children, while the possibilities are legion, the practicalities are relatively few. To give perspective to the following discussion we have reviewed all mediastinal masses encountered in the Royal Children's Hospital (RCH) between 1970 and 1988 with a view to establishing incidence of the various masses, their modes of presentation and management.

Anatomically the mediastinum is divided into superior, anterior middle and posterior components but this is somewhat arbitrary and not always of practical help. In the superior and anterior mediastinum lymphomas and teratomas predominate, in the middle, lymph node masses and in the posterior, neurogenic *tumours* and duplication *cysts* (Table 1). However, there are many exceptions to

Table 1. Mediastinal masses in children

	Benign	Malignant
Anterior and superior	Teratoma	Non-Hodgkin's lymphoma
	Cystic hygroma	Hodgkin's disease
	Haemangioma	Teratoma with yolk sac tumour
	Thymic cyst	Seminoma
		Desmoid
		Sarcoma
		Thymoma
Middle	Bronchogenic cyst (tracheal duplication cyst)	Hodgkin's disease
	Teratoma	Non-Hodgkin's lymphoma
	Plasma cell granuloma	Teratoma
	Cardiac rhabdomyoma	Rhabdomyosarcoma
		Other sarcomas
Posterior	Ganglioneuroma	Neuroblastoma
		Ganglioneuroblastoma
	Neurofibroma	Neurofibrosarcoma
	Enterogenous cyst	
	Teratoma (rare)	Sarcoma
	Lipoma	Liposarcoma
	Leiomyoma	Leiomyosarcoma

Table 2. Mediastinal masses in children in the Royal Children's Hospital 1970–1988

	Number	Percentage
Non-Hodgkin's lymphoma	34	28
Hodgkin's disease	29	24
Neuroblastoma	16	13.2
Ganglioneuroma	9	7.5
Duplication cysts	10	8.2
Teratoma	7	5.8
Neurofibroma	4	3.3
Lymphangioma	3	2.5
Mediastinal abscess	1	0.83
Thymic cyst	1	0.83
Pericardial cyst	1	0.83
Accessory lobe of lung	1	0.83
Inflammatory pseudotumour (plasma cell granuloma)	1	0.83
Fibromatosis	1	0.83
Neurofibrosarcoma	1	0.83
Carcinoid tumour (thymus)	1	0.83
Paravertebral Ewing's tumour	1	0.83
Total	121	

this and, especially with large masses, almost the entire mediastinum may be involved.

The relative incidence of the various lesions seems to vary considerably from series to series in the literature [5, 16, 17, 19, 25, 29] perhaps reflecting selection bias. There is also a wide difference between children and adults [24]. We believe the figures reported here are likely to be truly representative of the incidence in our community since the RCH is the largest tertiary *paediatric* institution in Victoria which deals with the majority of oncological and surgical thoracic problems in children. Indeed this fairly full ascertainment is one reason for publishing this present series, giving as it does a good idea of the relative frequency of the conditions likely to be encountered in the mediastinum of infants and children up to 16 years of age. The tumours, cysts and malformations in order of frequency in the present series of children are set out in Table 2.

The Malignant Lymphomas

The malignant lymphomas, non-Hodgkin's lymphoma (NHL) and Hodgkin's disease (HD), comprise the largest group in our series and the role of the surgeon in establishing the diagnosis can be crucial. While some cases of mediastinal lymphoma can be diagnosed by examination of pleural fluid or bone marrow, in many cases this is not possible and tissue diagnosis is required. It is vital that the tissue obtained by surgical means is handled in an optimal fashion.

The flow chart (Fig. 1) shows a plan for the sequence of investigations that should be performed in a child with a mediastinal mass and the surgeon's role in establishing the diagnosis in individual patients.

Tissue Biopsy

A pathologist should always be available to handle freshly removed biopsy material. Ideally, biopsy should be performed in the institution where the child will be treated; this should ensure that the proper investigations are arranged so that the optimal amount of information will be obtained from the excised tissue. Biopsy material may be subject to many investigative procedures and therefore is best done early in the day. The scheduling of elective biopsy cases for the end of the day is to be deplored.

Technique Removal

Although it may be considered presumptuous that a pathologist should offer advice on surgical technique, enough badly crushed and damaged lymph nodes and other pieces of tumour tissue have been seen by all practising pathologists to convince them of the need for this advice. There are many reasons why biopsy tissue is badly handled, not least of which is the tendency to give the job of biopsy to

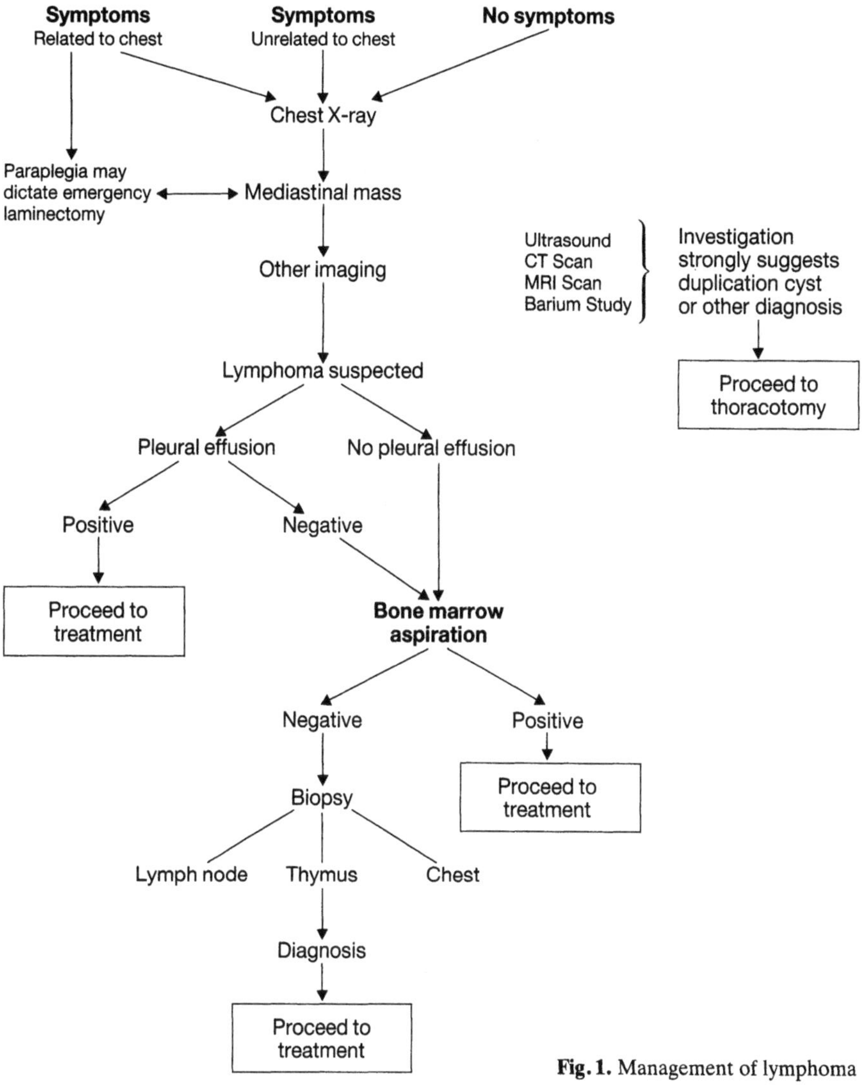

Fig. 1. Management of lymphoma

junior or inexperienced staff. Lymph node tissue is very delicate and friable and easily damaged and so everything should be done to ensure the tissue is excised in such a way that its diagnostic value is not impaired and in a nutshell this means with minimal handling.

Anaesthetic

General anaesthetics should always be employed in children undergoing a diagnostic lymph node or tumour biopsy. There is no place for local anaesthetic.

Biopsy Site

The site of biopsy should be chosen to provide adequate material with minimal operative interference. The incision should be large enough adequately to expose the lymph node or mass since minimal handling of tissue is the object of any diagnostic biopsy. Lymph nodes should be held in fine-toothed forceps by the capsule and never seized with haemostats or other crushing instruments. The temptation to cut open the node or tissue "to see what it looks like" should be resisted.

Equally, the pathologist should always use extreme care in cutting nodes or tumour tissue – a new razor blade is the best cutting edge to use, applied with a slicing motion to cut and not compress the tissue. The surgeon must wait while a sample is selected for immediate frozen section and good-quality cryostat sections are prepared and examined. If the specimen is adequate, then the surgeon can be notified and the wound closed. If the excised tissue is unsatisfactory, further material must be obtained; for example in early Hodgkin's disease peripherally placed nodes, although sometimes enlarged, are often not involved and deeper seated nodes must be removed; this should be done under the same anaesthetic so that the diagnosis can be firmly established at the one procedure. Apart from ensuring that the biopsy specimen is adequate for diagnosis, a second reason for performing an immediate frozen section on a lymph node is to provide fresh material for further studies; thus if the histology suggests NHL then fresh tissue can be section selected for surface marker studies and for chromosome analysis. If the frozen section shows HD, then since these studies are of no diagnostic benefit in this condition the material can be fixed and the laboratory saved the labour of unnecessary marker and cytogenetic studies.

In the event of there being no peripheral nodes to sample then the mediastinal mass itself must be biopsied. This can often be done through the suprasternal notch since the thymus is a neck organ as well as a mediastinal one (a fact that is sometimes not appreciated). Again frozen section is necessary to assess adequacy of the sample. If no tumour is found, then either a lateral thoracotomy or a midline sternotomy should be performed. In six instances in the present series in children with NHL and in four instances of Hodgkin's disease this was necessary, yielding diagnostic tissue that could not be obtained by other means.

Non-Hodgkin's Lymphoma

The commonest cause of a mediastinal mass in childhood is NHL [8, 22]. Children with this condition present in several ways, with both local and systemic symptoms, but the diagnosis is usually made when local symptoms become urgent and sometimes life-threatening. Symptoms and signs of superior vena caval obstruction, e.g. facial oedema, swelling and cyanosis; symptoms of respiratory obstruction, e.g. stridor, cough, respiratory distress, especially on lying flat, and enlargement of lymph glands in the neck, are the commonest local symptoms. While constitutional symptoms of general malaise, such as fever, night sweats and weight

Table 3. Non-Hodgkin's lymphoma

Age (years)	Sex	Symptoms	Signs	Chest X-ray	Pleural effusion	Method of diagnosis	Marrow involvement
1	M	Croup 4 months previously; recent wheeze, SOB, fever, lethargy	Lymph nodes not palpable, spleen enlarged	Large anterior mediastinal mass	+	Thoracotomy	○
1	M	Two weeks dyspnoea, stridor following croup, recent cyanosis	Stridor, chest retraction, lymph nodes not palpable	Large anterior mediastinal mass	○	Thoracotomy	○
1 2/12	M	Six months wheeze, two weeks pallor, increasing size R chest, lump in neck	Lymph node neck enlarged	Large mediastinal mass	+	Pleural fluid	○
2	M	Ten days enlargement of R testis, mass in groin	Right testis enlarged, lymph node groin enlarged	Large anterior mediastinal mass	○	Testis marrow	+
2 1/12	M	"Asthma" 5 days, anorexia 3 days, dyspnoea	Chest retraction, dullness to percussion	Large anterior mediastinal mass	+	Pleural fluid	○
3	M	One month wheeze and cough, anorexia, recent respiratory distress	Renomegaly, lymph node enlarged, spleen enlarged, trachea deviated R	Large anterior mediastinal mass	+	Lymph node	+
3	M	Tonsillitis, malaise, recurrent lump in neck	Cervical lymph node enlarged	Large anterior mediastinal mass	○	Lymph node	○
4	F	One month cough, weight loss	Cervical lymph node enlarged	Large anterior mediastinal mass	+	Pleural fluid	○
4	M	Seven weeks "croup", "asthma", weight loss, recurrent stridor	Signs of SVC, compression cervical node enlarged	Anterior mediastinal mass	+	Lymph node	○
5	F	Two months lump in neck, two weeks fever, night cough, dyspnoea	Cervical lymph node enlarged	Anterior mediastinal mass	+	Thoracotomy, pleural fluid	○
6	M	Flu-like illness 2 weeks, weight loss, anorexia	Lymph node enlarged, spleen enlarged, liver enlarged	Large nodular mediastinal mass	+	Marrow	+

Table 3 (continued)

Age (years)	Sex	Symptoms	Signs	Chest X-ray	Pleural effusion	Method of diagnosis	Marrow involvement
6	M	Pallor, weakness	Lymph node enlarged, spleen enlarged, liver enlarged	Mediastinal mass	○	Marrow	+
6	F	Swelling of face, persistent cough	SVC obstruction	Anterior mediastinal mass	○	Thoracotomy	○
7	F	Four weeks swelling neck, lethargy, anorexia	Cervical lymph node enlarged, thyroid enlarged	Anterior-superior mediastinal mass	○	Thyroid, lymph node	○
8½	M	Seven weeks swelling neck and face	Cervical lymph node enlarged	Anterior mediastinal mass	○	Lymph node	○ Constitutional chromosome abnormality
9	M	One week dry cough, anorexia, weight loss, dyspnoea, lumps in scalp	Liver enlarged, spleen enlarged, multiple scalp nodules	Anterior mediastinal mass	+	Scalp nodule	○
9	M	Six weeks cough, lethargy, shortness of breath	Cervical lymph node enlarged, veins visible chest	Anterior mediastinal mass	+	Thoracotomy	± equivocal
9	M	One week short history of face and neck swelling	Cervical lymph node enlarged, bilateral seventh nerve palsy	Large anterior mediastinal mass	○	Lymph node	+
10	M	Two weeks difficulty swallowing, noisy breathing dusky colour, facial swelling	Cervical lymph node enlarged, spleen enlarged	Anterior-superior mediastinal mass	+	Pleural fluid	○
10	M	Three weeks puffy face, cough, swelling in neck	Cervical lymph node	Anterior mediastinal mass with tracheal compression	○	Marrow	+
11	M	Four weeks "asthma", cough, dysphagia, bruising	General lymph node enlargment, liver enlarged, spleen enlarged	Lobulated anterior mediastinal mass	○	Marrow	+
11	M	Cough, stridor malaise	Cervical lymph node enlarged, SVC obstruction	Anterior mediastinal mass	○	Lymph node	○

11	M	Seven weeks malaise, anorexia, weight loss, 2 days SOB	Liver enlarged, lymph node enlarged, pleural effusion	Anterior mediastinal mass	+	Pleural fluid	+
11	M	Abdominal pain, malaise sweats	Cervical lymph node enlarged	Anterior mediastinal mass	○	Lymph node	○
11	M	Swelling and duskiness of face	Cervical lymph node enlarged	Anterior mediastinal mass	+	Pleural fluid	○
12	F	Two weeks progressive dyspnoea culminating in respiratory arrest	Cervical lymph node enlarged, axillary lymph node enlarged	Large anterior mediastinal mass	○	Lymph node	○
12	M	Ten days malaise, chest pain, shortness of breath and cyanosis	Cyanosis, SVC obstruction	Large anterior mediastinal mass	+	Thoracotomy	○
12	M	SOB on exertion, lump in neck	Cervical lymph node enlarged, SVC obstruction	Large anterior mediastinal mass	○	Marrow	+
12	M	Three weeks cough, SOB, chest pain	Pleural effusion, cervical lymp node enlarged, axillary lymph node enlarged	Large anterior mediastinal mass	+	Bronchoscopy	○
12	M	Fever, sweats, dry cough, SOB	Cervical lymph node enlarged, axillary lymph node enlarged	Anterior mediastinal mass	+	Pleural fluid, lymph node	○
13	F	Two weeks swelling of face, SOB, difficulty in swallowing	Cervical lymph node enlarged, axillary lymph node enlarged, spleen enlarged, liver enlarged	Anterior and middle mediastinal mass	○	Lymph node	○
13	F	Two weeks sore throat, malaise, 1 week lump in neck, 3 days stridor	Cervical lymph node enlarged	Superior mediastinal mass, tracheal deviation	○	Lymph node	○
16	F	Short history of rigors, and sweats (1 week)	General lymph node enlarged, kidney enlarged, liver enlarged	Anterior mediastinal mass	+	Submandibular gland	+
16	M	Lethargy, anorexia, supraclavicular lump	Supraclavicular lymph node enlarged	Anterior mediastinal mass	○	Lymph node	○

SOB, shortness of breath; SVC, superior vena cava

loss, may be present, in over half the children with NHL these systemic symptoms were absent or not noted in the history.

Often the history of obstructive symptoms is relatively short, reflecting no doubt the rapid growth of NHL in many children and its tendency to produce local symptoms before systemic illness is apparent.

In reviewing the variety of symptoms that were found in our own series, the terms croup and asthma occur quite frequently. These symptoms, reflecting compression of the trachea or bronchi, are relatively common in lymphoma as well as in HD (see below) and can delay the diagnosis. In almost all of the cases in our series, careful reading of the notes shows that the asthma or croup was atypical.

Nine of our 34 children with NHL presented under the age of 5 years, 9 between the ages of 5 and 10 years, and 14 between the ages of 10 and 15 years. Two children were 16 years old. There were 26 males and 8 females, and a pleural effusion was present in 17 of the 34 children. Bone marrow was positive in 11 of the 34 at the time of presentation with a large mediastinal mass. X-ray showed the mass to be in the anterior mediastinum, in the anterosuperior mediastinum or in the hilar region. The mass was often very large and it usually produced distortion, compression or displacement of the trachea and/or bronchi. Difficulty with swallowing or involvement of the oesopahgus was extremely rare.

Systemic symptoms – fever, night sweats, weight loss and malaise, occurred in 15 of the 34 children and obstructive symptoms in 18 of the 34. Bone marrow involvement at presentation was seen in 11 (Table 3). Histologically, all were diffuse lymphomas and when typing was performed the majority showed T-cell markers [4, 9].

Hodgkin's Disease

The second commonest cause of a large mediastinal mass in childhood is HD. While the distinction between HD and NHL is not always obvious in individual

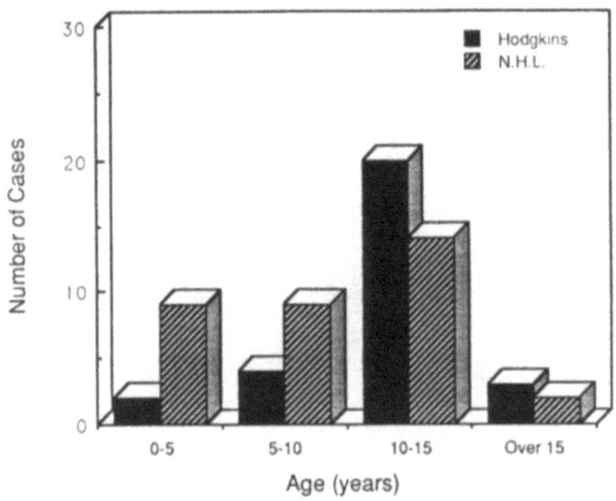

Fig. 2. Relative incidence of HD and NHL according to age

Table 4. Hodgkin's disease

Age (years)	Sex	Symptoms	Signs	Chest X-ray	Method of diagnosis	Pleural effusion	Marrow involvement	Pathology (type of Hodgkin's disease
4	F	Persistent cough following chest infection	Cervical lymph node enlarged, spleen enlarged	Superior mediastinal mass	Lymph node bx	○	○	LP
4	M	Two months swelling in neck	Cervical lymph node enlarged	Superior mediastinal mass	Lymph node bx	○	○	NS
7	M	Three months mass in neck, recent weight loss	Cervical lymph node enlarged	Bilateral hilar masses	Lymph node bx	○	○	NS
7	M	Nil	Incidental finding of enlarged lymph node in neck by school doctor	Prominent mediastinal and hilar masses with tracheal narrowing	Lymph node bx	○	○	MC
7	F	Six weeks fever, malaise, swelling in neck	Cervical lymph node enlarged	Superior and middle mediastinal widening	Lymph node bx	○	○	MC
9	F	Two days fever and vomiting, breathless when recumbent	Signs of SVC obstruction	Large anterior mediastinal mass displacing treachea backwards	Lymph node bx	+	○	NS
10	F	Weight loss, sweats, lump in neck	Cervical lymph node enlarged	Large mediastinal mass	Thoracotomy	+	○	NS
11	F	Two months lump in R neck	Cervical lymph node enlarged	Anterosuperior mediastinal mass	Lymph node bx	○	○	NS
11	M	Bilateral neck swelling, night sweats, anorexia	Cervical lymph node enlarged	Widened mediastinal mass L hilum	Lymph node bx	○	○	MC
11	F	Ten days L supra-clavicular mass	Cervical lymph node enlarged	Slight widening of superior mediastinum, multiple nodules both lungs	Lymph node bx	○	○	NS

Table 4 (continued)

Age (years)	Sex	Symptoms	Signs	Chest X-ray	Method of diagnosis	Pleural effusion	Marrow involve-ment	Pathology (type of Hodgkin's disease
11	F	Six weeks malaise, anorexia weight loss, night sweats, cough	Generalized lymph node enlargement	Bilateral hilar masses, loculated RML, pleural effusion	Lymph node bx (axillary)	+	+	NS
12	M	Six months lethargy, sweats, 6 weeks swelling neck	Cervical lymph node enlarged	Massive bilateral hilar enlargement	Lymph node bx, pleural fluid	+	+	LD
12	F	Three months pain L chest, 1 month lethargy and weight loss, 1 week dysphagia	Nil	Lobulated mass overlying cardiac shadow	Thoracotomy, bx, mediastinal mass	O	O	NS
12	F	Two months swelling in neck, anorexia	Cervical lymph node enlarged	Widened mediastinum, bilateral hilar masses	Lymph node bx	O	O	NS
12½	F	Twelve months lump neck, dry cough, recent SOB when flat	Cervical lymph node enlarged	Bilateral hilar masses	Lymph node bx	O	O	NS
13	M	Five weeks weight loss, 4 weeks shoulder pain, anorexia, SOB, sweats	Dullness to percussion R base	Huge anterior mediastinal mass	Thoracotomy, bx, mediastinal mass	+	O	NS
13	M	Six months mass in neck; 2 months sweats, weight loss, cough, SOB	Cervical lymph node enlarged	Bilateral hilar masses	Lymph node bx	O	O	NS
13	F	One month lethargy, 2 weeks neck lumps	Cervical lymph node enlarged	Superior mediastinal mass	Lymph node bx	O	O	NS
13	M	Two months lump in neck, recent lethargy, anorexia	Cervical lymph node enlarged	Large mediastinal mass with paratracheal component	Lymph node bx	+	O	LD

13	M	Two months lump in neck	Cervical and axillary lymph nodes enlarged	Mediastinal widening with narrowing of trachea	Lymph node bx (axillary)	○	+	NS
14	F	Two months cough, dyspnoea, sweats, lethargy, weight loss, 10 days swelling neck	Cervical lymph node enlarged	Widened mediastinum, trachea to right, bronchi narrowed	Lymph node bx	○	○	NS
14	F	Three weeks lump in neck	Cervical lymph node enlarged	Hilar masses	Lymph node bx	○	○	NS
14	F	Twelve months unwell	Cervical lymph nodes enlarged bilaterally	Hilar and anterior mediastinal masses	Thoracotomy, bx mass	○	○	NS
14	F	Eight weeks dry cough; 3 weeks lump in neck	Cervical lymph node enlarged	Anterior mediastinal mass, nodules both lungs	Lymph node bx	○	○	NS
14	F	One month lump in neck	Cervical lymph node enlarged	Bilateral hilar masses	Lymph node bx	○	○	NS
14½	F	Few weeks lump above L clavicle	Cervical lymph node enlarged	Large anterior mediastinal mass	Lymph node bx	○	○	NS
16	M	Three months fever, weight loss, lump in neck	Cervical lymph node enlarged	Bilateral hilar masses	Lymph node bx	○	○	NS
16	M	One month lump in neck	Cervical lymph nodes enlarged	Wide superior mediastinum with lobulated contour	Lymph node bx	○	○	NS
16	F	Bilateral neck lumps for 1 year, fever, malaise	Cervical lymph nodes enlarged	Bilateral hilar	Lymph node bx (axillary)	○	○	NS, developed T-ALL 3 years later

bx, biopsy; LD, lymphocyte depleted; LP, lymphocyte predominant; MC, mixed cellularity; NS, nodular sclerosis; RML, right middle lobe; SVC, superior vena cava; SOB, shortness of breath; T-ALL, T-cell acute lymphoblastic leukaemia

patients, in general children with HD are older (Fig. 2), more often have systemic symptoms of generalized illness with malaise, weight loss and night sweats and are less likely to have a pleural effusion. Very commonly they have enlarged lymph nodes in the neck which are usually able to be biopsied to provide a definitive histological diagnosis. Pressure symptoms, particularly acute pressure symptoms, are much less common in HD than in NHL and this is to be expected in view of the slower progression of this condition compared with malignant lymphoma. There were 29 children in our series and 17 of these presented with systemic symptoms, X-ray revealing the mediastinal mass.

Only two children were aged under 5 years, and four were aged between 5 and 10 years. The majority, 20 children, were aged between 10 and 15 years and there were 3 over 15 years. There were 11 males and 18 females. The diagnosis was made by lymph node biopsy in 25 of the 29 cases, 4 requiring thoracotomy. Radiologically the mass was in either the anterior mediastinum or the hilar region. The tumour edge was usually sharp and effusion was uncommon (6 of 29 children). Bone marrow trephine was positive in three children at the time of diagnosis, in one with lymphocyte-depleted type and two with nodular sclerosis. Bone marrow aspirate is usually negative. However, trephine is usually performed to stage the disease after the initial diagnosis has been established by other means. Histologically, 23 of the 29 cases showed the features of nodular sclerosis; in 3 the pattern was that of the mixed cellularity type, in two lymphocyte depleted and only one fulfilled the criteria for lymphocyte-predominant HD. In three children classified as nodular sclerosis, the macroscopic features were distinctive. In all three, the mediastinal tumours were very large, occupied predominantly the superior and anterior mediastinum and presented cauliflower-like nodular masses of tumour that projected from the surface. In two, the lung was also involved.

Clinical and pathological details are listed in Table 4.

Neuroblastoma

Neuroblastoma and ganglioneuroblastoma together comprised the third largest subgroup of mediastinal tumours in this series. It is well known that neuroblastomas arising in the thorax have a much better prognosis than those arising in the adrenal gland and abdomen whatever the age and this is borne out by the present series [1, 20]. This better prognosis may be due to the fact that the diagnosis is made earlier in thoracic neuroblastomas because of the frequent occurrence of spinal cord compression leading to paraparesis or paraplegia. However, this mode of presentation accounts for less than a third of the cases and there must be some other explanation; possibly tumours in this site are biologically different. We reported an earlier series of thoracic neuroblastomas from the RCH in 1983; so the present series includes some cases previously reported [10].

There were 18 children in this series. Ten were female and eight were male. Most of the children were infants. Ten were under the age of 1 year when diagnosed and five were less than 2 years. Only three were over 2 years of age, and the oldest child was 6, emphasizing the early onset of symptoms in children with thoracic neuroblastoma.

Six children presented with paraplegia, all aged 13 months or less. The paraplegia was usually of very rapid onset or at least was noticed by the parents over a short period. Wheeze, stridor and respiratory difficulty were major presenting symptoms for six children. These children were slightly older with the exception of one 1-day-old infant. Four were over the age of 1 year. Three children also had a Horner's syndrome at presentation; two of these had spinal cord compression.

In seven children the thoracic mass was an incidental finding only, discovered when the chest was X-rayed for either general symptoms or symptoms not related to the respiratory system or to weakness. The ages of these children ranged from 3 months to 6 years. In four enlarged lymph nodes were noted; in three, these were associated with other symptoms, and in one the enlarged nodes alone were the presenting feature.

In contrast to children with abdominal neuroblastoma, most of these children with thoracic neuroblastoma presented with local disease (stages I, II). Stage 4 disease was only encountered at presentation in four patients, three of them were infants, less than 1 year of age, and the fourth 3 years of age. Two had undifferentiated neuroblastoma, one had well-differentiated neuroblastoma and the eldest had well-differentiated ganglioneuroblastoma. All were treated by a combination of surgery and chemotherapy. One was the older 3-year-old child with ganglioneuroblastoma. One 3-month-old infant with metastatic liver disease died shortly after beginning chemotherapy. The youngest infant, who also died, had a very large mediastinal tumour at birth, with concomitant pulmonary hypoplasia. He died immediately following operative resection.

The other child in this series who died was a 1-year-old girl with stage III disease and spinal cord compression. She continued to deteriorate despite two decompressive laminectomies, a thoracotomy and chemotherapy. Histology showed undifferentiated neuroblastoma.

In general, the diagnosis of thoracic neuroblastoma is made histologically at the time of therapeutic resection. In this series, diagnosis was made at laminectomy in six children, at thoracotomy in nine, and in only one child, a baby of 9 months, was a diagnosis established by a lymph node biopsy (axilla). A summary of the clinical details of these 18 patients is shown in Table 5.

In all the cases, without exception, the mass lay in the posterior mediastinum, usually in one or the other paravertebral gutter, but often crossing the midline. In all cases, the mass was visualized radiologically on a plain chest X-ray. Calcification alone was visible in three children, calcification with erosion and splaying of ribs and/or widening of the intervertebral foramen in another three and rib changes alone without calcification in a further three. This suggests that calcification and widening or splaying of ribs or deformity of bone is a very helpful pointer in the radiological diagnosis of a neutral crest tumour. However, it must be cautioned that calcification and rib changes may also be seen in a benign mature ganglioneuroma (see below), and so radiological differentiation between neuroblastoma and ganglioneuroma is often not possible.

Table 5. Neuroblastoma

Sex	Age (years)	Symptoms	Signs	X-Ray	DX method	Catechol-amines	Histol-ogy	Outcome
M	1 day	Cyanosis and respiratory distress	Dullness to percussion, L chest	Left upper posterior mediastinal mass with erosion of ribs	Thoracotomy	ND	WNB	Died post-operatively
M	9 weeks	Two weeks not moving R arm, 1 week not moving L arm, leg weakness	Arms flaccid, legs weak, L Horner's syndrome	Left posterior mediastinal mass, block T5	Laminectomy, thoracotomy	Raised	UNB	Well
M[a]	3 months	Irritability, bilateral inguinal hernia	Legs weak, multiple skin nodules, lymph nodes enlarged, L Horner's syndrome	Left posterior mediastinal mass with calcification, ribs splayed, bone scan, uptake L posterior tibia	Laminectomy,	Raised	UNB	Well
F[a]	3 months	Diarrhoea with blood weight loss	Huge liver	Mass lower posterior thorax with calcification	Liver bx	Normal	UNB	Died shortly after beginning chemotherapy
M	4 months	Intermittent cough and wheeze	Nil	Left posterior mediastinal mass	Thoracotomy	Raised	GNB	Well
F	6 months	Six weeks irritability, screams when moved	Paraparesis, sensory deficient, neurogenic bladder	Right posterior superior mediastinal mass	Laminectomy, thoractomy	ND	WNB	Well, lower limb spasticity
M	7 months	Abdominal pain	Intussusception	(Routine X-ray) Posterior mediastinal mass	Thoracotomy	Raised	WNB	Well
F	8 months	Irritability, poor feeding, weight loss, cough	Café au lait spots	Right posterior mediastinal mass	Thoracotomy	Raised	GNB	Well
F	8 months	Six days unable to sit	VRD, flaccid, paraplegia, patulous anus	Bilateral posterior mediastinal masses, block T1–4	Laminectomy,	Slightly raised	UNB	Well

F	9 months	Three weeks irritability, crying when moved, legs weak	Paraparesis, lymph nodes enlarged	Left posterior paraspinal mass, speckled calcification, third rib eroded	Lymph node, axilla biopsy	Raised	WNB	(Recent case) Well
F	1 year	One month irritability, weakness in legs	Left Horner's syndrome, legs weak	Left apical mediastinal mass with erosion of second rib, block T4	Laminectomy, thoracotomy	ND	UNB	Died
M	13 months	Two weeks cough, wheeze, legs floppy	Paraplegia	Right posterior mediastinal mass with calcification, block T1	Laminectomy, thoracotomy	Raised	UNB	Well
F	14 months	Stridor shortly after birth	Reduced PN, R lung observed for 14 months without treatment	Superoposterior mediastinal mass with calcification	Thoracotomy	Raised	GNB	Postoperative Horner's syn-syndrome, well
M	20 months	Intermittent wheeze for most of life	Nil	Incidental chest X-ray finding of a posterior mediastinal mass notching ribs 1, 2, 3	Thoracotomy	Normal	WNB	Well
F[a]	3 years	One month fever, limp, L hip pain	Tender L hip cervical lymph nodes enlarged	Right posterior mediastinal mass, L hip bony metastases	Thoracotomy, lymph node biopsy	Raised	GNB	Dead
F	5 years	Recurrent URTI, wheeze	Cervical lymph nodes enlarged	Right posterior mediastinal mass, eroding ribs, calcification, air trapping R lobe	Thoracotomy, laminectomy	Raised	GNB	Well
F	6 years	Recurrent abdominal pain	Nil	Incidental chest X-ray finding of posterior mediastinal paravertebral mass	Thoracotomy	ND	GNB	Well
M	3 months		Left Horner's syndrome		Thoracotomy	Raised		Well, but paralysed L arm and atrophic chest

UNB, undifferentiated neuroblatoma; WNB, well-differentiated neuroblastoma; GNB, ganglioneuroblastoma; VRD, von Recklinghausen's disease; URTI, upper respiratory tract infection

[a] Those patients who presented with stage 4 disease

Urinary catecholamine estimation is a well-established useful diagnostic aid in the diagnosis of neuroblastoma/ganglioneuroblastoma; however, the correlation with prognosis is less well defined. Catecholamine estimations were performed on 14 of the 18 patients in this series. In 12, the catecholamines [3-methoxy-3-hydroxymandelic acid (MHMA), homovanillic acid (HVA), adrenaline, noradrenaline or dopamine] were elevated at initial presentation. Of the two children with normal levels, one was a 3-month-old infant with an undifferentiated tumour that had metastasized to the liver; this infant died shortly after beginning chemotherapy. The second patient aged 20 months had a well-differentiated tumour that was discovered incidently on chest X-ray performed because of persistent wheeze. Following surgical resection of this tumour, he remains well, 10 years later.

Other diagnostic procedures included CT scanning and barium swallow. Myelography was the diagnostic procedure of choice for the investigation of spinal cord compression [2, 6]. Bone marrow examination, skeletal survey, bone scan and liver function tests were important diagnostic aids in determining the presence or absence of metastatic disease.

The macroscopic appearance of neuroblastoma is characteristically purplish-red and fleshy. The cut surface usually is soft and friable and flecks of calcification may be visible. Histology of the resected tumour was typical of neuroblastoma in all cases; however, the degree of differentiation varied from those in which maturation to ganglion cells was a prominent feature (ganglio-neuroblastoma) to tumours that were completely undifferentiated. Review of the histology of the tumours at presentation (recurrent tumours were often more differentiated) showed that the majority in this small series were differentiating, i.e. contained areas where neurofibrillary material was prominent or where maturation to ganglion cells was easily recognisable. Eight children had ganglioneuroblastomas, five had well-differentiated neuroblastomas and the remaining five had undifferentiated neuroblastomas. Correlation of the histological appearance with survival, however, was relatively poor. Although two of the five children with undifferentiated neuroblastoma died, one of these had stage 4 metastatic disease at presentation. The other three are well following treatment. Of the eight ganglio-neuroblastomas, all survived except for one patient. However, this patient also had stage 4 disease with metastatic tumour involving her left femur; bone marrow examination was positive. Of the infants who survived, several had poorly differentiated tumours when they first presented, although material obtained at a later date from those in which further surgery was performed invariably showed more maturation. However, if this appearance of lack of differentiation in the very young (under 3 months of age at presentation) is discounted, then the findings from this series do support the conclusion reached from our large earlier series reported in 1983 [10], namely that undifferentiated tumours especially in children over the age of 1 year have a worse prognosis than tumours showing maturation. Stage at presentation is the other important prognostic factor [14]. This present series also confirms the well-recognized view that neuroblastomas arising primarily in the thorax have a much better prognosis than neuroblastomas arising in the abdomen.

Table 6. Ganglioneuroma

Sex	Age (years)	Symptoms	Signs	X-ray	Procedure	Pathology	Catechol-amine	Follow-up (years)
F	2	Incidental finding on chest X-ray for ? dislocated arm following trauma	Nil	Left paravertebral mass T4–T7, no calcification, thinning post-fifth rib	Left thoracotomy, 6-cm-diameter retropleural mass extending into fourth and fifth foramina, complete removal	Pale rubbery mass $5 \times 3 \times 2$ cm, typical GN	N	Well (14)
F	5	1½ years persistent dry cough, mild stridor, no response to anti-asthma agents	Nil	Large well-circumscribed R posterior mediastinal mass, erosion of fourth rib	Right thoracotomy, 10-cm mass with one small extension into foramen, complete removal	10×10-cm pale rubbery mass, typical GN	N	Well (6)
M	5	One week cough, anorexia fever, chest X-ray showed RML pneumonia plus posterior mediastinal mass	RML and RLL consolidation	RML and RLL pneumonia, posterior mediastinal mass, no bony erosion, not intraspinal (CT)	Right thoracotomy, complete removal	Firm tan rubbery mass $4 \times 3 \times 1$ cm, typical GN	N	Well (6)
M	5½	Six weeks dry cough	Nil	Large L posterior mediastinal mass, some intraspinal extension (CT)	Left thoracotomy mass arising from sympathetic chain, complete excision from chest, partial excision from spine	$8 \times 7 \times 2$ cm tan rubbery, typical GN	N	Well (6)
F	8	Two years intermittent sharp chest pains	Dull PN, L apex	L apical calcified mass in posterior mediastinum, no bony erosion or intravertebral extension	Left thoracotomy, well-circumscribed mass attached to sympathetic chain	Yellow rubbery mass $7 \times 5 \times 5.5$ cm, typical GN	N	Well (4)

Table 6 (continued)

Sex	Age (years)	Symptoms	Signs	X-ray	Procedure	Pathology	Cate-chol-amine	Follow-up (years)
F	9	Long history "asthma", recent SOB when recumbent, incidental finding on X-ray	Dull to percussion, L midzone and base	Left posterior mediastinal mass, erosion vertebral bodies, focal calcification	Left thoracotomy, very large paravertebral mass attached to sympathetic chain and intercostal nerves (T9–T11)	Lobulated creamy yellow mass 1476 g, typical GN	N	Well (12)
F	10	One month L-sided submammary chest pain, exertional dyspnoea	Diminished breath sounds, L apex	Large posterior mediastinal mass, speckled calcification, erosion of ribs and pedicles of T3, 4 and 5	Left thoracotomy, extension into third and fourth i.v. foramina, involvement of four intercostal N	10 × 7.5 × 7-cm mass, firm and rubbery, focal calcification, typical GN	Upper limit of normal	Well (12)
F	11	Incidental finding of chest mass on routine chest X-ray (clinical duodenal ulcer)	Nil	Left paravertebral mass T8–T9, focal calcification	Left thoracotomy, lobulated rubbery mass from T4–T8, sympathetic chain entered both ends	9 × 5 × 3-cm rubbery light tan mass, focal calcification	N	Well (12)
F	12	Cold dry red right hand since birth, X-ray to exclude cervical rib showed mass	Cold dry red fingers R hand, power normal	Right posterior mediastinal mass, splaying third and fourth ribs with notching	Right thoracotomy, 95% excision, some tissue left at apex and intervertebral foramina	Firm, rubbery mass, 12 × 8 × 2 cm, tan slightly gritty cut surface	N	Well (7), hand warm

GN, ganglioneuroma; PN, percussion note; RLL, right lower lobe; RML, right middle lobe; SOB, shortness of breath

Ganglioneuroma

There were nine cases of mature ganglioneuroma in this series (Table 6), seven females and two males. All patients were older than 2 years of age and in general older than the children with neuroblastoma. Thus ages ranged from 2 to 12 years. In all cases the tumour was located in the subpleural plane of the posterior mediastinum in the paravertebral region; six on the left side and three on the right. All tumours were quite large masses, with the smallest measuring approximately $4 \times 3 \times 2$ cm and the largest measuring $12 \times 8 \times 6$ cm (Table 6). Macroscopically all tumours were rounded or oval shaped, lobulated and well encapsulated. The cut surface tended to be firm and rubbery, with a homogeneous creamy-yellow tan or pink appearance. Focal calcification was present in many. Histologically all were typical, fully mature ganglioneuromas. Clinically the presenting features were mainly respiratory and in most cases symptoms had been present for several weeks. One patient presented with dry cough alone, another with intermittent chest pains and two with pneumonic consolidation, one child with both dry cough and stridor and another with both chest pain and shortness of breath on exertion. One 12-year-old boy presented with a cold dry right hand that had been noticed since birth; the mediastinal mass was seen on chest X-ray performed to exclude a cervical rib. In the last two patients the mediastinal masses were incidental findings on chest X-ray, one in a girl aged 12 years with a bleeding duodenal ulcer and another in a girl aged 2 years with a dislocated shoulder.

Physical examination was completely normal in five cases; in three signs were limited to the respiratory system, with decreased air entry and/or decreased percussion note and one patient already mentioned presented with a cool dry red hand. Chest X-ray was the single most useful investigation and in all cases the mass was adequately visualized. Other features commonly noted on chest X-ray included focal calcification, splaying of the rib spaces and/or erosion of ribs or vertebral bodies. CT scanning was occasionally of added value, showing evidence of intervertebral foramen invasion or intraspinal extension. In none of the cases was there evidence of metastatic disease and bone marrow examination was negative in all cases. Urinary catecholamine studies were performed in eight of the nine cases and these were completely normal in seven; the other case had elevated urinary levels of HVA and MHMA. All patients were treated by surgical excision alone. Complete excision was able to be obtained in eight of the nine cases. Attachment of the tumour to the thoracic sympathetic chain was specifically noted in the operation notes of four cases. On follow-up all patients have done well, with no evidence of recurrence.

Teratomas

In children the mediastinum is the fourth commonest site for teratomas after the ovary, the sacrococcygeal region and the testis. Mature and partially mature (immature) teratomas are the usual pathological types that occur in the mediastinum and pericardium. Mature teratomas are those with only histologically well developed tissues. Immature teratomas are those lesions reported to contain foci of embryonic mesenchyme, immature neuroectoderm and/or blastema [11]. Malignancy in teratomas takes the form of endodermal sinus tumour, also called yolk sac tumour; occasional ares of germinoma may be found in a mature or immature teratoma but this is much rarer, as is the occurrence of choriocarcinoma [11].

Of the seven cases in our series, five were classified as mature benign teratomas, the other two cases were histologically malignant, one was a mature teratoma with foci of yolk sac carcinoma and the other contained both differentiated and immature elements as well as foci of yolk sac carcinoma. This latter tumour was intrapericardial, the only one of this type encountered in our series.

Mature Teratomas

Of the five benign mature teratomas, three were in males and two in females. Most series report an even sex distribution [21]. The age ranged from birth to 13 years [birth, 1 months, 3 months, 13 years (×2)]. Three were located in the anterior or anterosuperior mediastinum, whereas two patients had tumours in the posterior mediastinum. (Other series have reported 3%–8% of benign teratomas arising in the posterior mediastinum [21]. Two tumours were left sided, two were right sided and one tumour was in the midline intimately related to the thymus. All the tumours were quite large with the smallest measuring approximately 6 cm in diameter and the largest measuring 17 × 15 × 9 cm. They were variably described as large, lobulated, well-circumscribed, partly encapsulated masses, partially solid and partially cystic. Many were locally adherent to surrounding mediastinal structures, making surgical resection more difficult. Histologically all tumours contained tissues derived from the three germinal layers. Most tumours contained mature ectodermal derivatives such as skin, pilosebaceous units and mature neuroglial tissue. Cysts lined by various epithelia, including stratified squamous, respiratory and mucinous epithelium were common. Other tissues commonly encountered included smooth muscle, fat and cartilage. In addition, liver tissue and retinal anlage were found in one case, pancreatic tissue in two cases and immature thyroid elements in another.

While histological features of the immature components of teratomas may be alarming, in the absence of yolk sac tumour elements, behaviour is almost invariably benign [2].

Clinically, the patients presented in two age groups – infants and adolescents. In the infant group, two patients presented with persistent respiratory distress from birth. On examination both infants were tachypnoeic with intercostal and subcostal retraction. Another 3-month-old infant presented with 2 months of hoarse dry cough and mild stridor with gradually increasing respiratory distress interfering with sucking. Examination revealed tachypnoea, mild intercostal and substernal retraction and decreased air entry over the left chest. A very different presentation was seen in two 13-year-old girls. Both had been perfectly well until they presented with vague chest symptoms. A chest X-ray demonstrated the mass; in one girl it was mediastinal; in the other it appeared on imaging to be within the left lower lobe. At operation, however, this mass was separate from lung and was attached via a long pedicle to the base of the pericardium, behind the thymus.

Chest X-ray was the most important diagnostic aid and this revealed the presence of the mass in all cases. Small flecks of calcium were common; however, bone or teeth were not visualized in any of our cases. Barium swallow was also performed in each case, revealing indentation or displacement of the oesophagus in two. Ultrasound examination was useful in one patient with a posterior mediastinal tumour, a pleural effusion and right lung collapse when the multicystic nature of the tumour was readily evident. CT was performed in one child and this showed the mass in the thymus. Alpha-feta-protein levels were not raised in any of these five cases.

It is well accepted that surgical excision via thoracotomy is the best means of diagnosing and treating benign teratoma [21]. Complete resection is preferred, and this was obtained in all cases; however, as these tumours were often locally adherent to surrounding mediastinal structures, complete excision was often difficult. A second thoracotomy was required in one infant. The postoperative courses were uneventful, apart from a huge chylous mediastinal collection in one case requiring subsequent needle aspiration. On follow-up, all patients are healthy, with no evidence of tumour recurrence.

Malignant teratomas

These remaining two cases have been reported previously but merit detailed description [3, 27]. One of the patients had Klinefelter's syndrome and first presented at 7½ years of age with precocious puberty. Endocrine studies were unhelpful, with normal basal levels of serum testosterone and serum-lutenizing hormone, and 24 h urinary gonadotrophin levels were also normal. A cranial CT scan was normal, but no chest X-ray film was obtained and he was lost to follow-up. Two and a half years later he presented with a 1-month history of anorexia, lethargy, night sweats, a dry cough and right-sided chest pain. On examination the trachea was deviated to the left and there was dullness to percussion with decreased air entry on the right side. His penis was adult in size, pubic hair was present, both testes were 3.5 ml in volume and he had bilateral gynaecomastia. Chest X-ray confirmed a large opacity in the right hemithorax which on ultrasound was found to be echogenic. Testicular ultrasound was normal. Bone scan was normal. The serum alpha-fetoprotein level was greatly elevated at 13000 μg/litre (normal is less than 12 μg/litre). The beta subunit of human chorionic gonadotrophin (beta-HCG) was also markedly elevated at 54.5 IU/litre (normal is less than 2 IU/litre). Plasma testosterone was in the adult range, luteinizing hormone was markedly elevated although follicle-stimulating hormone was low. At operation (right thoracotomy), a large multilobulated variegated mediastinal tumour was noted displacing the lungs laterally and indenting the diaphragm inferiorly. Biopsy showed a mostly differentiated teratoma but with foci of yolk sac carcinoma together with beta-HCG-positive cells. Complete macroscopic surgical clearance was subsequently obtained via a midline sternotomy. Postoperatively both alpha-fetoprotein and beta-HCG returned to within the normal range. Adjuvant chemotherapy was commenced with vinblastine, bleomycin and cisplatinum 1 week after surgery. Unfortunately, over the succeeding weeks, he developed increasing hepatosplenomegaly, generalized lymphadenopathy, increasing abdominal distension and marked haematological abnormalities. He was subsequently diagnosed as having malignant histiocytosis on biopsy of tissue removed at laparatomy. This case is interesting as it demonstrates the recognized potential of malignant teratomas containing beta-HCG-secreting cells to cause isosexual precocity. In addition it supports the recently recognized association between Klinefelter's syndrome and the development of extragonadal germ cell neoplasms, and between mediastinal germ cell tumours and haematological malignancy, usually of the monocytic histiocytic line [3].

In the other patient with yolk sac carcinoma elements the tumour was intrapericardial. This male infant first presented at 3 months of age with a short history of diarrhoea, shortness of breath and fever. On admission he was found to have signs of acute cardiac failure but no definite evidence of tamponade or constrictive pericarditis. Chest X-ray revealed a panthoracic shadow, not separable from the heart. Echocardiography suggested a large anterior pericardial effusion and urgent pericardiocentesis was performed under general anaesthesia. This yielded 20–30 ml serosanguinous fluid from which no microorganism or viral antigen was isolated. A pericardial biopsy showed signs of acute inflammation only. During this procedure and over the next 12–24 h there was severe impairment of myocardial function with increasing cardiorespiratory distress, hypotension and oliguria requiring intensive support with ventilation, inotropes and peripheral vasodilatation. The diagnosis of an intrapericardial tumour was only suggested at the time of subsequent CT scanning of the thorax. Alpha-fetoprotein levels were markedly elevated (1700 μg/litre). Skeletal survey and bone marrow examination were normal. Finally the thoracic cavity was explored via a median sternotomy. A large non-invasive bilobulated cystic tumour was found completely filling the pericardial cavity, displacing the heart and attached via a small pedicle to the anterior surface of the root of the aorta. Complete surgical macroscopic clearance was obtained. Postoperatively the infant's condition was markedly improved. Histological examination of the mass revealed, in varying proportions, an extraordinary variety of mature and immature tissues, including extensive sheets of primitive neuroglial tissue, primitive retina and tissue resembling nephroblastoma. In addition, small foci of yolk sac carcinoma were identified. It was thought that this malignant teratoma was likely to have a poor prognosis although the age of presentation was a probable favourable factor. It was decided that adjuvant chemotherapy or radiotherapy should not be used because of the likelihood of severe side effects. Alpha-fetoprotein levels returned to normal postoperatively and on review 1 year later he was alive and well with no evidence of tumour recurrence.

In other reported cases, as in our own, pericardial teratoma was seen most commonly in the neonatal period with evidence of severe cardiorespiratory distress [2, 31]. There is usually marked enlargement of the cardiac silhouette and it is the most common cause of pericardial effusion in the newborn [31]. Echocardiography, CT scanning and cardiac angiography are useful investigations in establishing the diagnosis prior to surgery. This neoplasm is lethal if the diagnosis is delayed and surgical treatment is not instituted.

Duplication Cysts

Benign congenital cystic lesions have been referred to by various names, including bronchogenic cyst, oesophageal duplication cyst, dorsal enteric cyst and foregut duplication cyst. They are all believed to constitute congenital abnormalities of division of the embryonic primitive foregut. The primitive foregut normally divides during the 5th week of fetal development. The tracheobronchial tree is derived from the ventral bud and the oesophagus from the dorsal component. Bronchogenic cysts may result when abnormal budding occurs in the ventral component and oesophagal duplications may result when this occurs in the dorsal component. Usually these duplications are thin-walled cysts containing thick viscid fluid. Histological examination of bronchogenic cysts usually reveals an internal lining of ciliated stratified columnar respiratory epithelium resting upon a wall composed of fibrovascular connective with variable amounts of smooth muscle cartilage and seromucous glands. Oesophageal duplications are usually lined by gastric or oesophageal mucosa and have a well-developed muscle wall with a myenteric plexus. Components of one system may also be found in anomalies of the other and so it is not unusual to find respiratory epithelium as a component of an oesophageal duplication.

These cystic masses usually occur in the posterior mediastinum. There may be associated anomalies of the lower cervical and upper thoracic vertebrae, including hemivertebrae, anomalies of segmentation and fusion, spina bifida and scoliosis. Although these mediastinal lesions usually lie very close to either the oesophagus or the tracheal bronchial tree, rarely is there a direct open communication.

In contrast to the situation in adults where these lesions are usually incidental findings, in children duplication cysts are usually symptomatic and in infants life-threatening respiratory complications may be the presenting features resulting from bronchial compression [13]. Symptoms include persistent cough, progressive dyspnoea, wheeze, stridor and cyanosis. Sometimes, compression of the oesophagus may cause dysphagia. The symptoms may be aggravated by crying or feeding. Very often the presenting feature is that of recurrent respiratory tract infections. Episodes may start quite early in life and may date from birth. Physical findings are usually confined to the respiratory system and include tachypnoea, audible wheeze, stridor, rhonchi, tracheal deviation consistent with mediastinal shift and relative differences in air entry or percussion note over the two lung

Table 7. Duplication cysts

Sex	Age (years)	Symptoms	Signs	X-ray	Procedure	Pathology	Diagnosis
M	5	Six weeks cough, rattly breathing, wheeze	Lingular pneumonia	Well-defined round mass, L paravertebral T10 level, lingular collapse	Left thoracotomy, posterior mediastinal subpleural cyst, no communication	$3.5 \times 2.0 \times 2.0$ cm mucous epithelium	Foregut duplication cyst
M	3/12	Poor weight gain, irritability, no respiratory symptoms	Right congenital glaucoma, no chest signs	Incidental chest X-ray showed large round mass R hemithorax, bilateral hyperinflation, abnormal segmentation and fusion C6, 7, T1–3	Right thoracotomy, posterior mediastinal cyst, fibrous connection to hemivertebra, no patent track	$4 \times 3 \times 2$ cm muscle ganglion cells, respiratory and mucus cells, no cartilage	Dorsal enteric duplication cyst
M	1	"Asthma" since 2 months, presented age 1 year with cough, stridor and wheeze	Febrile wheeze, stridor, hyperinflated chest	Posterior mediastinal mass at thoracic inlet with compression of mediastinal structures	Right thoracotomy, thin-walled cyst attached to trachea and part of tracheal wall	Respiratory epithelial seromucous glands, smooth muscle, no GC	Tracheal duplication cyst
F	1 1/12	Severe asthma attacks precipitating URTI	Decreased air entry	Bilateral hyperinflation, round mass, posterior mediastinal causing narrowing and compression of carina and L main bronchus	Right thoracotomy, cyst between trachea and oesophagus in midline	Thin cyst, respiratory epithelial seromucous glands, some muscle, no GC	Tracheal duplication cyst
F	7/12	Fever, wheeze, cough, treated for pneumonia but wheeze worsened	Wheeze and stridor, percussion note, reduced RUL	Right apical mediastinal mass 4 cm diameter, compressing oesophagus	Right thoracotomy, cyst adherent to midtrachea. Tracheal cartilage deficient at point of attachment	Thin 3.5-cm cyst, respiratory epithelial seromucous glands, fibrous wall	Tracheal duplication cyst
F	6	Multiple chest infections, 1 year cough, lethargy	NAD	Rounded mass at L hilum with fluid level	Left thoracotomy, cyst mediastinal above hilum, adjacent lung emphysematous	Mucus-filled cyst $6 \times 3 \times 3$ cm, respiratory epithelial seromucous glands, cartilage	Bronchogenic cyst

F	3/12	Cough, wheeze, cyanosis on feeding	Tachypnoea, retraction R bronchial areas	3-cm mass mid-mediastinum, bowing trachea anterior to R; L lung more lucent than R lung	Right thoracotomy, mass between carina and oesophagus 4 × 3 cm, close attachment to oesophagus	3.5 × 2.5 × 2.0 cm, respiratory epithelial sero-mucous glands, smooth muscle, no cartilage	Bronchogenic cyst
M	2	One year recurrent chest infection	Cough, wheeze, stridor	Rounded mid-mediastinum mass at L hilum constricting L main bronchus air trapping posterior displacement of oesophagus	Left thoracotomy, cyst above LMB attached to it	Cyst 4 × 3 × 2 cm, respiratory epithelial sero-mucous glands, some cartilage	Bronchogenic cyst
F	6/12	One episode of "bronchitis", 4 days cough, wheeze	Tachypnoea, trachea to R retraction, air entry reduced on L side	Mediastinal mass at level of carina with displacement of mediastinum, structures to R. Hyperinflated L lung	Left thoracotomy, cyst lying between posterior surface of LMB and MPA bifurcation attached to LMB	2 × 2 × 1 cm, respiratory epithelial sero-mucous glands, smooth muscle, cartilage	Bronchogenic cyst
F	10	One month dry cough	NAD	Left solid mediastinal mass level T8, 9 in front of vertebral bodies, no vertebral abnormality	Left thoracotomy, sub-pleural cyst fourth intercostal space, attached to oesophagus but no communication	1.3-cm cyst, mucus epithelium with some respiratory epithelium, muscle and GC	Foregut duplication cyst

GC, ganglion cells; LMB, left main bronchus; MPA, main pulmonary artery; NAD, no abnormality detected; RUL, right upper lobe; URTI, upper respiratory tract infection

fields. In infants, intercostal and/or sternal retraction may be prominent [13, 15, 23].

The plain chest X-ray is the most useful single investigation in establishing a diagnosis of bronchogenic cyst. It shows the cyst in the posterior mediastinum displacing or compressing the trachea, bronchi or oesophagus. One lung field may be hyperinflated, the other may be collapsed. There may be signs of mediastinal displacement. Barium swallow may demonstrate displacement or compression of the oesophagus. Bronchoscopy may be helpful in defining the extent of bronchial obstruction. Useful complementary investigations include CT scanning, echocardiography and tomography.

In our series, there were ten duplication cysts (Table 7), all within the posterior mediastinum, seven of which were purely bronchogenic and three of which were predominantly alimentary. The age at diagnosis ranged from 3 months to 10 years (3, 3, 6, 7, 13 months, 1, 2, 5, 6, 10 years). All patients were cured by surgical excision alone which was achieved via a thoracotomy. Nowadays the preferred treatment of duplications cysts is complete surgical excision and most patients are cured by this procedure. Of the bronchogenic cysts, four were located in the right and three on the left side. In our series, most common symptoms were cough, wheeze, stridor and recurrent chest infections. When patients presented with wheeze and cough a mistaken diagnosis of asthma or bronchiolitis was often made. One patient presented with a persistent dry cough only. Three patients presented with recurrent chest infections and two with acute pneumonia. In three children the duplication cysts were incidental findings on chest X-ray. In only three patients were there no abnormal respiratory signs. Plain X-ray directly revealed the presence of a mediastinal mass in nine of the ten patients and barium swallow was the single most useful investigation after chest X-ray.

Lymphangioma and Haemangioma

Lymphangioma

Most mediastinal lymphangiomas are thoracic extensions of cystic hygromas of the neck, causing symptoms at the same time as the cervical portion is visible and obvious, or causing problems some time after the cervical component has been excised or found as an incidental finding [7]. There were only three children with mediastinal lymphangioma in the 19-year span of the present series, indicating the rarity of this entity. All were under 1 year of age at presentation. In two, an obvious cervical component was noted at birth while in the third the presence of a mediastinal mass was not suspected until the infant was aged 10 months when she presented with 2 days of fever, cough, coryza and stridor culminating in respiratory arrest. X-ray showed a large anterior mediastinal mass with tracheal deviation to the right. An urgent thoracotomy revealed a multicystic lesion in the upper mediastinum encroaching on the right hemithorax. Some of the cysts were unroofed and partially excised and others were aspirated. Total removal was not attempted. Postoperatively she developed signs of bronchiolitis (respiratory syncytial virus was isolated). However, she quickly recovered from this and is now well. Both the other two children were noted to have cystic hygromas at birth and both were shown to have a mediastinal extension on X-ray. In one baby, no active treatment was given initially until the age of 7 months when rapid increase in the size of the neck mass together with fever and stridor developed. Partial excision of the neck mass was followed 4 months later by partial excision of the mediastinal component. The third infant presented at birth with fetal hydrops (diagnosed antenatally by ultrasound) together with a transluminable fluctuent mass on the right side of the neck. Ultrasound showed the neck lesion to be continuous with a mediastinal component which was also multicystic. Thoracotomy at 8 days of age revealed numerous cystic spaces in the upper right mediastinum which were only partially excised because of intimate relation with vessels and nerves.

The pathology of the excised tissue from all three cases showed lymphangioma with evidence of past haemorrhage and inflammation. Thus in all three cases it seems likely that complicating haemorrhage has led to the exacerbation of symptoms that precipitated the need for surgery. All three children have residual lymphangioma with the potential for growth and further complications such as haemorrhage and infection. From the experience of these three cases and previous examples seen before 1970, surgery of the mediastinal component of lymphangioma is reserved for complications and is essentially conservative with careful preservation of vital structures (e.g. phrenic nerve, recurrent laryngeal nerve and major vessels).

Brown et al. [7] in their review of 14 mediastinal lymphangiomas also concluded that limited conservative surgery was adequate treatment, and that radical surgery was neither necessary nor preferable.

Haemangioma

Pure haemangiomas either in the lung or the mediastinum presenting with mediastinal mass are extraordinarily rare; there was none in our series [12].

Neurofibroma

There were four neurofibromas with a mediastinal component in the series. Three of the patients were known to have von Recklinghausen's disease and only one showed no evidence of this condition. A brief outline of these childrens' histories follows:

Case 1: T. M. An 11-month-old boy who presented with a 2-week history of progressive loss of strength in the legs such that at the time of admission he had signs of paraparesis and a sensory level at T10. Chest X-ray showed a 3.0-cm mass in the left paravertebral gutter at the level of T9-T10 containing a streak of calcification. There was widening of the interspace between T9 and T10 with thinning of the left ninth rib. Myelogram shows a block from T9 to T11. Emergency laminectoma revealed a pink, fleshy extradural tumour and this was removed. Four months later the thoracic component was excised. He later developed kyphosis that was corrected by spinal fusion. He is otherwise well 10 years later and shows no evidence of von Recklinghausen's disease. Histology and electron microscopy showed neurofibroma.

Case 2: M. K. A 5½-year-old girl who presented with a knotted left supraclavicular mass of rubbery texture which had been noticed for 1 month. She had stigmata of von Recklinghausen's disease. A chest X-ray showed a large rounded mass in the upper anterior mediastinum in front of the trachea. An unusual coarse trabeculation of flat bones suggested marrow hyperplasia or infiltration. The child had a history of a bullous eruption at birth diagnosed on skin biopsy as urticaria pigmentosa. The supraclavicular mass was shown to be a plexiform neurofibroma of typical histological pattern. Two months later at elective thoracotomy (L. 5th rib) a grape-like mass of grey-pink tissue in the superior mediastinum was partially excised. The mass appeared to arise from the phrenic nerve and histologically was a typical plexiform neurofibroma. Sections of the rib showed extensive mast cell infiltration of the marrow. Her subsequent course has been complicated by recurrence of the neurofibroma in the neck and by renal artery and other stenoses associated with hypertension.

Case 3: J. M. An 11-year-old boy with known von Recklinghausen's disease was investigated for a cardiac murmur and shown on chest X-ray to have a huge right-sided posterior mediastinal mass that extended from the diaphragm to the apex of the pleural cavity. A smaller left-sided posterior mediastinal mass was also present.

Subtotal resection only was possible and the boy was followed up. Scoliosis developed and was corrected by a Dwyer's operation. He has recently developed neurofibrosarcoma in the thoracic mass and died at the age of 24 years.

Case 4: S. M. A 3½-year-old boy who presented with a swelling in the neck. Biopsy showed plexiform neurofibroma. Café au lait spots were present. Chest X-ray showed a mediastinal mass extending from C7-T1 but he had no symptoms. A diagnosis of von Recklinghausen's disease was made but no active treatment was given. At the age of 13 years, weakness and pain in the right arm developed together with pains in the chest. X-ray showed a very large mass which on biopsy proved to be fibrosarcoma. He died a few months later.

These children represent the usual spectrum of presentation and course of neurofibroma. The development of sarcomatous change in the mediastinal neurofibromas in von Recklinghausen's disease is also well known. Three of the children in our small series are included in a recent report [30].

Miscellaneous and Rare Mediastinal Masses

These comprise a mixed collection of inflammatory, developmental and neoplastic conditions, all rare and usually not all represented in the experience of a single institution. The cases we have seen that fall in this group are described briefly below.

Inflammatory Conditions

Mediastinal Abscess

Infection in the mediastinum is usually a fulminating process complicating perforating injuries of the oesophagus but may occasionally be more indolent, presenting with a mass, and not always with fever and leucocytosis. Infection can arise in the thymus but more commonly originates in hilar lymph nodes, the suppuration becoming localized and encapsulated so that a discrete mass forms.

Plasma Cell Granuloma (Inflammatory Pseudotumour)

A lesion of unknown etiology characterized by a localized proliferation of fibroblasts and blood vessels in which large numbers of plasma cells are found. These lesions usually occur in the lung but may involve the mediastinum. Excision is usually performed for diagnosis and is generally curative. One case has been seen at the RCH but occurred before 1970.

Developmental Conditions

Thymic Cyst

This is a rare lesion resulting from cystic degeneration of the epithelial component of the thymus. The cyst is lined by cells that commonly show squamous metaplasia [28]. One case was seen in a boy aged 5 years with a neck mass that also had a mediastinal component.

Pericardial Cyst

These are usually small, incidentally discovered, lying anteriorly or in the costophrenic angle. They are lined by mesothelial cells and contain serous fluid [28].

Extralobar Pulmonary Sequestrations can present with a middle or posterior mediastinal mass that may mimic a duplication cyst. They are usually angular in outline lying close to the diaphgram. In our experience most occur in association with diaphgramatic hernia and are an incidental finding at operation.

Thymic Hyperplasia, so called, is not an entity. The normal thymus can be quite large in young infants and can be misinterpreted as enlarged when it is in fact quite normal. The thymus may weigh up to 50 g at postmortem in normal infants and completely fill the anterior mediastinum.

The thymus in *myasthenia gravis* is rarely enlarged.

Tumours

In the *anterior mediastinum, germinomas* have been described but are very rare [18, 22]. There was none in the present series.

Thymomas [6, 28] seem to be very rare in childhood also, with only one example in the whole experience of the RCH, a girl of 4 years. This case was seen before 1970.

Fibromatosis. Desmoid tumours may occur anywhere in the body, producing a slowly growing mass that involves adjacent structures causing compression and distortion. One example was seen in the present series, in a girl of 9 months, who presented with a mass in the upper anterior mediastinum following a median sternotomy for repair of a ventricular septal defect. In spite of several attempts at excision, total removal proved impossible. The tumour relentlessly enlarged and led to the child's death at 2½ years of age from respiratory obstruction and failure. Histology showed fibroblasts in a dense collagenous stroma.

Carcinoid Tumour of the Thymus

An 11-year-old boy with a 4-week history of cough and wheeze not responding to anti-asthma treatment was shown on chest X-ray to have a huge anterior mediastinal mass. The mass was biopsied and the nature of the tumour was uncertain. He was given a course of chemotherapy with no response. Because of this lack of response subtotal resection via a median sternotomy was performed and histology, cytochemistry and electron microscopy established the diagnosis of malignant carcinoid tumour. In spite of further therapy he died 1 year later. Necropsy was not performed.

Middle Mediastinum

Cardia tumours are rare and whilst they are strictly situated in the mediastinum they are usually diagnosed by other means and are not usually considered to be mediastinal tumours as such.

Rare *sarcomas* have been described arising in the mediastinum, for example rhabdomyosarcoma, liposarcoma and fibrosarcoma. Diagnosis can only be made at thoracotomy although the diagnosis may be suspected by examining pleural fluid if involvement of the lung has occurred from local spread.

Posterior Mediastinum

Neurofibrosarcoma either arising de novo or from malignant change occurring in a pre-existing mediastinal plexiform neurofibroma is a rare tumour in the paediatric age. Only one example was seen in the present series in a boy with von Recklinghausen's disease who presented with an asymptomatic neck mass shown on biopsy to be plexiform neurofibroma. X-ray showed a mediastinal mass. He remained asymptomatic until the age of 13 years, when he developed pain and weakness in the right arm. The mediastinal mass had enlarged and on biopsy was now neurofibrosarcoma. It could not be excised and the child died. This case together with four others is the subject of a recent report [30].

Ewing's tumour of the vertebrae can produce a soft tissue shadow in the paravertebral region. Collapse or erosion of bone is usually evident, making the diagnosis of a bone tumour likely. One presumed case occurred in the present series in a boy aged 7 years who presented with lower back pain for a few weeks. X-ray showed a paraspinal mass at level of T8 together with partial collapse of T8. Histology showed a small round cell tumour with typical imprint cytology of Ewing's tumour. Urinary catecholamine estimation was in the normal range and immunocytochemistry was negative for lymphoma. Ewing's tumour, although often thought of as a tumour of long bones, can arise in vertebrae and ribs and should always be considered in the differential diagnosis of a child with a posterior mediastinal mass.

References

1. Adam A, Hochholzer L (1981) Ganglioneuroblastoma of the posterior mediastinum. Cancer 47:373–381
2. Aldousany AW, Joyner JC, Price RA, et al (1987) Diagnosis and treatment of intrapericardial teratoma. Pediatr Cardiol 8:51–53
3. Beasley SW, Tiedemann K, Howat A, et al (1987) Precocious puberty associated with malignant thoracic teratoma and malignant histiocytes in child with Klinefelter's syndrome. Med Pediatr Oncol 15:277–280
4. Bleyer WA, Sather H, Coccia P, et al (1986) The staging of childhood acute lymphoblastic leukemia: strategies of the Children's Cancer Study Group and a three-dimensional technic of multivariate analysis. Med Pediatr Oncol 14 (5):271–280
5. Bower RJ, Kiesewetter WB (1977) Mediastinal masses in infants and children. Arch Surg 112:1003–1009
6. Bowie PR, Teixeira OHP, Carpenter B (1979) Malignant thymoma in a nine-year-old boy presenting with pleuropericardial effusion. J Thorac Cardiovasc Surg 77:777–781
7. Brown LR, Reiman HM, Rosenow EC, et al (1986) Intrathoracic lymphangioma. Mayo Clinic Proc 61:882–892
8. Bunin NJ, Hvizdala E, Link M, et al (1986) Mediastinal nonlymphoblastic lymphomas in children: a clinico-pathologic study. J Clin Oncol 4:154–159
9. Callihan TR, Berard CW (1982) Childhood non-Hodgkin's lymphomas in current histologic perspective. Perspect Pediatr Pathol 7:259–277
10. Carachi R, Campbell PE, Kent M (1983) Thoracic neural crest tumours, a clinical review. Cancer 51:949–954
11. Carter D, Bibro MC, Touloukian RJ (1982) Benign clinical behaviour of immature mediastinal teratoma in infancy and childhood. Cancer 49:398–402
12. Cohen AJ, Sbaschnig RJ, Hochholzer L, et al (1987) Mediastinal haemangiomas. Ann Thorac Surg 43:656–659
13. Eraklis AJ, Griscom NT, McGovern JB (1969) Bronchogenic cysts of the mediastinum in infancy. N Engl J Med 281:1150–1155
14. Evans AE (1980) Staging and treatment of neuroblastoma. Cancer 45:1799–1802
15. Grafe WR, Goldsmith EI, Redo SF (1966) Bronchogenic cysts of the mediastinum in children. J Pediatr Surg 1:384–393

16. Haller JA, Mazur DO, Morgan WW (1969) Diagnosis and management of mediastinal masses in children. J Thorac Cardiovasc Surg 58:385–393
17. Heimburger IL, Battersby JS (1965) Primary mediastinal tumours of childhood. J Thorac Cardiovasc Surg 50:92–103
18. Hurt RD, Bruckman JE, Farrow GM, et al (1982) Primary anterior mediastinal seminoma. Cancer 49:134–140
19. King RM, Telander RL, Smithson WA, et al (1982) Primary mediastinal tumours in children. J Pediatr Surg 17:512–520
20. Kinnier-Wilson LM, Draper GJ (1974) Neuroblastoma, its natural history and prognosis. A study of 487 cases. Br Med J 3:301–307
21. Lewis BD, Hurt RD, Payne WS, et al (1983) Benign teratomas of the mediastinum. J Thorac Cardiovasc Surg 86:727–731
22. Mullen B, Richardson JD (1986) Primary anterior mediastinal tumours in children and adults. Am Thorac Surg 42:338–345
23. Opsahl T, Berman EJ (1962) Bronchogenic mediastinal cysts in infants: case report and review of the literature. Pediatrics 30:372
24. Ovrum E, Birkland S (1979) Mediastinal tumours and cysts: a review of 91 cases. Scand J Thorac Carciovasc Surg 13:161–168
25. Pokorny WJ, Sherman JO (1974) Mediastinal masses in infants and children. J Thorac Cardiovasc Surg 68:869–875
26. Punt J, Pritchard J, Pincott JR, Till K (1980) Neuroblastoma: a review of 21 cases presenting with spinal cord compression. Cancer 45:3095–3101
27. Skillington PD, Brawn WJ, Edis BD, et al (1987) Surgical excision of primary cardiac tumours in infancy. Aust NZ J Surg 57:599–604
28. Welch KJ, Tapper D, Vawter GP (1979) Surgical treatment of thymic cysts and neoplasms in children. J Pediatr Surg 14:691–697
29. Whittaker LD, Lynn HB (1973) Mediastinal tumours and cysts in the pediatric patient. Surg Clin North Am 53:893–904
30. Wijesinha SS, Lugg PC, Cole WG, Myers NA (1989) Neurofibrosarcoma – a compilation of von Recklinghausen's disease. Pediatr Surg Int 3:193–198
31. Zerella JT, Halpe DCE (1980) Intrapericardial teratoma – neonatal cardiorespiratory distress amenable to surgery. J Pediatr Surg 15:961–963

Unusual Varieties of Diaphragmatic Herniae

K. B. Stokes

Summary

Unusual varieties of diaphragmatic herniae can be classified into two major groups, congenital and acquired. The late-presenting Bochdalek herniae often present difficulties in diagnosis which may lead to inappropriate treatment. The prime example is the herniated stomach, which is mistaken for a tension pneumothorax. Strangulation is a rare, but an important, complication of Bochdalek herniae. A number of techniques for closure of large diaphragmatic defects are described with recommendation of those procedures which can be performed rapidly and effectively in a critically ill infant.

The literature concerning eventration is confusing due to different definitions of the condition by different authors. It may be difficult to distinguish preoperatively between this condition and congenital diaphragmatic hernia with a sac. Such distinction is often not important as the decision for intervention is based on evaluation of clinical and radiological considerations. The majority of Morgagni herniae are asymptomatic and only rarely does strangulation supervene. There is a small group of infants with Morgagni hernias who present in early infancy with respiratory symptoms.

Paralysis of the diaphragm due to phrenic nerve palsy recovers spontaneously in the majority of patients. The selective use of diaphragmatic plication for this condition is widely accepted, but the decision and appropriate timing for surgical intervention is often difficult. The results of surgery are very good both in the early postoperative period and also on long-term follow-up.

The diagnosis of traumatic diaphragmatic hernia is often overlooked in the presence of other major injuries. The danger of strangulation of contents of this hernia is ever present and repair should be undertaken without delay once the diagnosis is made.

Zusammenfassung

Seltene Varianten der Zwerchfellhernie können in 2 Gruppen eingeteilt werden: angeborene und erworbene. Die spät manifest werdenden Bochdalek-Hernien bereiten diagnostische Schwierigkeiten, die zu inadäquater Behandlung führen können. Hauptbeispiel ist der prolabierte Magen, der für einen Spannungspneumothorax gehalten werden kann. Strangulationen sind seltene, aber schwerwiegende Komplikationen der Bochdalek-Hernie. Es wird eine Reihe von Techniken zum Verschluß großer Zwerchfelldefekte beschrieben, insbesondere Verfahren, die schnell und effektiv beim kritischen Säugling eingesetzt werden.

Die Literatur zur Eventeration ist widersprüchlich, da verschiedene Autoren verschiedene Definitionen dieses Krankheitsbildes geben. Die Unterscheidung zwischen einer Eventeration und einer Zwerchfellhernie mit Bruchsack kann präoperativ Schwierigkeiten bereiten; sie ist aber häufig auch nicht nötig, da die Operationsindikation aufgrund klinischer und radiologischer Kriterien gestellt wird.

Children's Specialist Centre, Royal Children's Hospital Melbourne, Flemington Road, Parkville 3052, Victoria, Australia.

Progress in Pediatric Surgery, Vol. 27
Myers and Angerpointner (Eds.)

In der Mehrzahl der Fälle kommt es bei Morgagni-Hernien nicht zu Symptomen, und nur selten tritt eine Strangulation ein. Eine kleine Gruppe von Kindern mit Morgagni-Hernien zeigen respiratorische Symptome in der frühen Säuglingszeit.

Eine Zwerchfellrelaxation aufgrund einer Läsion des N. phrenicus bildet sich bei der Mehrzahl der Patienten spontan zurück. Die elektive Zwerchfellraffung ist als Behandlung der Relaxation weitgehend anerkannt, jedoch können Entschluß zur Operation und zeitliche Planung Schwierigkeiten bereiten. Die operativen Ergebnisse sind sowohl in der frühen postoperativen Phase als auch im Langzeit-Follow-up sehr gut.

Eine traumatische Zwerchfellhernie kann bei Vorliegen anderer größerer Verletzungen leicht übersehen werden. Dabei besteht immer die Gefahr der Strangulation der herniierten Organe, weshalb die operative Korrektur ohne Verzögerung durchgeführt werden sollte, sobald die Diagnose gestellt ist.

Résumé

Les hernies diaphragmiques de type peu courant peuvent être classées en deux groupes principaux: hernies congénitales ou acquises. Le diagnostic de la hernie de Bochdalek, qui se tard, est souvent compliqué et cela peut entraîner un traitement inadéquat. L'exemple le plus courant est la hernie de l'estomac qui peut être confondue avec un pneumothorax suffocant. L'étranglement est une complication rare mais très grave de la hernie de Bochdalek. Les auteurs décrivent un grand nombre de techniques de fermeture des vices diaphragmatiques étendus et en recommandent certaines permettant une intervention rapide et efficace dans le cas d'enfant en état critique.

La littérature sur l'éventration prête souvent à confusion car les différents auteurs ne sont pas d'accord sur la définiton. Il peut s'avérer difficile, avant toute intervention, de distinguer cette affection d'une hernie diaphragmatique congénitale avec sac. Toutefois, cette distinction est souvent sans grande importance, vu que la décision d'intervenir est fondée sur l'évaluation (l'appréciation) des données cliniques et radiologiques.

Le majorité des hernies de Morgagni sont asymptomatiques et un étranglement ne se produit que rarement. Un petit groupe d'enfants seulement, avec hernie de Morgagni, présenta des symptômes respiratoires dès la petite enfance.

La paralysie du diaphragme due à une paralysie du nerf phrénique guérit spontanément dans la plupart des cas. On est en général d'accord pour pratiquer une plication diaphragmatique dans ces cas. Il est souvent difficile de savoir quand exactement pratiquer cette intervention. Les résultats de l'intervention sont très bons, qu'il s'agisse de la période directement postopératoire ou des patients suivis à long terme.

Le diagnostic de hernie diaphragmatique traumatique est souvent rendu difficile par la présence d'autres traumatismes majeurs. Le danger d'étranglement du contenu de cette hernie est toujours présent et il faut intervenir aussitôt après l'établissement du diagnostic.

Introduction

In recent literature related to the topic of "diaphragmatic hernia" the emphasis has been directed towards the challenging problem of management of the newborn infant afflicted with the typical congenital Bochdalek (posterolateral) diaphragmatic hernia.

The emphasis in this article will be away from this group of patients and will address the less common varieties of diaphragmatic herniae, both congenital and acquired. This group of conditions comprises a variety of quite different entities, which often present difficulties in diagnosis and controversy concerning the correct management.

The conditions to be discussed are classified as follows:

A. Congenital Lesions of the Diaphragm

1. Bochdalek (posterolateral) diaphragmatic hernia
   a) Unusual modes of presentation
      α) Late-presenting Bochdalek hernia
      β) Strangulated Bochdalek hernia
      γ) Bilateral Bochdalek herniae
      δ) Rare modes of presentation
   b) Large diaphragmatic defects, including agenesis
2. Eventration of the Diaphragm
3. Morgagni (retrosternal) diaphragmatic hernia
4. Central (septum transversum) diaphragmatic hernia
5. Para-Oesophageal hiatus hernia

B. Acquired lesions of the diaphragm

1. Paralysis of the diaphragm due to phrenic nerve palsy
2. Traumatic diaphragmatic hernia

Bochdalek Posterolateral Diaphragmatic Hernia

Unusual Modes of Presentation

Late-Presenting Bochdalek Hernia

Between 5% and 10% of Bochdalek herniae present after the neonatal period [5]. The clinical and radiological features of patients with Bochdalek herniae presenting after the neonatal period may be difficult to interpret and may result in diagnostic delay and inappropriate treatment for mistaken diagnosis. Berman et al. [5] reported a series of 26 patients with late-presenting hernias and 16 (62%) were misdiagnosed. Mistaken diagnoses included pneumonia, pleural effusion, congenital lung cysts and pneumothorax. Particular emphasis is directed towards the mistaken diagnosis of pneumothorax for a herniated distended stomach on the left side [5]. This had led to the insertion of a chest tube into the distended viscus. A similar trap is the "pleural effusion" on either side, where a drain tube has also been inappropriately inserted. Delay in diagnosis is well recognized with right-sided Bochdalek herniae which have languished under the mistaken diagnosis of right lower lobe pneumonia or pleural effusion [5, 35].

Investigations

Plain X-ray of Chest and Abdomen. Demonstration of a distended stomach herniated into the left chest cavity is readily achieved by passage of a nasogastric tube into the viscus (Figs. 1, 2). Detection of a right-sided Bochdalek hernia may be

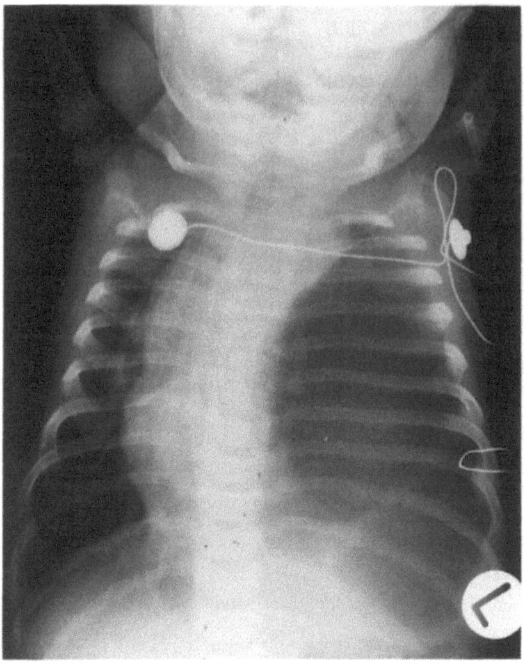

Fig. 1. Chest X-ray of infant with large air-containing cavity in the left hemithorax. Is it due to a pneumothorax or is it a distended stomach?

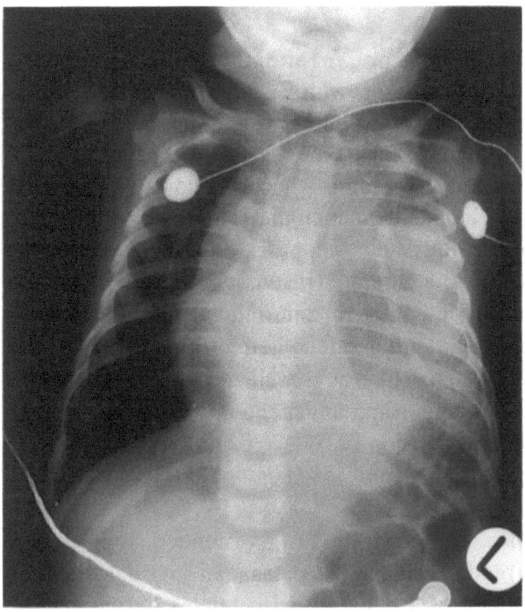

Fig. 2. The diagnostic problem is readily solved by the insertion of a nasogastric tube into the viscus, demonstrating it to be stomach which has herniated through the Bochdalek diaphragmatic hernia

difficult as it may masquerade as persistent right lower lobe pneumonia or pleural effusion in the neonatal period. Further investigations may be required to help resolve the problem. It should be emphasized that previous chest X-rays may be normal and the diagnosis cannot be dismissed on the basis of normal early chest X-rays.

Barium Meal. Barium studies may be necessary to demonstrate the presence of stomach or intestine in the chest cavity.

Ultrasound and Radionucleotide Imaging. Ultrasound and radionucleotide imaging may be of use, particularly in demonstrating the presence of liver through the diaphragmatic defect [30].

Management

Surgical repair of the hernia is advised without delay. Berman et al. [5] reported two previously asymptomatic children who died as a result of cardiorespiratory arrest, possibly due to mediastinal compression by herniated viscera. There is also the risk of volvulus or strangulation of the herniated viscera.

Strangulated Bochdalek Hernia

Strangulation of herniated viscera is a rare complication of Bochdalek herniae. The diagnosis should be apparent in the presence of bilious vomiting, radiological evidence of intestinal obstruction, together with a respiratory illness and chest X-ray signs of pneumonia, pleural effusion or the presence of air fluid levels [21]. Surgery is advised through a subcostal incision to permit complete evaluation of peritoneal contents. Reduction of the hernia may be difficult and it may be necessary to enlarge the diaphragmatic defect by a radial incision to allow safe reduction of the hernia. This technique should also allow preservation of the phrenic nerve.

Bilateral Bochdalek Herniae

Fortunately, this combination is extremely rare. There are 11 recorded cases in the literature [11] and in only 1 of these was the correct diagnosis made before operation or autopsy. Only three of the reported cases have survived. Usually, left-sided herniation is easily diagnosed on preoperative X-ray of the chest and abdomen, but detection of the right-sided hernia may be difficult because the right hemithorax is opacified with compression of the right lung associated with mediastinal shift towards the right side. As a routine, at operation for Bochdalek herniae, the contralateral diaphragm should be carefully examined to exclude a defect. This implies that repair is usually performed through a subcostal transabdominal approach. Bilateral absence of the diaphragms has been reported [47].

Rare Modes of Presentation

Bochdalek herniae may rarely present in the following ways:

- Hydrops foetalis and hydramnios associated with congenital diaphragmatic hernia [31]

- Intrathoracic torsion of the spleen [46]
- Gastric volvulus
- Failure to thrive [13]
- Incidental discovery of an intrathroacic kidney [10, 24]

Familial incidence of congenital diaphragmatic hernia is rare. The condition has been described in siblings [2, 45] and, extremely rarely, in identical twins [50].

Large Diaphragmatic (Bochdalek) Defects Including Agenesis

Most Bochdalek herniae consist of relatively small defects in the diaphragm which can be readily closed by primary suture repair. In some cases, the defect is a little larger and the posterior muscle leaf is relatively small, but significant tissue can be unravelled from the posterior chest wall to enable satisfactory suture repair to be made.

Occasionally, however, the diaphragmatic defect is very large, representing significant deficiency in the diaphragm, or there may be complete agenesis. Very rarely, bilateral agenesis occurs and Toran and Emery [47] reported such a case where only the muscular crura of the oesophageal hiatus were represented.

Closure of large diaphragmatic defects represents a technical challenge to the surgeon. This challenge is superimposed on the almost invariable presence of severe pulmonary hypoplasia and the latter problem may determine survival. Choice of the technique is guided by that procedure which can be performed quickly and safely in a critically ill infant. Numerous techniques to achieve closure of the defect have been reported, in both experimental series and the clinical situation, and range from the use of organs and tissues in the immediate vicinity of the defect to the use of soft tissue abdominal wall flaps or prosthetic materials.

Visceral Closure

Techniques which have been used include suturing of the liver to the edge of the defect [27], suturing of renal fascia [51] and suturing of stomach and other viscera to the margins of the defect. Such visceral closure is usually inadequate.

Muscle and Musculoskeletal flaps

The subcostal transabdominal incision is the favoured approach for repair of congenital diaphragmatic herniae. Via this incision, flaps from the anterior abdominal wall may be fashioned to close large defects.

Muscle Flaps

Such flaps consist of the transversus abdominis and the internal oblique muscle after separation from the external oblique muscle. This flap is swung posteriorly and sutured to the posterior muscle rim of the defect or to the rib cage directly [40].

Musculoskeletal Flaps

A flap consisting of intercostal muscles and ribs forming the costal margin on the side of the defect is separated from the overlying skin and subcutaneous tissues and is hinged posteriorly. The edge of this flap is sutured to the posterior edge of the defect or the rib cage posteriorly. Local flap closure has the advantage of adequately closing the defect with living adjacent tissue and the procedure can be performed effectively and quickly. Another option is closure with a pedicled abdominal muscle flap, but such a procedure involves more dissection and, accordingly, takes a longer time to complete [6, 39]. The musculoskeletal flap is recommended as a quick and effective means of closing large defects in critically ill patients. Its only disadvantage in the long term is possible chest wall deformity on the side of the repair and the spleen is no longer protected under the costal margin in left-sided repairs.

Prosthetic Closure

An increasing range of prosthetic materials has been used to close large defects, in both the clinical and experimental settings. Preserved dura and pericardial heterografts have been used to achieve secure closure of large diaphragmatic defects [17]. However, future use of such heterografts is uncertain because of possible transmission of slow virus infections. Prosthetic materials which have been used for repair include Marlex mesh, Silastic (Dacron-reinforced silicone elastomer) and Goretex[1] cardiovascular patch (polytetrafluorothylene) [12, 28].

In experimental studies, Newman et al. [28] compared the use of Goretex, Silastic and muscular flap closure of large defects in puppies. The Goretex prosthesis was associated with tissue incorporation and there was satisfactory function demonstrated on fluoroscopy in the early postoperative period. On the other hand, Silastic implants became encased in a fibrous capsule without evidence of adherence. Inflammation and calcification were also observed histologically in this group. The conclusion from this study is that Goretex is currently the favoured prosthetic material to use for closure of large diaphragmatic defects.

Eventration of the Diaphragm

The literature on this topic is confusing because different authors have defined the condition in different ways. Some have used the term to encompass both congenital and acquired (paralytic) disorders. However, the original definition of Beclard [3] should apply exclusively to congenital lesions and diaphragmatic palsy should be discussed as a separate entity.

Eventration is characterized by elevation of an attenuated, but otherwise intact, diaphragm and is the result of incomplete development of the muscular portion of the diaphragm. It is often difficult to distinguish eventration from a

[1] Goretex, trademark of W.L.Gore & Associates, Inc., North Elkton, MD 21921.

diaphragmatic hernia with a sac, since such sacs often have a few fibres of muscle between the serosal layers.

The difference is that, in addition to possessing three layers, an eventration as stated by Beclard [3] must possess a large base and involve the entire hemidiaphragm [9, 38]. If one portion of the hemidiaphragm is normal in location and muscle thickness, and another bulges into the chest, it is a hernia and not an eventration or partial eventration. Obviously, there will be difficulty in distinguishing between the two entities on occasions, and such distinction is often of academic interest only, as the important practical consideration is the need for intervention based on evaluation of clinical and radiological considerations. Eventration of the diaphragm may involve either the right or left diaphragm, or it may be bilateral. If eventration is severe, interference with lung development may be as severe as with a typical Bochdalek hernia.

Associated Congenital Anomalies

Eventration is often accompanied by other congenital anomalies such as abnormal pulmonary segmentation, congenital heart disease, cerebral agenesis and chromosomal anomalies. These various associated anomalies contribute significantly to morbidity and mortality of patients with eventration.

Clinical Features

Symptoms

The symptoms associated with eventration range from the patient being asymptomatic to severe respiratory compromise. The symptoms, which are predominantly respiratory and occasionally gastrointestinal, may develop at any age.

Respiratory Symptoms

Severe Respiratory Distress. The infant may develop severe respiratory distress in the newborn period if the eventration is severe. Large eventrations may seriously impair ventilation since the newborn infant depends primarily on diaphragmatic respiration.

Recurrent Respiratory Infections

Poor Exercise Tolerance

Gastrointestinal Symptoms

Left-sided diaphragmatic eventration, in particular, may be associated with gastrointestinal disturbance. Such symptoms include intermittent vomiting, postprandial pain and bloating and failure to thrive. Gastric volvulus has resulted in necrosis of the stomach.

Clinical Signs

Signs associated with an eventration include varying degrees of respiratory embarrassment, mediastinal shift to the opposite side and flaring of the costal margins.

Investigations

Chest and Abdominal X-ray
Eventration of the diaphragm is represented as smooth elevation of the hemidiaphragm, but the diaphragmatic outline may be obscure on plain radiology, making the distinction from a diaphragmatic hernia difficult. The diagnosis may be obscured in the infant who is on positive pressure ventilation, which displaces the diaphragm to the normal position. The diagnosis should be considered when it is difficult to wean a baby off the respirator.

Fluoroscopic Examination of the Diaphragm
Will Demonstrate Paradoxical Movement

Ultrasound Imaging of the Diaphragm
This modality can be used to demonstrate the attenuated, elevated diaphragm together with paradoxical movement. Other investigations which may be useful in elucidating the diagnosis include contrast peritoneography, pneumoperitoneum and radionucleotide scanning of the liver and spleen [32]. Also, ventilation and perfusion scans of the lungs may provide useful information concerning impaired lung function, as a guide to management of this condition.

Differential Diagnosis

1. Congenital diaphragmatic hernia
2. Paralysed diaphragm due to phrenic nerve palsy
3. Supradiaphragmatic mass lesion

Treatment

Eventration may not require surgical intervention if it is not intruding significantly into the thoracic cavity and is not associated with adverse symptoms. However, surgery is indicated in the following circumstances:

1. a) Respiratory distress which requires continuing ventilatory support
   b) Repeated pulmonary infections
   c) Respiratory compromise associated with feeding difficulty and failure to thrive
2. Large eventration: The displaced diaphragm can potentially interfere with lung function and postnatal development, and on these grounds surgical intervention may be warranted.

Surgery

The procedure performed is plication of the diaphragm with careful preservation of the phrenic nerve. Phrenic nerve preservation is best achieved via a thoracotomy when it is possible readily to identify the point of entrance of the nerve into the diaphragm and directly trace its main branches in their peripheral course. However, the abdominal (subcostal) approach is recommended in bilateral cases or where predominant symptoms are related to the gastrointestinal tract. This enables the abdominal viscera to be directly assessed. Plication is achieved by means of a row of non-absorbable sutures, placed parallel to the branches of the phrenic nerve. Alternatively, a radial or peripheral incision may be made in the diaphragm and the edges overlapped and sutured with non-absorbable suture material.

Bilateral Eventration of the Diaphragms

This entity is relatively rare and in the past has been associated with almost uniform mortality. Rodgers and Hawks [38] reviewed the English literature and reported a total of 28 patients with bilateral eventration. Their review disclosed that this combination is associated with an extremely high mortality rate. However, they reported a personal series of three patients who underwent successful treatment of this anomaly with bilateral plication of the diaphragm. Bilateral eventration always produces significant respiratory embarrassment. These infants exhibit similar pathophysiological responses to infants with congenital diaphragmatic herniae and associated pulmonary hypoplasia.

Treatment

The aim of treatment is early surgery provided there is no potentially lethal associated congenital anomaly. Early bilateral repair via transabdominal subcostal incisions allows ready access to both diaphragms and satisfactory plications.

Morgagni (Retrosternal) Diaphragmatic Hernia

Introduction

This anomaly was first described by Morgagni [25] in 1761. Morgagni was Professor of Anatomy at Padua University. He reviewed congenital diaphragmatic herniae to that date, and described the defect that bears his name. He discovered the hernia as an incidental finding at autopsy in an adult.

Incidence

Morgagni herniae constitute between 2% and 4% of large series of congenital diaphragmatic herniae [1].

Anatomy

Morgagni defects occur at the junction of the septum transversum, anterior chest wall and the lateral component of the diaphragm. The failure of fusion between the central and lateral portions of the diaphragm leaves a gap immediately behind the xiphoid process. The hernia occurs as a midline defect, although some authors have described a hernial defect on either the right or the left side of the midline, or bilaterally. A peritoneal sac is nearly always present. Rarely, there is direct communication with the pericardium [9, 18, 34].

Contents of the Hernia

The most common contents include colon and omentum. Less commonly liver, small intestine, stomach and spleen are encountered in the sac.

Associated Anomalies

Morgagni herniae diagnosed in childhood are commonly associated with other congenital anomalies [34]. Such anomalies include congenital heart disease, genitourinary anomalies, exomphalos and trisomy 21. Also there is a definite association with mental retardation. The anomaly may be seen as part of Cantrell's pentalogy [8, 42, 48]. Morgagni herniae are usually asymptomatic and discovered incidentally on routine chest X-ray. A small number of patients present in infancy with respiratory distress similar to that seen in Bochdalek herniae at a similar age [34]. Complications of Morgagni herniae are uncommon. In particular, bowel obstruction and strangulation are rarely reported in the literature, although such complications are commonly stated indications to justify elective repair of the Morgagni defect [19]. Except for evidence of respiratory compromise in the child presenting in infancy, or rarely gastrointestinal symptoms and signs associated with obstruction, physical examination contributes little to the diagnosis in this condition.

Investigations

Chest X-ray

The presence of intestinal loops above the diaphragm, immediately behind the xiphisternum, confirms the diagnosis of this condition. However, if the viscus above the diaphragm is solid, a Morgagni hernia is difficult to distinguish from an anterior mediastinal mass or lung pathology.

Contrast Studies of the Gastrointestinal Tract

Contrast studies will confirm the presence of intestinal content in the Morgagni hernia.

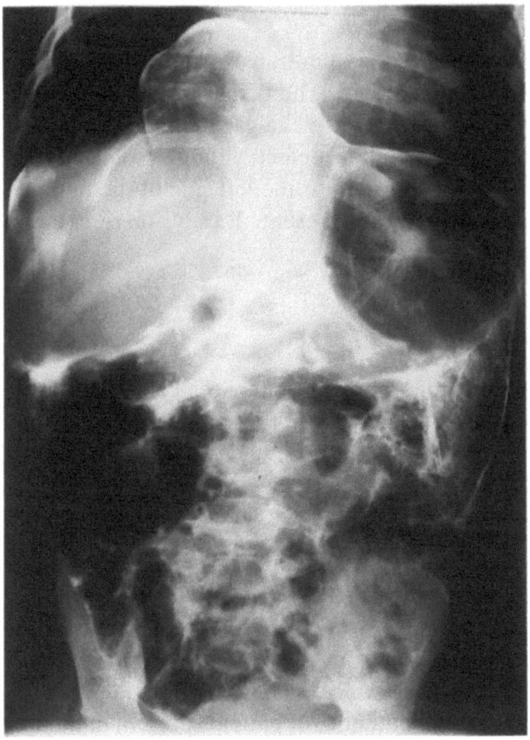

Fig. 3. Contrast peritoneography can be usefully employed to demonstrate a Morgagni hernia and distinguish it from other mediastinal masses

Ultrasound

Radionucleotide Liver Spleen Scan

Ultrasound and liver spleen scan may be helpful in demonstrating the presence of liver in the hernia.

Contrast Peritoneography and Pneumoperitoneography

Contrast peritoneography and pneumoperitoneography have been used to help demonstrate the anatomy of Morgagni hernias (Fig. 3).

Surgical Treatment

Very satisfactory exposure of such herniae is achieved through an upper midline abdominal incision. The sac is excised and the edge of the defect is sutured to the costal margin and the xiphoid process. The abdominal approach also allows satisfactory repair of the unusual bilateral herniae. The only serious reported complication following repair is pneumopericardium in several instances [19]. This complication is almost always fatal. If the pericardium is entered during dissection of the sac, it should be drained to an underwater seal.

Central (Septum Transversum) Diaphragmatic Hernia

This hernia is usually associated with a large atypical central opening in the area of the diaphragm formed by the septum transversum. Such herniae account for 1%–2% of all congenital diaphragmatic defects [52].

Associated Congenital Anomalies

Associated anomalies are common and include defects of the anterior abdominal wall, pericardium and sternum and may be associated with the complete pentalogy of Cantrell [52]. Gastrointestinal anomalies such as malrotation may also occur.

Clinical Features

Central herniae usually present in early infancy with varying degrees of respiratory distress.

Investigations

Plain-X-Ray of Chest and Abdomen

The hernia may present as an apparently solid right-sided paracardiac mass. Alternately, multiple central mediastinal air-filled loops of bowel will be apparent.

Contrast Studies

Contrast Studies of the gastrointestinal tract will identify intestinal contents in the hernia.

Pneumoperitoneography or Contrast Peritoneography

Pneumoperitoneography or contrast peritoneography may be useful in delineating the diaphragmatic defect, particularly in association with a paracardiac mass.

Radionucleotide Scan

Radionucleotide scan may readily demonstrate a portion of the liver wedged into a central diaphragmatic defect.

Treatment

Thorough investigation is recommended with this type of defect to exclude significant associated anomalies such as congenital cardiac anomalies. The presence of an exomphalos may influence the plan of management. Usually the diaphragmatic defect will demand priority and the exomphalos can be treated on its merit, with attention to avoiding further respiratory compromise.

The transabdominal approach for repair is recommended. Wesselhoeft and De Luca [52] reported a series of eight patients with central diaphragmatic herniae, six of whom are alive and well 6 months to 10 years following surgery. One of the deaths occurred in an infant with pentalogy of Cantrell after attempted mesh prosthesis closure of the exomphalos. The diaphragmatic defect could not be closed because of severe cardiac irregularities.

Para-Oesophageal Hiatus Hernia

This type of hernia is rare in childhood.

Anatomy

In contrast to the more common sliding hiatus hernia, the oesophagogastric junction is usually situated beneath the diaphragm. There is a peritoneal sac extending through the hiatus alongside the lower oesophagus and the greater curvature of the stomach extends up into the sac in the chest.

Clinical Features

Regurgitation of food is the usual presenting symptom and is usually due to obstruction of the distal oesophagus related to compression by the herniated stomach. Severe vomiting may herald the development of volvulus and strangulation of the herniated stomach.

Diagnosis

Chest X-ray

The diagnosis is usually suggested by the presence of an air fluid level in the lower chest, frequently just to the right of the cardiac shadow (Fig. 4).

Barium Meal

Contrast studies of the upper gastrointestinal tract confirm the diagnosis and accurately demonstrate the anatomy of the hernia, with the gastro-oesophageal junction usually situated below the diaphragm (Fig. 5).

Treatment

Surgical repair is indicated when the diagnosis is made because of the potential complication of strangulation of the stomach in the hernia. The left subcostal

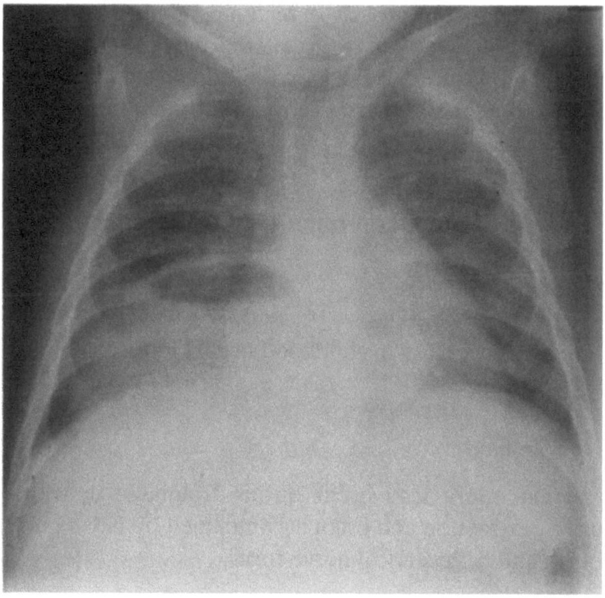

Fig. 4. Plain chest X-ray demonstrates a single large air fluid level to the right of the cardiac shadow, due to the presence of a large para-oesophageal diaphragmatic hernia

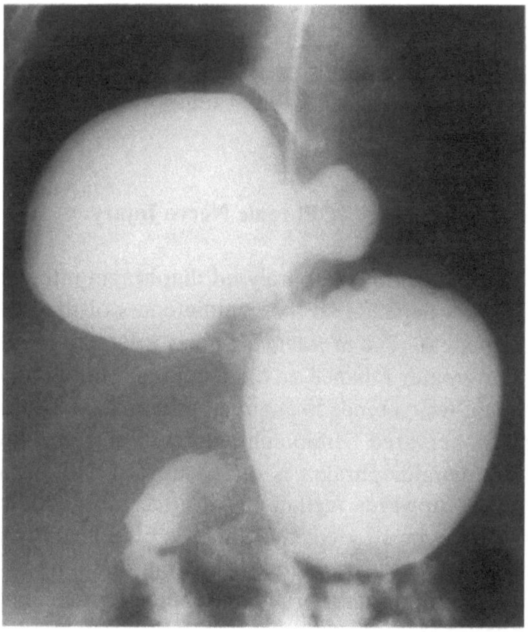

Fig. 5. Contrast study confirms the air fluid level in the chest to be a loculus of stomach in the chest, alongside the lower oesophagus

transabdominal approach is recommended. The hernia is reduced and the sac resected, followed by repair of the oesophageal hiatus with interrupted, non-absorbable sutures. If the gastro-oesophageal junction is normally situated below the diaphragm and there is normal intra-abdominal oesophageal length, there is no indication for adding a fundoplication to the procedure.

Paralysis of the Diaphragm Due to Phrenic Nerve Palsy

Aetiology

Phrenic nerve palsy in childhood occurs most commonly in infancy due to several possible causes.

Birth Trauma

Traction injury may occur during traumatic delivery, usually associated with breech extraction and often accompanied by Erb's palsy, with injury to the third, fourth and fifth cervical nerve roots.

Trauma

Surgical Trauma. Direct injury to the nerve may occur during operations on the heart or mediastinal structures [49].

Insertion of Intercostal Drain Tubes. This entity has been described in infants suffering from respiratory distress syndrome, complicated by development of a tension pneumothorax. Diaphragmatic paralysis becomes apparent after insertion of the drain tube and is presumably due to direct trauma from the tube. The paralysis in this instance is often temporary so that surgical intervention may not be necessary [9, 33].

Pathophysiology of Phrenic Nerve Injury

Whether or not the paralysed diaphragm interferes significantly with respiratory function depends on the completeness of the phrenic nerve palsy and the age of the patient. The problem is poorly tolerated in infants and young children, due to their greater reliance on the diaphragm for ventilation and a more mobile mediastinum, which tends to augment paradoxical diaphragmatic movement. As the normal innervated hemidiaphragm contracts and lowers with inspiration, the paralysed hemidiaphragm is drawn upwards by negative intrathoracic pressure and pushed upwards further by positive intra-abdominal pressure. The mediastinal shift may be so great that there is little air movement in and out of the trachea. Most airflow is back and forth from one lung to the other. In older patients the mediastinum is more rigid and there is much less tendency for the mediastinum to shift.

Modes of Presentation

1. Respiratory distress
2. Recurrent pneumonia
3. Difficulty weaning from the ventilator

Investigations

1. Elevation of the affected diaphragm is demonstrated on plain chest X-ray.
2. Fluoroscopy demonstrates paradoxical movement of the paralysed diaphragm.
3. Ultrasound may be used to demonstrate paradoxical diaphragmatic movement. As mentioned with eventration of the diaphragm, the diagnosis may be obscured in diaphragmatic paralysis when the patient is requiring ventilator support which maintains the diaphragm in the normal position.

Differential Diagnosis

Congenital Eventration of the Diaphragm. A careful history will usually provide the clue to distinguishing this entity and acquired nerve palsy.

Congenital Diaphragmatic Hernia (Bochdalek), with a Sac. This entity can usually be distinguished on fluoroscopy where there is no movement of the herniated contents in the chest.

A Mass Lesion in the Chest

Treatment

Eighty per cent of patients with phrenic nerve injury will recover function spontaneously [49]. Those who do not recover and remain symptomatic are candidates for plication of the diaphragm.

In experimental animals plication has been shown significantly to improve respiratory mechanics after phrenic nerve division [22]. These results are also mirrored in the clinical setting where plication has been demonstrated to lead to a marked improvement in ventilatory function as evidenced by dramatic reduction in duration of intubation and the need for ventilation [20].

Although the selective use of plication has been accepted for phrenic nerve palsy, the actual decision to intervene surgically and the appropriate timing for such intervention is often difficult. Langer et al. [20] in a review of this topic recommend an arbitrary period of 3 weeks non-operative management, recognizing that spontaneous recovery is common within the first 2–3 weeks following the injury. A supportive period of longer duration, such as 4–6 weeks, might be appropriate for particular situations such as phrenic nerve palsy associated with intercostal drain tube insertion. This condition has a very high chance of spontaneous recovery within this period.

It should be noted that patients with phrenic nerve palsy who do not improve considerably when on positive pressure ventilation are likely to have significant parenchymal lung disease together with possible cardiac disease and are unlikely to have a good result following plication.

Surgical Technique

A thoracic approach is recommended so that the phrenic nerve can be readily identified and its branches preserved. The technique by which plication is achieved has been described for repair of diaphragmatic eventration.

Results of Diaphragmatic Plication

Langer et al. [20] reviewed 23 cases of plication over a 10-year period. They achieved a very good response in 20 of the 23 patients. Thirteen of the 16 patients who underwent operation because of inability to wean off the ventilator were weaned after an average duration of 2 days postoperatively. All four patients with recurrent pneumonia and all three patients with respiratory distress were extubated on the average 2 days postoperatively. The three patients in the ventilator-dependent group who did not respond as rapidly to plication had persistent congestive heart failure. However, one of these patients was extubated 9 days after plication and was well subsequently.

Stone et al. [44] reported a small long-term review of patients following plication for phrenic nerve palsy. They reported return of diaphragmatic function in six patients reviewed for varying periods ranging from 1 to 7 years postoperatively.

Traumatic Diaphragmatic Hernia

This injury is seen uncommonly in children and is usually the result of severe compressive injury to the abdomen and chest. This is usually the result of a motor vehicle accident, either as passenger or pedestrian. Attention to other injuries such as head injuries, pneumothorax or fractures may lead to the diaphragmatic hernia being overlooked. Suspicion of the injury may be obscured by the presence of other pathology such as a haemopneumothorax. The injury may occur on either side.

Clinical Features [26]

Acute Symptoms

The symptoms associated with this injury are usually non-specific and include respiratory distress, chest pain and abdominal pain.

Vague, Persisting Symptoms Related to the Chest and Abdomen

Delayed Presentation

Previously unrecognized cases may present later with acute symptoms associated with a complication of the hernia such as strangulation of its herniated content.

Investigations

Chest X-Ray

The diagnosis of this condition is suggested by one or more of the following radiological signs:

1. Elevation of the diaphragm or loss of all or part of its contour. Herniation of the stomach may be readily demonstrated by passage of a nasogastric tube into the herniated viscus.
2. Presence of a gas-containing or solic viscus above the diaphragm.
3. Shift of the mediastinum.

Contrast Study of the Gastrointestinal Tract
Contrast may delineate the presence of stomach or intestine in the chest.

Ultrasound

Ultrasound studies together with a liver-spleen radionucleotide scan may helpful in demonstrating herniation of a solid viscus into the chest.

Associated Injuries

As previously mentioned, the diaphragmatic injury is usually just one of numerous injuries. These include pulmonary contusion which is often associated with rib fractures and haemopneumothorax. There may also be associated injuries to the liver and spleen. Fractures of long bones are common. Contents of traumatic diaphragmatic hernias include stomach, colon and small intestine together with the spleen on the left side. Contents in right-sided herniae include the liver and colon.

Treatment

The danger of strangulation is always present in association with traumatic diaphragmatic herniae and repair should not be delayed once the diagnosis is established. Surgical repair is recommended via a subcostal abdominal approach on the side of the defect and this provides adequate exposure and access for repairing the damaged diaphragm as well as recognition and appropriate treatment of accompanying intra-abdominal injuries. Repair is achieved with interrupted non-absorbable suture material.

References

1. Anderson KD (1986) Congenital diaphragmatic hernia. In: Welch KJ et al (eds) Pediatric surgery, 4th edn, vol 1. Yearbook Medical, Chicago, pp 589–601
2. Arai T, Hirai J, Kitahara J, et al (1976) Congenital diaphragmatic hernia in two successive siblings. Jpn J Soc Pediatr Surg 12:571–578
3. Beclard E (1829) Cited by J Cruveilhier. In: Atlas d'Anatomie Pathologique, vol 1, Book 17, Plate V. Paris, p 2
4. Benjamin DR, Juul S, Siebert JR (1988) Congenital posterolateral diaphragmatic hernia, associated malformations. J Pediatr Surg 23:899–903
5. Berman L, Stringer D, Ein S, et al (1988) The late presenting pediatric Bochdalek hernia, a 20 year review. J Pediatr Surg 23:735–739
6. Bianchi A, Doig CM, Cohen SJ (1983) The reverse lattissimus dorsi flap for congenital diaphragmatic hernia repair. J Pediatr Surg 18:560–563
7. Campbell DN, Lilly JR (1982) The clinical spectrum of right Bochdalek hernia. Arch Surg 117:341–344
8. Cantrell JV, Haller JA, Ravitch MM (1958) A syndrome of congenital defects involving the abdominal wall, sternum, diaphragm, pericardium and the heart. Surg Gynecol Obstet 107: 602–614
9. Collins DL (1980) Diaphragmatic hernia. In: Holder TM, Ashcraft KK (eds) Pediatric surgery. Saunders, Philadelphia, pp 227–239
10. De Castro FY, Schumaker H (1969) Asymptomatic thoracic kidney. Clin Pediatr 8:279
11. Furuta Y, Makamura Y, Miyamoto K (1987) Bilateral congenital posterolateral diaphragmatic hernia. J Pediatr Surg 22:182–183
12. Geisler F, Gotlieb A, Fried D (1977) Agenesis of the right diaphragm repaired with Marlex. J Pediatr Surg 12:587–588
13. Golladay ES, Katz JR, Katz H, et al (1981) Delayed presentation of congenital posterolateral diaphragmatic hernia, a dramatic cause of failure to thrive. J Pediatr Surg 16:503–505
14. Gonzales R, Heiss W (1984) Bilateral diaphragmatic hernia. Z Kinderchir 39:339–340
15. Gray SW, Skandalakis JE (1972) Embryology for Surgeons. Saunders, Philadelphia, pp 359–374
16. Holder TM, Ashcraft KW (1979) Congenital diaphragmatic hernia. In: Ravitch MM et al (eds) Pediatric surgery, vol 1. Yearbook Medical, Chicago, pp 432–445
17. Hutson JM, Azmy AF (1985) Preserved dura and pericardium for closure of large abdominal wall and diaphragmatic defects in children. Ann R Coll Surg Engl 67:107–108
18. Janneck C, Ekersparre WV, Wesener G (1983) Congenital intrapericardial diaphragmatic hernia: a case report. Z Kinderchir 38:31–33
19. Kimmelestiel FM, Holgersen LO, Hilfer C (1987) Retrosternal (Morgagni) hernia with small bowel obstruction secondary to a Richter's incarceration. J Pediatr Surg 22:998–1000
20. Langer JC, Filler RM, Coles J, et al (1988) Plication of the diaphragm for infants and young children with phrenic nerve palsy. J Pediatr Surg 23:749–751
21. Lynch JM, Adkins JC, Wiener ES (1982) Incarcerated congenital diaphragmatic hernias with bowel obstruction (Bochdalek). J Pediatr Surg 17:537–540
22. Marcos JJ, Grover FL, Trinkle JK (1974) Paralysed diaphragm – effect of plication on respiratory mechanics. J Surg Res 16:523–526
23. McCollum C, Anyanwu CH, Umeh BUC, et al (1987) Management of traumatic rupture of the diaphragm. Br J surg 74:181–183
24. Moazzenadea AR, Khodadadian R, Potter RT (1977) The intrathoracic kidney. J Thorac Cardiovasc Surg 73:480–482
25. Morgagni GB (1769) Seats and causes of diseases. Translated by B Alexander. A Millar A and T Cadell, London, p 205
26. Myers NA (1964) Traumatic rupture of the diaphragm in children. Aust NZJ Surg 34:123–127
27. Neville WE, Glowes GH (1954) Congenital absence of hemidiaphragm and use of a lobe of liver in its surgical correction. Arch Surg 69:282–290

28. Newman BM, Jewett TC, Lewis A, et al (1985) Prosthetic materials and muscle flaps in the repair of extensive diaphragmatic defects, an experimental study. J Pediatr Surg 20:362–367
29. Newman BM, Afshani E, Kapp MP, et al (1986) Presentation of congenital diaphragmatic hernia past the neonatal period. Arch Surg 121:813–816
30. Nussbaum AR, Ben Ami T, Treves S, et al (1987) Diagnosis of delayed onset right sided congenital diaphragmatic hernia using ultrasonic and radionuclide imaging. Pediatr Surg Int 2: 149–156
31. Omenaca F, Quero J (1976) Right diaphragmatric hernia with fetal ascites. J Pediatr Surg 11:97–98
32. Otherson HB, Lorenzo RL (1977) Diaphragmatic paralysis and eventration, newer approaches to diagnosis and operative correction. J Pediatr Surg 12:309–315
33. Philipps AF, Rowe JC, Raye JR (1981) Acute diaphragmatic paralysis after chest tube placement in a neonate. Am J Radiol 136:824–825
34. Pokorny WJ, McGill CW, Harberg FJ (1984) Morgagni hernias during infancy, presentation and associated anomalies. J Pediatr Surg 19:394–397
35. Puri P, Gorman W (1987) Natural history of congenital diaphragmatic hernia, implications for management. Pediatr Surg Int 2:327–330
36. Ramenofsky ML, Luck SR (1980) Diaphragmatic anomalies. In: Raffensperger JG (ed) Swenson's paediatric surgery. Appleton Century Crofts, New York, pp 675–690
37. Refsum JS, Nordshus T (1981) Late presentation of left sided congenital diaphragmatic (Bochdalek) hernia. Z Kinderchir 34:279–283
38. Rodgers BM, Hawks P (1986) Bilateral congenital eventration of the diaphragms, successful surgical management. J Pediatr Surg 21:858–864
39. Rosenkrantz JG, Cotton EK (1964) Replacement of left hemidiaphragm by a pedicled abdominal muscular flap. J Thorac Cardiovasc Surg 48:912–920
40. Simpson JS, Gossage JD (1971) Use of abdominal wall muscle flap in repair of large congenital diaphragmatic hernia. J Pediatr Surg 6:42–44
41. Schoemaker R, Palmer G, Brown JW, et al (1981) Aggressive treatment of acquired phrenic nerve paralysis in infants and small children. Ann Thorac Surg 32:251–259
42. Spitz L, Bloom KR, Milner S, et al (1975) Combined anterior abdominal wall, sternal, diaphragmatic, pericardial and intracardiac defects. A report of 5 cases and their management. J Pediatr Surg 10:491–496
43. Stahl GE, Warren WS, Rosenberg H, et al (1981) Congenital right diaphragmatic hernia, a case report and review of the literature. Clin Paediatr 20:422–425
44. Stone K, Brown JW, Canal MD, et al (1987) Longterm fate of the diaphragm surgically plicated during infancy and childhood. Ann Thorac Surg 44:62–65
45. Thomas MP, Stern LM, Morris LL (1976) Bilateral congenital diaphragmatic defects in two siblings. J Pediatr Surg 11:465–467
46. Thorup J, Pederson P, Nielsen O (1986) Late return of function after intrathoracic torsion of the spleen in congenital diaphragmatic hernia. J Pediatr Surg 21:722–724
47. Toran N, Emery JL (1981) Congenital bilateral absence of the diaphragm. Thorax 36:157–158
48. Toyama WM (1972) Combined congenital defects of the anterior abdominal wall, sternum, diaphragm, pericardium and heart, a case report and review of the syndrome. Paediatrics 50: 778–792
49. Watanabe T, Trusler GA, Williams WG, et al (1987) Phrenic nerve paralysis after pediatric cardiac surgery: retrospective study of 125 cases. J Thorac Cardiovasc Surg 94:383–388
50. Watanatittan S (1983) Congenital diaphragmatic hernia in identical twins. J Pediatr Surg 18:628
51. Weinberg J (1938) Diaphragmatic hernia in infants: surgical treatment with use of renal fascia. Surgery 3:78–86
52. Wesselhoeft CW, De Luca FG (1984) Neonatal septum transversum diaphragmatic defects. Am J Surg 147:481–485
53. Woolley MM (1977) Delayed appearance of a left posterolateral diaphragmatic hernia resulting in significant small bowel necrosis. J Pediatr Surg 12:673–674

Current Status of Cardiac Surgery in Childhood

R. B. B. Mee

Summary

In the 50 years since Gross (1938) obliterated a patent ductus arteriosus, congenital cardiac surgery has come of age, synchronized with the world explosion in microtechnology and space age materials. The late 1960s and early 1970s saw Barratt-Boyes pioneering complete intracardiac repairs on infants with congenital heart disease employing modifications of the Kyoto technique (Shirotani) for profound hypothermia and circulatory arrest. The past 10–15 years have been marked by the more widespread dissemination of increasingly safe techniques, and the application of progressive incremental refinement to the entire management package of complex congenital heart disease. Many innovative methods and concepts have been added to the therapeutic armamentarium of the congenital heart team. Currently, transplantation adds the prospect of "second chance", and in the future may constitute preferred primary management in certain complex forms of congenital heart disease. In the Western world the concept of "frequency sensitivity" and the value of rationalizing congenital heart surgery facilities, such that a single unit manages a population of 8–12 million, is established, though not necessarily widely accepted and acted upon.

High-volume, low-risk units emerge such that operative mortality, despite the high acceptance rate of complex problems and high rates of neonatal and infant complex repairs, has dropped below 5%. Paradoxically, the so-called simple closed surgery (neonatal coarctation, shunts and other palliative procedures in complex congenital heart disease) retain relatively high risk and must be regarded as one of the areas of challenge over the next 5–10 years.

Zusammenfassung

Seit dem ersten operativen Verschluß eines persistierenden Ductus Botalli durch Gross (1938) ist in den letzten 50 Jahren die Chirurgie angeborener Herzfehler aus den Kinderschuhen herausgewachsen, parallel zur explosiven Entwicklung der Mikroelektronik und neuer Materialien in der Raumfahrttechnik. Die späten 60er und frühen 70er Jahre sahen die Pioniertaten von Barratt-Boys, der zur intrakardialen Korrektur bei Kindern mit angeborenen Herzfehlern Modifikationen der Kyoto-Technik (Shirotani) der profunden Hypothermie und des Herzstillstandes einsetzte. Die letzten 10–15 Jahre waren gekennzeichnet durch eine breit gefächerte Weiterverbreitung von immer sicherer werdenden Methoden und einer zunehmenden Verfeinerung des gesamten Managements komplexer angeborener Herzfehler. Viele innovative Techniken und Konzepte kamen zum Instrumentarium der Behandlungsteams hinzu. Gegenwärtig verbessert die Herztransplantation die Aussichten auf eine „zweite Chance" und mag in der Zukunft das derzeit noch favorisierte primäre Management bei manchen komplexen angeborenen Herzfehlern ersetzen. Zur Zeit wird in der westlichen Welt das Konzept der Konzentration auf einzelne, rationalisierte Operationszentren für angeborene Herzfehler realisiert, so daß ein einzelnes Zentrum

Director Victorian Paediatric Cardiac Surgical Unit, Royal Children's Hospital Melbourne, Flemington Road, Parkville 3052, Victoria, Australia.

Progress in Pediatric Surgery, Vol. 27
Myers and Angerpointner (Eds.)

eine Population von 8–12 Mio. Einwohnern versorgt, wenngleich dieses Konzept nicht notwendigerweise allgemein anerkannt oder umgesetzt werden muß.

Demgemäß entstehen Zentren mit hoher Kapazität und niedriger Risikostufe, so daß die operative Letalität trotz gehäuft vorkommender komplexer Probleme und hoher Operationsfrequenzen komplizierter Herzfehler bei Neugeborenen und Säuglingen unter 5% gefallen ist. Paradoxerweise bleibt bei sogenannten einfachen, geschlossenen Operationen (Aortenisthmusstenose, Shunts und andere palliative Methoden bei komplizierten Herzfehlern) ein relativ hohes Risiko bestehen, was als eine der Herausforderungen während der nächsten 5–10 Jahre angesehen werden muß.

Résumé

Durant les 50 années qui suivirent l'intervention de Gross (1938) l'oblitération du canal artériel, la chirurgie des affections cardiaques congénitales a eu le temps d'arriver à maturité avec l'aide des progrès fulgurants en microtechnologie dans le monde entier et des matériaux inventés pour la conquête spatiale. A la fin des années 60 et au début des années 70, Barrat Boyes commença à effectuer des corrections intracardiaques complètes sur des enfants présentant des malformations du coeur. Pour ce faire, il modifia la technique de Kyoto (Shirotani) pour assurer une hypothermie profonde et un arrêt de la circulation. Durant les 10 on 15 dernières années, les techniques sont devenues de plus en plus courantes, fiables et d'une subtilité toujours plus poussée offrant dès lors tout un éventail pour le traitement des affections cardiaques congénitales. A l'heure actuelle, la transplantation a ajouté la conception d'une "seconde chance" et il se pourrait qu'à l'avenir elle constitue le traitement primaire de choix pour certaines formes d'affections cardiaques congénitales complexes. Dans le monde occidental, on a reconnu l'importance d'une organisation rationelle des centres de chirurgie cardiaque et une seule unité peut maintenant répondre aux besoins d'une population de 8–12 millions, en dépit des réticences qui peuvent encore exister dans ce domaine.

Ces unités, équipées pour traiter un grand nombre de patients en réduisant les risques à un minimum malgré la complexité des problèmes qui se posent et le nombre élevé d'interventions à pratiquer sur les nouveaux-nés et les petits enfants, sont parvenues à faire baisser la mortalité en dessous de 5%. Paradoxalement, on constate que la chirugie dite simple, à coeur fermé (coarctation chez les nouveaux-nés, dérivation et autres techniques palliatives pour traiter les affections cardiaques congénitales complexes), est toujours relativement à haut risque et c'est dans ce domaine que des progrès se doivent d'être faits dans les 5 à 10 années à venir.

Introduction

The importance of cardiac surgery in childhood is epitomized by the fact that in approximately 1% of all live births congenital heart disease is present. With the improved resolution available today, ultrasonographic evaluation of the fetus frequently results in the diagnosis being made before birth. Fifty years have elapsed since the modern era of cardiac surgery was ushered in by Robert Gross [1], who was the first surgeon to obliterate blood flow through a patent ductus arteriosus. Extracardiac operations have continued to play an important role in the management of aortic arch anomalies and in enabling appropriate shunts to be constructed in selected cases of cyanotic congenital heart disease, but as time has passed a wide variety of intracardiac procedures have been devised permitting correction of lesions previously regarded as inoperable. Thus in the 50 years from 1938 to 1988 paediatric cardiac surgery has come of age and this is therefore an opportune time to review its current status. To do this some general observations will be made followed by discussion of individual lesions. Both the general observations and the comments regarding the various forms of congenital cardiac anomalies are based upon the experience at the Royal Children's Hospital, Melbourne. A particular feature of the cardiac surgery unit at this institution is that it can be defined as a low-risk centre and apart from other factors it has become possible to undertake complex repair procedures in the neonatal or early infant age groups. During the past 11 years more than 5500 operations have been performed for babies, infants and children with congenital cardiac anomalies.

General Observations

Congenital heart disease is present in approximately 1% of all live births and of these between 10% and 95% will eventually undergo surgery after referral depending on the nature of the referral centre. In most forms of congenital heart disease, morbidity and mortality accrue as a function of time, the rate of accrual being, in turn, a function of the actual cardiac abnormality.

Untreated, 90% of all patients with transposition of the great vessels are dead within 1 year [2]. On the other hand, untreated secundum atrial septal defect (ASD) is associated with a life expectancy of about 55 years [3], with slowly progressive pulmonary vascular obstructive disease, cardiac dilatation and arrhythmias.

Provided repair can be achieved safely early in life, there is a powerful incentive to do so as early as possible. Multiple incremental improvements in the entire management programme for congenital heart disease, have, over the relatively short history of cardiac surgery, resulted in progressively better results. This is particularly true in major congenital heart centres exposed to large numbers of referrals, such that currently published literature [4] refers openly to "high-risk" and "low-risk" centres. It is no real surprise that there is an inverse relationship in the western world between management risk in congenital heart surgery and in the actual number of cases handled by an institution. Best results are documented from institutions with the highest clinical work load for each member of the management team, making this a highly "frequency sensitive" field of medicine. In the low-risk major institutions a common feature which has evolved is complex repair in the neonatal or early infant age group, especially where there is support from broad-based expertise in "small body technology".

An earlier concept in the surgical management of congenital heart disease was "wait until the patient is larger". The reason at the time was clear. There were significant difficulties in management of small babies, and open heart surgery on babies under the age of 1 month carried a mortality of 60%–70% even in the best hands. Much of this risk was attributed to the insult of cardiopulmonary bypass alone, but in retrospect it was also clear that accurate fast surgical repair was hampered by poor lighting, lack of magnification, inferior suture materials and clumsy operating tools. In addition preoperative invasive diagnosis created its

Table 1. Complications of delaying repair

1. Pulmonary vascular obstructive disease
2. Progressive myocardial hypertrophy (stenotic lesions)
a) Increased operative risk
b) Arrythmias
3. Progressive myocardial damage (volume loading)
a) Left to right shunts
b) Regurgitant valvular lesions
4. Progressive mechanical damage
a) Jet lesions
b) Endocarditis
c) Fibrosis
5. Recurrent lung infections
6. Cumulative effects of venous mixing (arterial desaturation)
a) Acceleration of pulmonary vascular disease
b) Polycythaemia, thrombosis and embolism
c) Brain abscess

own problems and postoperative care was imprecise and poorly conceptualized. Survival after neonatal or infant surgery was often marred by recurrent lesions due to uneven growth, at a time when reoperation was deemed just too difficult.

On the other hand, deferring repair until a late date incurred the risk of permanent damage from complications of the original lesion, making long-term survival or quality of life disappointing (Table 1).

The era of exaltation from achieving survival after a difficult operation has given way to management planning aimed at the best possible chance of early survival, late survival and maximizing the chances of quality survival for each particular lesion or combination of lesions. Much credit for such refinement must be attributed to the analytical statistical approach promulgated by the University of Birmingham, Alabama (Kirklin, Blackstone). The congenital heart disease management team must lift its sights beyond responsibility for survival to the end of the paediatric age (14–15 years), to adulthood. This alone is a good argument for congenital heart disease management to be considered as a continuing contract throughout the patient's life, and not to consider it as a disease that somehow alters in terms of expertise and support needs at the age of 15 years.

Of great importance in the overall management of congenital heart disease is correct timing of initial surgical intervention, good follow-up data and reintervention for any residual or recurrent lesion before irreversible complications occur. Sound management planning for each patient clearly requires an early comprehensive and accurate diagnosis with simultaneous assessment of other major organ systems. In a community well endowed with obstetricians and paediatricians, early referral for comprehensive assessment becomes the cornerstone for optimalizing overall management. Subsequently, a close and understanding liaison between the referral centre and paediatricians and general practitioners allows for timely patient return for further assessments and interventions.

As more children with "repaired" complex congenital heart disease graduate from the paediatric age group, there is a growing need for a well-designed follow-up clinic, again monitoring progressive residual defects (valve stenosis or incompetence, conduit failure, baffle obstruction or arrhythmias), connected back to a centre where further intervention in these often high-risk difficult patients can be achieved with maximum safety. In short, an initial major investment in resources, time and effort should remain well protected and supervised throughout. For this reason, in our paediatric hospital, dispensation is given to treat overage patients with complex congenital cardiac anomalies.

Two-dimensional echo with Doppler and colour flow mapping often provides adequate data for management decision making, particularly in the neonatal group. In our institution 95% of neonates proceed to surgery on the basis of ultrasound diagnosis.

Recent Advances

Recent advances that have contributed to improved results are many and include:

1. An increased level of awareness amongst obstetricians, paediatricians and general practitioners of the early signs of congenital heart disease and the need for early referral.

2. Accepting the concept of the fetus as a patient.

3. Two-dimensional ultrasound aided by Doppler and colour flow mapping permit early, accurate and usually comprehensive diagnosis both outside and within the referral centre. Cardiac catheterization, which is a significantly greater insult to a severely ill infant, can then be limited to certain cases and confined in its scope to elicit only one or two items of critical information not available from non-invasive studies. An increasingly close liaison between surgeons and cardiologists ensures pursuit of relevant diagnostic information.

4. Intravenous prostaglandin E_1 (PGE_1) infusion or oral PGE_2 is now available more widely, can be given early at point of presentation to reopen the ductus arteriosus, and allows transport of the neonate to the referral centre in a much improved condition. Rapid deterioration of the neonate soon after birth is almost always due to duct closure threatening a duct-dependent pulmonary or systemic circulation.

5. Transport of profoundly ill neonates or infants over very long distances is an area of tremendous advance in many countries including Australia. Such infants can be flown the thousands of kilometres across Australia safely within a support capsule providing high-quality ventilation support, monitoring and accurate infusions of PGE_1, inotropes, vasodilators and other appropriate drugs.

6. Rapid access to multidisciplinary assessment of other organ systems allows for improved management decisions without undue therapeutic delay.

7. The subspeciality of cardiac anaesthesia has led to the accumulation of experience and expertise amongst a limited number of anaesthetists able to deliver appropriate anaesthesia for each anatomical and haemodynamic combination of complex heart disease and to minimize the trauma of multiple instrumentation sites for monitoring.

8. Cardiopulmonary bypass and physiological manipulation of the small baby has improved dramatically. The more gentle membrane oxygenators are now almost routinely used, allowing longer periods of bypass with less insult. Appropriate perfusion pressures and flows for given body size are better understood and more precisely achieved. In-line continuous monitoring of arterial and venous O_2 saturations, pH and PCO_2 have permitted continuous fine adjustment of cardiopulmonary bypass and maintenance of closer to ideal biochemistry, while the newer precision roller and centrifugal pumps deliver flows accurate to within 1%. Advances in cardioplegia content and delivery have enhanced myocardial protection during the sometimes necessary long periods of myocardial ischaemia for complex repairs.

9. In the operating room there have been singular advances in suture materials and ergometrically designed precision small instruments. High-quality non-obstructive magnification supported by high-intensity fibre optic lighting have certainly enhanced the quality and accuracy of surgical repair and reconstructions. Concentration of experience amongst a limited number of active surgeons has contributed enormously to general expertise, knowledge and “on-table” decision making and execution.

10. “Small body” technology, knowledge and expertise in the intensive care unit has advanced very rapidly, providing the whole body physiological support and minute by minute fine adjustments necessary for good survival rates even after a flawless surgical repair. Appropriate ventilators and precision, safe, low-volume infusion pumps are just one part of this advance.

11. Follow-up is an extremely important part of overall management of CHD, especially after complex neonatal repair, where differential growth patterns in repaired areas may lead to quite rapidly progressive life-threatening lesions, best dealt with before myocardial or pulmonary decompensation occurs.

Principles of Management

On the whole principles of management are simple:
1. Early accurate diagnosis.
2. A decision on whether or not an operation is required at the time of referral or best deferred until later.
3. A consultative approach on the nature of the operation to be performed, including the decision on initial palliation or a haemodynamic repair.

Good surgical decision making can only be achieved with a realistic detailed knowledge of the capabilities of the management team. A thorough familarity with the team's results to date, and which way these results are trending, is a cornerstone of this decision making. Some management teams are more or less able to handle small bodies. Surgeons vary in their speed and accuracy. Surgical decision making therefore becomes a contractural affair with the patient, in which the surgical team must *know* within a very narrow range the actual probability of the operation producing a survivor and the risk of irreversible non-lethal complications.

Current Management Programmes and Expectations in Congenital Heart Disease

In this chapter, a single unit's management approach and results are shown to illustrate current trends and expectations in a low-risk institution handling a large volume of congenital heart disease (CHD) at the Royal Children's Hospital, Melbourne.

A total of approximately 700 operations (370–430 on cardiopulmonary bypass and 300–330 without bypass) are currently performed yearly. We expect 96%–97.5% of operations to result in the patient leaving the hospital alive or surviving the first 30 days (Table 2). Less than 3% of patients progress to death without surgical intervention and this includes those cases of hypoplastic left heart syndrome that do not undergo palliation. The majority of those not having surgery, where death is the chosen alternative, are those with complex multiorgan defects in whom mental retardation is known to be highly likely (e.g. proven dysmorphic syndromes and significant chromosomal abnormalities). The recommendation to do nothing is usually given to support parents who have already made a concordant decision based on accurate and forthright counselling.

Patent Ductus Arteriosus

Four categories are defined:
1. The premature respirator-dependent patient with evidence of a persisting large duct after non-surgical attempts at closure have failed (indomethecin). The

Table 2. Results of cardiac surgery

		1978	1979/1980	1981/1982	1983/1984	1985/1986	1987/1988
		All cardiac surgery under 6 months of age 1978–1988					
Under 1 month	Open	7 (4) (57%)	20 (8) (40%)	25 (5) (20%)	31 (7) (19%)	108 (9) (8%)	138 (12) (9%)
	Closed	27 (4) (15%)	64 (9) (14%)	115 (7) (6%)	90 (8) (9%)	153 (9) (6%)	198 (9) (5%)
1–6 months	Open	1 (1) (100%)	20 (4) (20%)	61 (7) (11%)	96 (4) (4%)	89 (2) (2%)	134 (7) (5%)
	Closed	21 (1) (5%)	35 (0) (0%)	51 (2) (3%)	65 (2) (3%)	73 (1) (1%)	85 (3) (4%)
Total	Open	8 (5) (62%)	40 (12) (30%)	86 (12) (14%)	127 (11) (9%)	197 (11) (6%)	272 (19) (7%)
	Closed	48 (5) (10%)	99 (9) (9%)	166 (9) (5%)	155 (10) (6%)	226 (10) (4%)	283 (12) (4%)
		All cardiac surgery over 6 months of age 1978–1988					
	Open	150 (10) (7%)	397 (15) (4%)	351 (8) (2%)	342 (7) (2%)	461 (11) (2%)	544 (17) (3%)
	Closed	54 (0) (0%)	152 (0) (0%)	201 (4) (2%)	292 (5) (2%)	306 (3) (1%)	294 (3) (1%)
		All ages, all surgery					
		260 (20) (7.7%)	688 (36) (5.2%)	804 (33) (4.1%)	916 (33) (3.6%)	1190 (35) (2.9%)	1393 (51) (3.6%)

Note the important increase in open heart surgery under 6 months of age

Open, surgery performed on cardiopulmonary bypass; *Closed*, surgery performed without cardiopulmonary bypass
( ), Death within 30 days

Table 3. Patent ductus arteriosus 1979–1988: surgical closure

	1979	1980	1981	1982	1983	1984	1985	1986	1987	1988	Total
Prematurity and under 1 month	11 (2)	16 (2)	15	12	20	23	20	23	34 (1)	28	202 (5)
1–6 months	3	2	6	7	2	3	4	1	1	4	33
Over 6 months	35	27	25	22	26	25	19	22	23	19	243
Total											478 (5)

( ), Known death within 30 days: none due to patent ductus arteriosus (PDA) ligation or complication of PDA ligation

actual risk of surgical closure is miniscule, but late survival is closely related to birth weight and the state of the lungs at the time of operation.

2. Non-respirator-dependent infants with a large duct presenting with cardiomegaly, plethora, congestive heart failure (CHF) and failure to thrive. The risk of duct closure by double ligation is negligible and should be performed on that admission.
3. Older infants or children presenting with a small duct of minimal or mild haemodynamic significance should be doubly ligated at negligible surgical risk. A persistently patent small ductus carries very little risk to the baby or preschool child but the incidence of endocarditis increases with age to about 0.5%/year. In adult life a patent ductus may become calcified and aneurysmal presenting a much more *difficult* and risky surgical problem.
4. Late presentation of a large hypertensive duct is almost unknown in our practice, and requires careful assessment of pulmonary vascular resistance (fixed and labile) and possibly a lung biopsy before deciding on operability. Ablation of the ductus may be a high-risk procedure, requiring careful postoperative intensive care management and a guarded long-term prognosis. Appropriate early management avoids this unnecessary tragedy (Table 3).

Coarctation of the Aorta

The risk in this condition is governed by the degree of coarctation and the degree of complexity of associated cardiac anomalies or the absence thereof. The most severe coarctation is haemodynamically equivalent to interruption of the aorta with distal aortic flow duct dependent. Postnatal duct closure precipitates catastrophic clinical deterioration, acidosis and death within a matter of hours. In the presence of duct closure an emergency exists with the only chance of survival being immediate referral and surgery, still with a high probability of renal failure and other abdominal organ damage. Early institution of PGE_1 infusion and reopening of the duct restores descending aortic perfusion, allowing correction of acidosis, general stabilization and a very much more optimistic outlook for aortic repair.

A new cohort of patients is surviving because of early PGE_1 use. In 1979 in our unit no cases of neonatal coarctation repair were recorded. Currently, we expect about 20–30 cases/year to undergo surgery. The majority of these have been acidotic at presentation, often within 24 h of birth. The survival rate exceeds 90%. We assume no change in incidence, but in 1979 the sickest neonates were not referred early enough and a few with less severe coarctation or persisting patent ductus survived for postneonatal repair.

Coarctation of the aorta may be classified as (a) *simple,* (b) ventricular septal defect *(VSD) and coarctation* and (c) *coarctation with complex intracardiac abnormalities.* In *simple* coarctation with an otherwise normal heart, we expect 98% survival following neonatal repair. In other cases of coarctation with an intact interventricular septum or pressure-limiting VSD, survival is almost entirely dependent on the adequacy of the systemic ventricle. Small-sized left ventricle, stenotic inlet or outlet has an important influence on survival. On the other hand, unimpeded systemic inlet and outlet even in the presence of a univentricular heart results in a survival expectancy of greater than 95%. The other principal determinant of survival is the aortic arch. In simple coarctation the arch is usually well formed. In coarctation combined with VSD or in the complex coarctation group, arch hypoplasia is common and if severe must be corrected at the same time as the coarctation; otherwise descending aortic blood flow will be inadequate to support tissue perfusion. Failure to attend to arch repair has been the commonest error in this group. A possible "rule of thumb" is that for full confidence in adequate descending aortic flow, the diameter in millimetres of the arch should be equivalent to body weight in kg + 1.

Coarctation repair is achieved by excision and end-to-end anastomosis [5] with short segment narrowing, and by subclavian flap repair [6] when the aortic isthmus is also narrow. Distal arch narrowing is repaired by reverse subclavian aortoplasty [7] combined with resection of the coarctation and end-to-end anastomosis; or by left carotid aortoplasty retaining aortic to carotid continuity, combined with subclavian flap repair of the coarctation; or by coarctation resection and anastomosis of the descending aorta to the underside of the aortic arch overlapping the origin of the left carotid (extended Crafoord). When hypoplasia involves the proximal arch (between innominate and left carotid arteries) arch reconstruction is more readily achieved from the front using cardiopulmonary bypass.

The need for re-operation in coarctation can be traced to many factors, including inadequate initial repair, or a failure of growth of the repaired segment. If the latter, the risk of re-operation probably correlates inversely with the body weight at the time of initial repair.

Indications for repair in non-life-threatening coarctation are evolving. Presentation with congestive heart failure is considered an indication in our institution. If CHF has not been a problem, our preference is to repair by the age of 1 year of age. Milder coarctation may not be diagnosed until later in life. On the whole the operative decision is then based on the anatomical appearance on angiography,

Table 4. Coarctation of the aorta 1979–1988 surgical repair

Under 1 month	153 (11) [13]
1–6 months	64 (6) [0]
Over 6 months	198 (0) [0]

Neonatal coarcation repair

Simple	VSD + coarctation	Complex coarctation	Total
52 (1) [0]	54 (3) [5]	47 (7) [8]	153 (11) [13]

( ), Death within 30 days. Causes: inadequate relief of aortic obstruction; hypoplastic LV and mitral valve stenosis; uncontrolled acidosis and preoperative anuria
[ ], Late death.
Note: patients with small LV/mitral valve, 18 (6) [5]

and on right arm blood pressure at rest and in response to exercise. Delayed repair appears to increase the risk of persistent or early development of systemic hypertension [8] (Table 4).

Atrial Septal Defect

Since progressive damage to the heart and lungs in this condition is slow, early repair is not critical. However, once diagnosed there is now little merit in waiting until the customary 4–5 years of age. If diagnosed early the anxiety of several years wait by the parents is probably not necessary. The risk of repair of secundum ASD is very small. However, primum ASD associated with mitral incompetence is more difficult technically and the possibility exists that very early repair, even though exact, may lead to later mitral valve distortion due to uneven growth of the septal component of the mitral valve during the most rapid growth period. Repair of sinus venosus ASD with partial anomalous pulmonary venous drainage to the superior vena cava (SVC) requires division of the lower SVC into two channels. Larger-sized patients makes it relatively easy to septate the SVC without

Table 5. Atrial septal defect 1979–1988: surgical closure. Primum ASD, secundum ASD, sinus venosus defect

	1979	1980	1981	1982	1983	1984	1985	1986	1987	1988	Total
Under 1 month	–	–	–	–	–	–	–	–	–	1	1
1–6 months	–	–	1	–	1 (1)	–	–	1	1 (1)	–	4 (2)
Over 6 months	41	27	28	25	31	18	22	36	43 (1)	44	310 (1)
Total											315 (3)

( ), Death within 30 days. Three patients all under 1 year of age. Symptomatic. Causes. Primum ASD with small LV and coarctation aorta, PDA; respirator dependent, cardiomyopathy with secundum ASD; diminutive left coronary cusp with coronary stenosis, infarction producing an obstructive channel. Primum ASD and sinus venosus defect in the absence of developing pulmonary hypertension may reasonably be scheduled for repair prekindergarten. ASD presenting in infancy with marked symptoms may need repair but one should look very carefully for other problems (e.g. myocardial dysfunction, coronary ostium stenosis) (Table 5).

Ventricular Septal Defect

It is probable that 30% of perimembranous VSDs close spontaneously sufficiently quickly to avoid permanent damage to the lungs. A policy of waiting for spontaneous closure must be accompanied by frequent examinations to measure VSD size and assess pulmonary blood flow and resistance. It is a mistake simply to interpret signs of diminishing pulmonary blood flow as evidence of a closing VSD. The same changes occur without VSD closure, but with increasing pulmonary vascular resistance. As the current risk of isolated perimembranous VSD closure after the age of 3 months is less than 1%, the threshold for surgical closure is lower and the risk to the lungs of prolonged conservative management is reduced. When a large perimembranous VSD is complicated by additional abnormalities then the need for early repair on symptomatic grounds is more likely, except when the only additional abnormality is of moderate but not severe right ventricular outflow tract obstruction which serves to protect the pulmonary circuit from excessive flow and pressure. In actual fact, however, in our experience, resection of right ventricular outflow tract (RVOT) muscle or the addition of pulmonary valvotomy has not added to surgical risk.

Other VSD types may warrant a variety of management plans. A large inlet VSD or outlet VSD is unlikely to close spontaneously and surgery can be scheduled within the first 3 months of life. Outlet VSDs (supracristal) may become haemodynamically smaller by virtue of a prolapsing right or left aortic cusp resulting in progressive aortic valve distortion and incompetence. It is prudent to intervene early in these cases. Large midmuscular VSDs may close spontaneously and may be managed on similar lines to perimembranous VSDs, advocating closure by 3–4 months, if evidence indicates persistence of a substantial VSD.

Table 6. Simple and complex or multiple VSDs 1979–1988: surgical closure

	1979	1980	1981	1982	1983	1984	1985	1986	1987	1988	Total
Under 1 month	–	–	1 (1)	–	1	–	2	10	9	8	31 (1)
1–6 months	–	2	9	7 (1)	13 (1)	18 (1)	10	16 (1)	36	17	128 (3)
Over 6 months	44 (1)	48	49	41 (1)	41 (1)	31	47 (1)	42 (1)	57	41	441 (5)
Total											600 (9)

( ), Death within 30 days. Principal causes: surgical damage in complex cases; pulmonary vascular obstructive disease

Multiple muscular VSDs present a difficult surgical problem in terms of early definitive intervention. If a large pulmonary blood flow is evident and persists beyond 6–8 weeks, then our policy is to apply a pulmonary artery band via a midline sternotomy and attempt ventricular septation and band removal when the band is outgrown (usually after 2 years of age). During this time some of the VSDs may have closed spontaneously, but at the same time the lungs have been protected from pulmonary vascular obstructive disease (Table 6).

Total Anomalous Pulmonary Venous Drainage

The anomalous drainage is (a) *supracardiac* via a vertical vein joining the leftward end of the innominate vein or directly to the superior vena cava. In 30% of cases drainage is obstructed. (b) *Infracardiac* via a vertical vein draining through the ductus venosus to the hepatic veins, directly to the portal system, or directly to the IVC. In 95% of cases drainage is obstructed. (c) *Intracardiac* usually via the coronary sinus to the right atrium or directly to the right atrium, and in 20% of cases drainage is obstructed. Mixed varieties of total anomalous pulmonary venous drainage (TAPVD) occur but are rare. In all cases, left heart filling is via an ASD which may be restrictive, so that with either restrictive ASD or obstructed TAPVD systemic cardiac output is low, with additional pulmonary congestion or oedema in the latter condition. We believe corrective surgery should be performed (connecting the pulmonary venous confluence to the left atrium, dividing the vertical vein and closing interatrial communications) on referral, and as an emergency in the presence of low systemic output or pulmonary congestion. Pulmonary resistance may rise very rapidly. The principal determinant of survival,

Table 7. Total anomalous pulmonary venous drainage, 1979–March 1989, surgical repair

	Obstructive	Non-obstructive	Total
a) Anatomical and physiological factors			
Supracardiac	9	13	22
Cardiac	3	12	15
Infracardiac	18 (1) [2]	1	19 (1) [2]
	30 (1) [2]	26	56 (1) [2]
	Obstructive		
b) Age			
Under 1 month	36 (1) [2][a]		
1–6 months	16		
Over 6 months	4		
	56 (1) [2]		

( ), Death within 30 days. Causes: death on table (1979); high pulmonary resistance
[ ] Late death. [a] Cause: both from progressive fibrosis; pulmonary veins

short or long term, is the pulmonary circuit, predicating a management protocol aimed at lowering pulmonary resistance. In approximately 5% of TAPVD after a successful operation there is rapidly progressive and fatal diffuse fibrotic obliteration of pulmonary veins [9, 10] (Table 7).

Complete Atrioventricular Septal Defect (Complete Atrioventricular Canal)

In this condition, the centre of the heart is missing with continguous atrial and ventricular septal defects and a single inlet valve variously straddling both ventricles and with various degrees of regurgitation. Down's syndrome contributes 85% of the cases in our series. In most cases right and left ventricular pressures are equalized, ensuring a high pulmonary blood flow under high pressure, and tending to early development of pulmonary vascular obstructive disease. Most patients are dead, inoperable or marginally operable by the age of 2 years [11, 12]. Repair, which is complex and difficult, involves septating the heart with one patch, in which case straddling leaflets are divided and re-attached to the patch; *or* by using two patches placed above and below the atrioventricular valve (AV) leaflets (our preference). In addition the left-sided AV valve (mitral) usually needs to be repaired to reduce incompetence. Our preference is to repair by 2–3 months of age or earlier if severe congestive heart failure is a problem. After infant repair the reoperation rate for recurrent severe mitral incompetence or repair dehiscence is quite high (10% in our series) [13] (Table 8).

Tetralogy of Fallot

The outlet septum of the heart is dislocated forwards and to the left, creating a large malalignment VSD (which will not close spontaneously), bringing the aortic valve ring into a position overriding the VSD, and narrowing the right ventricular outflow tract (RVOT), which in turn results in RV hypertrophy – completing the

Table 8. Complete atrioventricular canal 1978–1988, surgical repair

	Single-patch technique		Two-patch technique								
	1978	1980	1981	1982	1983	1984	1985	1986	1987	1988	Total
Under 1 month		1	–	–	–	–	2	4 (1)	–	–	6 (1)
1–6 months		2 (1)	6	2	8	7	11	11	14	17	76
Over 6 months		12 (3)	9	8 (1)	6	9	14	23	19 (1)	4	92 (2)
Total		15 (4)									174 (3)

( ), Death within 30 days. Principal causes: surgical imprecision; pulmonary vascular obstructive disease

Table 9. Tetralogy of Fallot 1981–1988

	1981	1982	1983	1984	1985	1986	1987	1988	
	Trans right atrial approach								
Under 6 months	2	–	2	1	2	3	4 (1)	4	18 (1)
Over 6 months	12	22	14	33	26	29	60	35	231 (1) [1]
Total									249 (2) [1]
	Palliation by shunt during era of transatrial repair								
Under 1 month	2	1	–	2	–	1	1	1	8
1–6 months	3	1	5	5	–	3	3	4	24
Over 6 months	2	6	7	7	8	5	3	4	42
Total									74 (0)

( ), denotes death within 30 days; causes, pulmonary vascular disease; mitral stenosis and small LV
[ ], denotes late death; cause, pulmonary vascular disease

tetrad. RVOT obstruction may be at subpulmonary valve level, at pulmonary valve level, at main pulmonary artery level, at pulmonary artery bifurcation level or involving branch pulmonary arteries. In some cases obstruction at all levels is present. In our view, it is the nature of the RVOT obstruction which dictates the management plan. The standard form of repair involves a right ventriculotomy (transverse if the pulmonary valve ring is of normal size, or vertical and extending through the pulmonary valve ring if the latter is smaller than normal) [14]. The VSD is patched through the right ventriculotomy, and the RVOT is repaired usually by a pericardial patch, if the incision is vertical, and the patch may need to extend distally into stenotic branch pulmonary arteries. When a patch extends across the pulmonary valve ring, the pulmonary valve is variously incompetent. An incompetent pulmonary valve is not as innocent as once thought, with late development of RV dilatation and dysfunction (10–20 years) now being identified more and more. For this reason we have adopted the transatrial approach in an attempt to preserve the RV function as much as possible. The VSD patch repair and RVOT resection are performed via the right atrium and tricuspid valve. A pulmonary valvotomy is performed through the main pulmonary artery and if the pulmonary valve ring is small the incision is carried across the annulus for a few millimetres, exactly in a commissure to preserve the pulmonary valve cusps. Early repair (in the first few months) can be advocated if RVOT obstruction is mild and pulmonary blood flow is high (acyanotic tetrad) or in infancy as a primary procedure in the presence of severe subpulmonary muscular obstruction but well-formed pulmonary valve ring and central pulmonary artery system. When obstruction is severe and the pulmonary valve ring or central pulmonary artery system is small then we prefer the initial procedure to be a shunt (creating a connection between the systemic arterial tree and the central pulmonary artery system). Our preference is a Goretex shunt between the right subclavian artery and right pulmonary artery. It is known that the increased flow from shunting through the pulmonary arteries encourages growth of the pulmonary artery tree and the pulmonary valve ring, such that later repair may entail a smaller or no patch across the pulmonary valve ring. Our policy is to proceed to repair in all cases by 12–18 months. In our experience the risk of shunting in tetralogy of Fallot is very low and the total cumulative risk of our management protocol (primary repair or shunt followed by later repair and subsequent reoperations for residual defects) has resulted in a combined early and late mortality of about 1% in the 9 years since the transatrial approach was adopted (Table 9). In our series the incidence of transannular RVOT patching is 64% compared with 90% or more when the exclusive policy is primary infant repair [15].

Truncus Arteriosus

There is a single outlet valve connected to the aortic root, from which arise the pulmonary arteries, with origins common or slightly separated or completely separated. A pulmonary artery or part thereof may arise from the aortic arch or descending aorta (hemitruncus). Physiologically, the pulmonary circuit is exposed to high pressure and flow throughout systole and diastole, enhancing rapid development of pulmonary vascular obstructive disease. Congestive heart failure develops early and is severe in almost all cases. Occasionally, when CHF is transient or unimpressive, the baby thrives, and, an ominous outlook can be envisaged, because of early elevation of pulmonary vascular resistance. Palliation by individual pulmonary artery banding is difficult, imprecise and accompanied by poor immediate and late results. Untreated, 90% of patients die within the 1st year [16]. The best option, although a technical and physiological challenge, is complete repair preferably by 2–3 months of age. About 20% of patients diagnosed in the neonatal period cannot be supported at home or in hospital for this period and require intensive care support, including intermittent positive pressure ventilation.

In this subgroup, many have additional significant cardiac or non-cardiac problems such as truncal valve incompetence or stenosis, coronary ostial stenosis, interrupted aortic arch (type B) or atrioventricular valve incompetence. Complete repair in this subgroup is clearly more hazardous and falls in the salvage category.

Table 10. Truncus and hemitruncus arteriosus 1979–1988, surgical repair

	1979	1980	1981	1982	1983	1984	1985	1986	1987	1988	Total
Under 1 month (includes prematurity)		2 (1) [1]	1 (1)	–	–	1	3 [1]	–	2	3	12 (2) [2]
1–6 months		1	1	5	5*	5**	4*	1	2	1 (1)	25 (1)
Over 6 months	1 (1)	3*	–	2	1 (1)	1	2	3* [1]	2	1	16 (2) [1]

( ), Death within 30 days. Causes: prematurity; truncal valve incompetence; pulmonary vascular obstructive disease; coronary ostial stenosis; tracheomalacia
[ ], late death
Each *asterisk* represents a hemitruncus patient: (0) [1]
Six patients had truncus and interrupted aortic arch: (0) [0]

Despite this, delaying repair once ventilation is required for severe CHF carries no merit. If repair is delayed beyond 6 months an increasing number of patients develop established elevation of pulmonary vascular resistance, making postoperative management difficult or impossible and decreasing the hope of return to normal resistance in those surviving repair.

Repair entails transventricular patch closure of the VSD, direct suture of the ASD through the right atrium, detachment of the pulmonary arteries from the trunk, reconstruction of the right and left pulmonary artery connection if necessary and insertion of a valved conduit between the right ventriculotomy and the pulmonary arteries. Our preference is to use a valved Dacron conduit during initial infant repair and subsequently to replace this by a further Dacron-valved conduit or an aortic or pulmonary homograft conduit.

Our results (Table 10) illustrate the hazard of forced repair in the 1st month of life (including prematurity), the relative safety of elective repair and possibly the hazard of late repair. Conduit replacement, in general, has been safe (no deaths in 40).

Transposition of the Great Arteries

This condition is incompatible with life unless there is some connection between right and left sides of the heart to permit mixing of pulmonary and systemic venous blood.

1. *In simple transposition of the great arteries (TGA)* the interventricular septum is intact or virtually so. Profound cyanosis is present soon after birth and accentuated by duct closure. Initial patient survival is dependent on the size of the atrial septal defect. Palliation by balloon atrial septostomy (BAS) performed with ultrasound guidance in the Intensive Care Unit (ICU), or under X-ray control in the catheter laboratory, results in a dramatic rise in aortic oxygen saturation in most patients, allowing delay of repair by atrial switch (Mustard or Senning) until 3–4 months of age, or anatomical repair by arterial switch at a convenient time in the neonatal period (our preference is the 2nd week of life). In some patients (about 10%), BAS is inadequately effective, so PGE_1 infusion is commenced with the opening ductus resulting in volume priming of the left atrium and enhanced mixing at atrial level. This situation usually signals the need for atrial or arterial switch as an urgent procedure within the subsequent 1–2 days. Atrial switch entails insertion of a new atrial septum (pericardium, Dacron or Goretex) configured in such a way that systemic venous blood is redirected through the mitral valve and thence, as is normal, to the pulmonary artery; and pulmonary venous blood is redirected to the tricuspid valve and thence to the aorta via the right ventricle (Mustard procedure 1963) [17]. Such a baffle may result immediately or later in obstruction to systemic or pulmonary venous flow. In the Senning procedure (1959) [18] the same principle is pursued, but baffling is achieved by rearranging the atrial walls and septal remnant, creating a living baffle with growth potential. Obstruction of venous return is rare after this technically more difficult

Table 11. Simple and complex TGA and DORV 1979–1988; primary surgical repair

	1979	1980	1981	1982	1983	1984	1985	1986	1987	1988	Total
Atrial repair (Senning)	21 (3)	19	21 (1)	16 (1)	8	10	8	1	–	1	105 (5)
Arterial switch (Jatene)	–	–	–	–	9 (1)	10 (2)	24 (1)	33	28	34	134 (4)
Total											239 (9)

( ), Death within 30 days. Principal causes: Small RV or LV; Coronary artery damage
TGA, transposition of great arteries; DORV, double outlet right ventricle

Table 12. Simple TGA 1983–1988, surgical repair by primary arterial switch

1st week (urgent)	2nd week (elective)	3–4 weeks	4–6 weeks	6–8 weeks	Over 8 weeks	Total
22	44	11	2	2	1	83 (0)

( ), Death within 30 days
TGA, transposition of great arteries

procedure. Both forms of atrial switch exhibit a time-related increasing incidence of atrial arrhythmias due largely to a damaged or deteriorating sino-atrial node. In a small number (10% in 10 years) of "atrially" repaired simple TGA, progressive RV failure and tricuspid valve incompetence is observed. An increasing number of centres are now opting for neonatal anatomical repair [arterial switch Jatene (1975)] [19] as the treatment of choice for simple TGA. Arterial switch entails division of the duct, ascending aorta and main pulmonary artery (MPA), translocation of the coronary arteries from the aortic root to the proximal MPA, pericardial patch repair of the two resulting defects in the aortic root, passing the distal ascending aorta behind the pulmonary artery bifurcation (Le compte procedure) [20], anastomosis of the distal ascending aorta to the proximal MPA (now bearing the coronary arteries), end-to-end anastomosis of the reconstructed proximal aorta to the distal MPA and direct suture of the ASD. This is a long and difficult operation with coronary translocation representing a critical step. Delaying arterial switch beyond 1–2 months (2 months in our opinion) results in involution of the left ventricle which is connected to the low-pressure pulmonary circuit, and the risk that after arterial switch the left ventricle will be inadequate to support the systemic circulation. Late referral of simple TGA can be managed, however, by "retraining" the LV by MPA banding usually accompanied by a systemic to pulmonary shunt to ensure adequate pulmonary blood flow [21]. "Retraining" of the left ventricle in the small infant may take as little as 2 weeks (Boston Children's Hospital, personal communication) (Tables 11, 12).

2. With *complex transposition* (TGA and VSD with or without coarctation of the aorta) atrial repair can be achieved but the late results are disappointing in terms

Table 13. Transposition of great arteries and VSD, 1983–1988: surgical repair by arterial switch

Number patients	49 (2) [0]
Weight at operation 1.6–15 kg (median, 4 kg)	
Age at operation, 4 days–7 years, (median, 3.2 months)	
Associated cardiac anomalies and risk	
Hypoplastic RV	5 (1)
RVOTO	6
LVOTO	6 (1)
Coarctation	8 (1)
Interrupted aortic arch	3
Crisscross AV connection	2
Posterior TGA	1
Situs inversus	1
TAPVD to cs	1
Left juxtaposed appendages	1
Jehovah's Witness	1

RVOTO/LVOTO, right/left ventricular outflow tract obstruction; TAPVD, total anomalous pulmonary venous drainage

Table 14. Double-outlet right ventricle and subpulmonary or double committed VSD: 1983–1988 repair by arterial switch

Number patients,	8 (2) [0]
Main VSD type and risk	
Subpulmonary	3 (1)
Doubly committed	2
Uncommitted	3 (1)
Additional VSDs	1 (1)
Other cardiac anomalies and risk	
Hypoplastic left ventricle	1 (1)
Coarctation	3
LVOTO	1
RVOTO and coarctation and arch hypoplasia	2

LVOTO/RVOTO, left/right ventricular outflow tract obstruction; VSD, ventricular septal defect

Table 15. Post Mustard/Senning right ventricle dysfunction and tricuspid incompetence: two-stage conversion to arterial switch

Stage 1:	"Retraining" LV by banding main pulmonary artery			
	Twelve patients	1	Two banding attempts	(0) [1]
		11	Bands applied	(0) [1]
Stage 2:	Take down Mustard/Senning then arterial switch			
	Seven patients	(1) [1]		

( ), Early death; [ ], late death

of the higher incidence of RV dysfunction and tricuspid incompetence. Arterial switch, which is the same as for simple TGA but with additional VSD closure, is now the generally preferred approach. Arterial switch should be achieved by 2–3 months of age (possibly earlier) and may need to be preceded by coarctation repair with or without MPA banding (our preference is not to band the MPA unless there are multiple VSDs). When coarctation is associated with severe hypoplasia of the aortic arch or if interruption is present, then our preference is to operate as soon as the patient is stabilized on PGE_1 infusion, reconstructing the aortic arch, performing the arterial switch and closing the VSD and ASD along with resection of subaortic stenosis if present – all simultaneously via a midline sternotomy (Table 13).

3. There is a subgroup of patients with double-outlet right ventricle, subpulmonary VSD or doubly committed subaortic and subpulmonary VSD having physiology similar to TGA with VSD and managed by the same protocol (Table 14).

4. In patients who have undergone an atrial repair and subsequently developed RV dysfunction and TI, a two-staged conversion to an arterial switch has been performed [22]. Initially the MPA is banded to "retrain" the LV, and, at a later date, the band is removed, the atrial repair reversed and an arterial switch performed. The remaining viable alternative is heart transplantation (Table 15).

5. In a difficult to manage subgroup of neonates presenting with single ventricle, TGA, subaortic stenosis, coarctation with severe hypoplasia of the aortic arch, or arch interruption and who have a duct-dependent descending aortic blood flow, simultaneous arterial switch, aortic arch reconstruction and atrial septectomy has been performed at our institution in an attempt adequately to palliate with a view to a modified Fontan procedure at a later date. There were five neonates with one early death and one late death. The hazard of the arterial switch operation varies considerably from centre to centre. In general, it has only been the high-throughput (low-risk) institutions which have so far achieved an early mortality similar to the considerably less taxing atrial repairs.

Single Ventricle or Univentricular Heart and the Fontan Concept

Debate continues on what does and does not consitute a ventricle, and, surprisingly, whether "single ventricle" has the same meaning as "univentricular heart". Nevertheless, there is a disparate group of hearts in which it is considered impossible to achieve a biventricular repair. There are many different reasons for making this decision, and it is best made as early as possible. In the surgical management of a single useful ventricle, the aim of palliation is to ensure adequate but not excessive pulmonary blood flow. In addition, unobstructed systemic outflow from the ventricular mass and unobstructed pulmonary venous return to the ventricular mass must be ensured during palliation. If early and subsequent palliative procedures are well conceived and executed each patient may then fulfil the criteria controlling eligibility for a Fontan-type "repair" (Fontan, 1971) [23]. The Fontan concept demonstrates that provided total resistance to flow of blood from MPA to the ventricular cavity is normal or near normal and that the ventricular mass has near normal diastolic compliance and contractility, then the distal pulmonary artery without a valve may be connected directly to the systemic venous atrium, which has been isolated from the ventricle by various methods of atrial neoseptation. Systemic venous blood will then flow continuously through the lungs, without a pump, with a mean pressure of between 8 and 14 mmHg. Some straying from these strict preoperative criteria can be tolerated, but the price is usually a higher systemic venous pressure. Different patients clearly tolerate a given venous pressure differently, but it can be generally stated that a post Fontan

Table 16. Modified Fontan operation: 138 patients 1979–1988

	Number	Early death	Late death	Cumulative mortality
Tricuspid atresia	27	0	4 (15%)	4 (15%)
Double inlet ventricle	58	4 (7%)	5 (9%)	9 (16%)
Pulmonary atresia intact ventricular septum	12	2 (17%)	0	2 (17%)
Hypoplastic right ventricle, VSD, straddling AV valve	12	1 (8%)	0	1 (8%)
Heterotaxia	11	1 (9%)	1 (9%)	2 (18%)
Double outlet right ventricle	7	1 (14%)	0	1 (14%)
Hypoplastic left heart syndrome	2	1 (50%)	0	1 (50%)
Others	9	1 (11%)	1 (11%)	2 (22%)
Totals	138	11 (8%)	11 (8%)	22 (16%)

VSD, ventricular septal defect

venous pressure exceeding 16 mm Hg carries a less favourable long-term prognosis. The Fontan procedure and its many modifications results in separation of systemic and pulmonary circuits, full oxygen saturation of systemic arterial blood and volume unloading of the single ventricle. The true longevity of single ventricle patients managed by the Fontan principle is unknown. At worst it is an ingenious and effective form of palliation (Table 16).

Many other forms of congenital heart disease demand their own particular management protocols involving primary repair or initial palliation followed by repair.

Transplantation

An important number of patients on follow-up after repair exhibit less than normal cardiac function, due to recurrent or residual defects, or irreversible complications of the original lesion complex (e.g. pulmonary vascular obstructive disease, or ventricular or valve dysfunction).

With the addition of heart and heart/lung transplantation, patients with end-stage problems unmanageable by conventional surgical interventions are offered a second chance. The results of transplantation in children have lagged behind those in adults but are steadily improving, with encouraging results emerging in the neonatal group of heart transplants (Bailey, Loma Linda, personal communication, 1989; 40 of 44 surviving).

Heart/lung transplantation, however, is more difficult and the long-term results less promising than heart transplantation alone. Approximately 50% of survivors of heart lung transplantation exhibit some degree of obstructive bronchiolitis. The aetiology of this complication is uncertain, but chronic rejection is probably important. In addition, chronic low-grade infection and poor preservation of the lungs during the preimplantation ischaemic period may also be contributory.

Improved donor lung preservation and more specific control of rejection can be expected in the future, extending the application of heart/lung, single lung or double lung transplantation.

References

1. Gross RE, Hubbard JP (1939) Surgical ligation of a patent ductus arteriosus. Report of first successful case. JAMA 112:729
2. Keith JD, Neill CA, Vlad P, Rowe RD, Chute AL (1953) Transposition of the great vessels. Circulation 7:830
3. Campbell M (1970) Natural history of atrial septal defect. Br Heart J 32:820
4. Norwood WI, Dobell AR, Freed MD, Kirklin JW, Blackstone EH, Congenital Heart Surgeons Society (1988) Intermediate results of the arterial switch repair: a 20 institution study. J Thorac Cardiovasc Surg 96:854
5. Crafoord C, Nylin G (1945) Congenital coarctation of the aorta and its surgical treatment. J Thorac Surg 14:347
6. Waldhausen JA, Nahrwold DL (1966) Repair of coarctation of the aorta with a subclavian flap. J Thorac Cardiovasc Surg 51:432
7. Hart JC, Waldhausen JA (1983) Reversed subclavian flap angioplasty for arch coarctation of the aorta. Ann Thorac Surg 36:715
8. Clarkson PM, Nicholson MR, Barratt-Boyes BG, Neutze JM, Whitelock RM (1983) Results after repair of coarctation fo the aorta beyond infancy: a 10–28 years follow-up with particular reference to late systemic hypertension. Am J Cardiology 51:1481
9. Fleming WH, Clark EB, Dooley KJ, Hofschire PJ (1979) Ruckman RN, Hopeman AR, Sarafian L, Mooring PK (1979) Late complications following surgical repair of total anomalous pulmonary venous return below the diaphragm. Ann Thorac Surg 27:435
10. Sano S, Brawn WJ, Mee RBB (1989) Total anomalous pulmonary venous drainage. J Thorac Cardiovasc Surg 97:886–892
11. Berger TJ, Blackstone EH, Kirklin JW, Bargeron LM Jr, Hazelrig JB, Turner ME Jr (1979) Survival and probability of cure without and with surgery in complete atrioventricular canal. Ann Thorac Surg 27:104
12. Newfeld EA, Sher M, Paul MH, Nikaidoh H (1977) Pulmonary vascular disease in complete atrioventricular canal defect. Am J Cardiol 39:721
13. Weintraub R, Brawn WJ, Venables AW, Mee RBB (1990) Two patch repair of complete atrioventricular septal defect in the first year of life: results and sequential assessment of atrioventricular valve function. J Thorac Cardiovasc Surg 99:320
14. Kirklin JW, Ellis FH Jr, McGoon DC, DuShane JW, Swan HFC (1959) Surgical treatment of tetralogy of Fallot by open intracardiac repair. J Thorac Surg 37:22
15. Castenada AR, Norwood WI (1983) Fallot's tetralogy. In: Stark J, Leval M de (eds) surgery for congenital heart defects. Grune and Stratton, London
16. Kirkland JW, Barratt-Boyes BG (1986) Cardiac surgery. Wiley, New York, pp 928
17. Mustard WT (1964) Successful two-stage correction of transposition of the great vessels. Surgery 55:469
18. Senning A (1959) Surgical correction of transposition of the great vessels. Surgery 45:966
19. Jatene AD, Fontes VF, Paulista PP, Souza LCB, Neger F, Galantier M, Sousa JE (1975) Successful anatomic correction of transposition of the great vessels. A preliminary report. Ar. Bras Cardiol 28:461
20. Lecompte Y, Zannini L (1981) Hazam E, Jarreau MM, Bex JP, Tu TV, Neveau JY (1981) Anatomic correction of transposition of the great arteries. J Thorac Cardiovasc Surg 82:629
21. Yavoub MH, Radley-Smith R, Maclaurin R (1977) Two-stage operation for anatomical correction of transposition of the great arteries with intact ventricular septum. Lancet I:1275
22. Mee RBB (1986) Severe right ventricular failure after Mustard or Senning operation. Two-stage repair: pulmonary artery banding and switch. J Thorac Cardiovasc Surg 92:385
23. Fontan F, Baudet E (1971) Surgical repair of tricuspid atresia. Thorax 26:240

An Approach to the Management of Chest Wall Deformities

N. A. Myers

Summary

Chest wall deformities are seen frequently in children and adolescents. Fortunately, the deformity is usually mild and the only therapeutic requirement is patient and family reasurance. If the deformity is more severe, consideration must be given to surgical correction. Although sophisticated studies have shown that cardiopulmonary function may be limited by funnel chest, the findings are rarely of clinical significance and, therefore, with few exceptions, operations will be performed for cosmetic and/or psychological reasons. In order to be able to manage patients with chest wall deformities appropriately, clarity of thinking is essential in relation to classification, symptomatology and treatment options. Before reaching a final decision regarding operation, several interviews may be required. In order to assess the final result, long-term follow-up is mandatory.

Zusammenfassung

Brustwanddeformitäten sind häufig bei Kindern und Jugendlichen. Glücklicherweise sind die Deformitäten gewöhnlich nur wenig ausgeprägt, und die einzige therapeutische Maßnahme ist Beruhigung von Patienten und Familien. Wenn die Deformität schwerer ist, muß die chirurgische Korrektur ins Auge gefaßt werden. Obwohl ausgeklügelte Untersuchungen ergeben haben, daß die kardiopulmonale Funktion durch die Trichterbrust eingeschränkt sein kann, haben diese Befunde jedoch kaum klinische Bedeutung, und somit werden – mit einigen wenigen Ausnahmen – die Operationen aus kosmetischen und/oder psychologischen Gründen durchgeführt. Um Patienten mit Brustwanddeformitäten optimal betreuen zu können, ist eine Klarheit des Denkens in bezug auf Schweregrad, Symptomatik und therapeutische Ziele nötig. Bevor eine endgültige Entscheidung für eine Operation getroffen wird, sind manchmal wiederholte Gespräche erforderlich. Um das endgültige Resultat beurteilen zu können, ist ein Langzeit-Follow-Up zwingend notwendig.

Résumé

Les déformations du thorax se rencontrent fréquemment chez les enfants et les adolescents. Heureusement, la déformation est en général peu importante et le traitement consiste essentiellement à rassurer le patient et la famille. Si la déformation est grave, il faudra envisager une intervention chirurgicale de correction. Bien que des études poussées et compliquées aient démontré que la fonction cardio-pulmonaire peut être entravée par la présence d'un thorax en entonnoir, les résutalts ont rarement une portée clinique et les interventions sont le plus souvent pratiquées pour des raisons esthétiques ou psychologiques. Pour un traitement approprié des déformations du sternum, il faut faire le point avec précision sur la classification, la symptomatologie et les

Royal Children's Hospital Melbourne, Flemington Road, Parkville 3052, Victoria, Australia.

Progress in Pediatric Surgery, Vol. 27
Myers and Angerpointner (Eds.)

options thérapeutiques. Avant de prendre la décision finale d'une intervention, des consultations répétées peuvent s'imposer. Pour pouvoir juger des résultats, il est indispensable de suivre le patient à long terme.

Introduction

In order to manage chest wall deformities adequately it is necessary to have clear-cut ideas regarding classification and the natural history of these deformities. In addition, the clinician who is called upon to care for children with chest wall deformities must be aware of the needs of the parents of the child as well as the child himself. Many of the patients are adolescent and an additional requirement is to be aware of and sensitive to the specific needs of the adolescent.

In 1977, Ravitch [40] in a superb monograph pointed out that when he originally became interested in the subject, "the general impression... was that these deformities were rare, that they were physiologically unimportant and that... this was of no consequence since no methods were available for their treatment". Ravitch continued as follows: "All three counts have long since proved to be fallacious".

At an earlier stage, in 1956, Koop [27] had commented as follows: "In spite of the number of recent additions to the surgical literature on pectus excavatum it would seem that there is no agreement concerning the etiology of this thoracic defect, no uniformity of opinion concerning the physiological deficits produced by the funnel chest, no established indication for operation, no critical cardiac or pulmonary function tests to establish such indications and no little confusion concerning the age for operation if and when surgical treatment is indicated".

From a very large experience at the Royal Children's Hospital, Melbourne, we would agree with Koop and with two of Ravitch's premises, namely that the deformities occur frequently and that treatment is available, but we feel that there is little evidence to support the contention that they are physiologically important. Like others who have seen many children – and adults – with a chest wall deformity we have several anecdotal experiences indicating subjective improvement in cardiorespiratory function and lessening of the frequency of intercurrent respiratory infections following corrective surgery for pectus excavatum but there is little objective data to support the subjective impressions.

We have carried out respiratory function tests in many patients but have found little correlation between the severity of the deformity and the results of such tests. However, review of the literature certainly demonstrates a variation in views expressed regarding the physiological effects of chest wall deformities, particularly those of the depression type [2, 4, 6, 8, 13, 21, 28, 30].

Although many contributions in the literature do refer to the physiological effects of chest wall deformities, particularly funnel chest, and describe the results of treatment of large series of patients managed surgically, it is not the purpose of this article to add to the literature in this way. Rather, the object of this article is to consider an approach to treatment and reflect on the evolution surgical treatment has undergone in our institution. This is of particular importance in view of the emotive issues which surround the subject and the need to introduce an objective approach to the problem when so much of the patients' and the physicians' attitude is subjective.

Aspects to be considered in this article are:
1. Classification
2. Decision making
3. Surgical options
4. The uncommon varieties of chest wall deformity

Classification

Chest wall deformities may be *primary* or *secondary;* although the majority of patients who present for opinion regarding the shape and appearance of their chest have a primary deformity it is essential to take a complete history and make a complete physical examination to ensure that the deformity is not secondary to and/or associated with an underlying disorder. However, it is necessary to stress that, even if the deformity is secondary, if it is symptomatic consideration can and should always be given to surgical correction although careful case selection and analysis of all factors is essential.

Primary Chest Wall Deformities

Reference will be made later to the less frequently observed anomalies such as cleft sternum, bizarre rib deformities and the like. Primary deformities are basically of three types:

1. Depression deformities
2. Protrusion deformities
3. Deficiency deformities

Depression Deformities (Pectus Excavatum)

This is the group seen most frequently; the deformity is characterized by a triad of features, namely sternal depression, lateral sulci and costal margin eversion. Although the most significant element of this triad is the sternal depression, which is of course associated with parasternal depression to a varying degree, the costal margin eversion may also be a very significant feature and add to the overall cosmetic disability. The deformity may be symmetrical or asymmetrical; if the latter some degree of sternal rotation will be present.

In the early years of life inspiratory retraction of the sternum and adjacent costal cartilages is a frequent finding in the depression deformity group; this can be quite alarming to parents but they can certainly be reassured that the retraction will ultimately cease. In providing such reassurance it is important to add that it is quite impossible to predict the ultimate residual deformity. It is possible that the degree of inspiratory retraction may reflect the presence of laryngomalacia which is itself a self-limiting condition.

As with all chest wall deformities a clinical classification is also relevant; firstly in relation to symptoms and, although in many patients in whom the deformity is not severe the condition is asymptomatic, in others symptoms are present. However, these are rarely truly physical and as has previously been mentioned there is little objective data to support the existence of a significant physiological disturbance. The rarity of physical symptoms is balanced by the frequency of emotional symptoms resulting from the cosmetic disability which the deformity causes. This immediately leads one to the second area in the clinical classification and this is perhaps the key to the whole problem – the key which unlocks the decision making. Regardless of the type, or for that matter, the aetiology, chest wall deformities may be:

1. Mild
2. Moderate
3. Severe

Simple though this may sound, in practice it is often far from simple; thus, a chest wall deformity may appear to be mild to the patient but severe to the parents, and the physician whose opinion has been sought may have different views again. It is a well-recognized fact that there is a genetic predisposition, and involvement of other members of the family is frequent. This is of particular significance in the

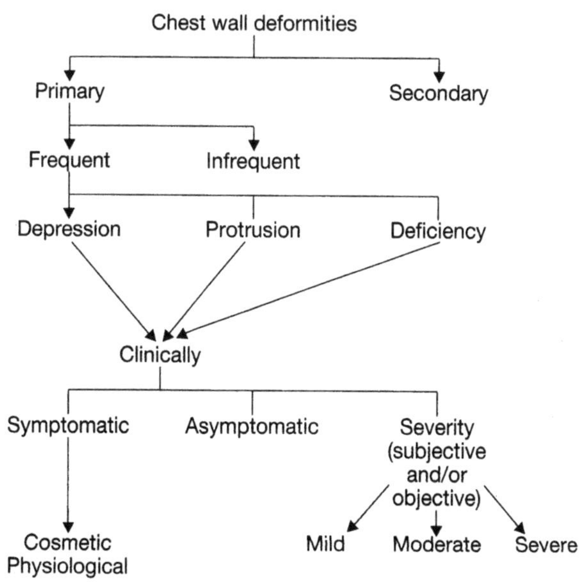

Fig. 1. An approach to the evaluation of chest wall deformities

parent who has had a deformity "all his life" and either plays down the deformity in the next generation or expresses the view that if treatment is available the child should be given the opportunity for this.

The algorithm (Fig. 1) summarizes the above and provides a preliminary approach to areas yet to be covered.

In summary, therefore, depression deformities:
1. Are the most frequent deformities
2. Have a genetic predisposition
3. Are associated with inspiratory retraction (up to the age of 4 years or thereabouts)
4. Have an unpredictable natural history
5. May be mild, moderate or severe
6. Assessment is largely subjective

Protrusion Deformities

"The chest becomes sharp pointed, not broad and becomes affected with difficulty in breathing and hoarseness" – Hippocrates [18]. The description of many of the features of funnel chest are relevant to the group of deformities known as "pigeon chest". A relatively large number of such deformities are secondary, not primary, and in particular are secondary to congenital heart disease and such respiratory disorders as asthma. However, the majority who present for cinical evaluation and opinion do not have an underlying condition which has led to the development of the deformity. Subjectively, as with depression deformities, this group may be mild, moderate or severe, but there are significant differences between the two groups. These differences occur despite the fact that the same skeletal elements are involved – sternum, costal cartilages and to a certain extent the ribs. The first difference to be noted is that there are two definite and distinct types of pigeon chest and these can be referred to as "high" or "low". Simplistically the two types have been distinguished as the "pigeon-pigeon" when a high deformity exists, or "human-pigeon" when a low deformity is present. Ravitch [38, 39] distinguished the two types as follows: "the arcuate kind which we call the pigeon breast, and other kind which is a regular chicken breast". Welch and Vos [48] described high deformity as chondromanubrial or arcuate deformity, and the more frequent "low" type as chondrogladiolar. Pickard [35] used the descriptive term "pouter pigeon-like deformity" for the chondromanubrial type; in all large series the low deformity or "human-pigeon" is the more frequent type and in this group the severity of the deformity is largely related to the extent of the forward protrusion of the sternum but this may be added to by the so-called "pinching in" of the lower costal cartilages, a feature which needs to be taken into account if surgical correction is undertaken. Lateral X-ray of the chest also indicates the degree of protrusion and reveals a normally ossified sternum with several sternebrae. Not so in the high protrusion group (Fig. 2) where a lateral radiograph usu-

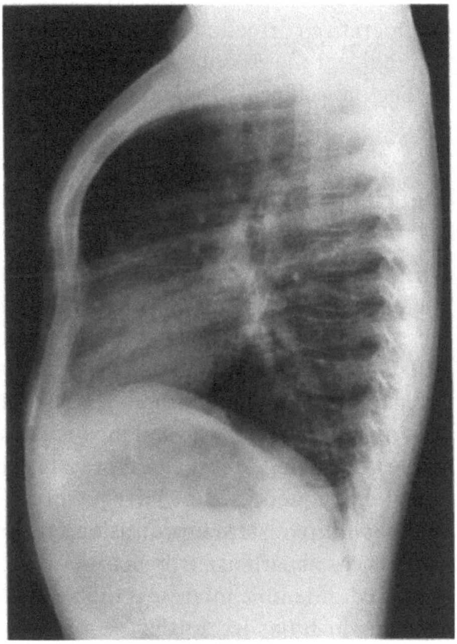

Fig. 2. High-protusion deformity: lateral X-ray (Currarino-Silverman syndrome)

ally reveals a "one-piece" sternum without the normal segmentation. This feature has been well documented by Schamberger and Welch [44] (who give credit to Currarino and Silverman [9]). It is tempting to suggest that this abnormality in ossification is of some aetiological significance. With the high protrusion there is inevitably a compensatory depression below this; not only does this lead to some descriptive diagnostic confusion, but it may also have therapeutic significance when operative correction is performed.

A second point of differences between the "funnels" and the "pigeons" relates to symptomatology; the only symptom in the protrusion is the cosmetic disability [35] and this is important in counselling because the suggestion that the deformity may interfere with activity or longevity of life can be categorically denied.

Finally, there is a third difference – in a significant number of children with a relatively severe low deformity spontaneous improvement occurs but this may take longer than in the funnel chest group and in general terms surgery should not be considered for pigeon chest before the age of 9 years. In babies with cranio-facial asymmetry thoracic wall asymmetry may also be present with parasternal elevation; the prognosis in this group is excellent in that in the course of time complete resolution of the deformity occurs.

In summary,
1. Pigeon chest is common but less so than funnel chest
2. Two major types occur – "low" and "high"

3. The "high" type is almost invariably associated with a short fused sternum
4. Operative correction is available but should certainly not be considered until it is evident that spontaneous improvement will not occur
5. The only clinical problem is the cosmetic disability

Deficiency Deformities

These are the least common of the primary deformities; the name is derived from the obvious fact that certain elements of the chest wall are deficient – specifically, ribs, costal cartilages and part of the pectoralis major. Depending upon the extent of the deformity a lung hernia may or may not be present – an alarming situation for parents who may become overanxious and overprotective towards the child. The nipple is hypoplastic and the breast anlage is also deficient so that in the post-pubertal female the ipsilateral breast is absent and there will be anticipated emotional consequences. Not infrequently there is an associated costosternal abnormality with parasternal protrusion on the ipsilateral or contralateral side and/or various costal cartilage irregularities.

Of considerable interest is the associated hand anomaly which varies in severity but which has led to the use of the eponymous nomenclature, Poland's syndactyly, for the syndrome. The original description by Alfred Polland [36] has been well documented by Ravitch [40], who reproduced Poland's original description in toto and also quoted Thomson [45], who had summarized the situation with great clarity as follows:

Under such dissimilar headings as congenital defect of the pectoral muscles, unilateral amazia, malformation of the chest wall, congenital hernia of the lungs etc. a large number of cases have been described which present in common a congenital unilateral deficiency of the structures of the front of the thorax. The salient features of these cases vary in different instances according partly to the point of view of the observer who reports them and partly to the extent of the defect...

...In all of the cases there is a congenital lateral defect of some of the structures on the front of the chest. This defects varies considerably in depth and also in extent but always mainly implicates the lower pectoral region. The structures deficient are as follows:
1. The hair in the mammary and axillary regions
2. Subcutaneous fat over the pectorals
3. The nipple and breast
4. The pectorals and some other adjacent muscles
5. The costal cartilages and anterior ends to ribs
6. The hand and forearm"

Clinically the major problem as far as the chest wall deformity is concerned is cosmetic but there may well be other problems, especially the lung hernia and the hand deformity. Treatment will need to be individualized and may require the involvement of a plastic surgeon if specific hand surgery is considered necessary. With recent developments in microvascular surgery the additional help of a surgeon skilled in this field may also be required.

In summary, therefore, deficiency deformities are:

1. Uncommon and vary in severity.
2. May require surgical correction which is best carried out when the child becomes self-conscious as a result of the deformity.
3. Latissimus dorsi transfer has provided a satisfactory alternative or addendum to earlier operative procedures.
4. Breast replacement by prosthesis will be required in affected female patients.
5. Hand deformity may accompany the chest wall deformity (Poland's syndrome).

Decision Making

With very few exceptions, the decision to operate on a patient with a chest wall deformity will depend upon the cosmetic appearance. There are two major exceptions – firstly, if a funnel chest is associated with cardiac insufficiency, corrective surgery should be undertaken, and secondly in the deficiency deformity group the presence of a lung hernia is a positive indication for surgery at some stage. These exceptions are rare and in more than 95% of operations performed for chest wall deformities the indication is cosmetic. It follows that the surgeon involved in the care of the child or adolescent with a chest wall deformity must have a very balanced view and express a very sympathetic approach to the child and his parents. Not infrequently various opinions have been expressed regarding the significance and management of the deformity prior to the interview with the surgeon – these opinions vary in keeping with the personal views of the physicians; some will have expressed the view that operation is not indicated whereas others will have given a diametrically opposite opinion. Few unfortunately will have the courage not to prejudge. Despite this the surgeon must assume prejudging has not occurred and, having taken the personal history of the patient and made relevant enquiries regarding the family history, the most important facet of the consultation follows and that is a frank and often prolonged discussion regarding the child's condition. If possible the word "deformity" should be avoided and the same applies to the term "abnormality"; it has been found that "chest wall condition" is an adequate and satisfactory phrase. Each situation needs to be individualized – at times the discussion should be conducted with the patient in the office, at times part or all of the interview is best conducted with the patient in an adjoining room.

There is nothing specific in this approach – it should apply throughout all paediatric surgical consultations. If the patient is adolescent then he or she should certainly remain throughout the entire consultation and discussion because their views are vital as far as decision making is concerned.

The surgeon should as soon as possible make it clear that there are three persons involved in the decision making; and in order of importance these are – the patient, the parents and the surgeon himself. Clearly, the involvement of the patient will vary; in the baby and toddler, involvement will be nil but will subsequently increase with increasing age and will become of paramount importance in the preadolescent and adolescent periods. Another early area of discussion

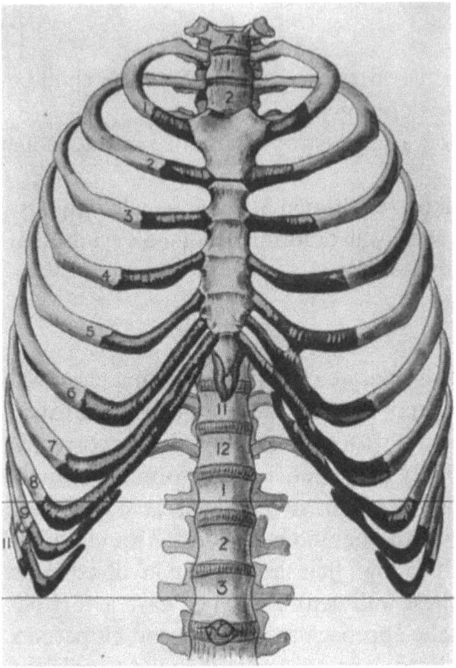

Fig. 3. Skeleton of thorax [34]. (Reproduced by kind permission of Longman Group Ltd., Edinburgh)

should address the cause of the problem; this is an area frequently overlooked but is of considerable significance to the family and possibly to the patient although the latter is more likely to be concerned regarding the natural history and treatment. A simple explanation which may or may not be valid but which is very helpful in counselling parents and children is that at some stage the costal cartilages grow too quickly and as a consequence the sternum is either pushed inwards (pectus excavatum) or outwards (pigeon chest or pectus carinatum). It is useful to have a diagram of the skeleton of the chest wall (Fig. 3) and this can act as a basis for discussion regarding cause and treatment. It is also useful to have copies of this diagram, use it during the discussion and give it to the patient and/or parents at the conclusion of the interview.

Basically, decision-making centres on the two possibilities – observation or surgery. The role of physiotherapy and allied methods of treatment may require some discussion; although the early literature contains references to the value of certain exercises, it is generally agreed that these have little or no effect on the deformity but attention to posture may be of some benefit.

In approaching a decision regarding management it is helpful to introduce or reintroduce the classification into mild, moderate and severe and although this is largely, almost completely, subjective, it is helpful. There can be little argument that the management of the patient with a mild deformity is non-operative and at the other end of the scale that subject to patient and parent attitudes it is very reasonable to advise operation for the severe deformity. This leaves perhaps the largest group – the "moderate" deformities – and here considerable judgement is required; not infrequently the best course to follow is to give a complete explanation of the nature of the deformity, indicate the possible natural history and discuss the treatment. Having done all this, the suggestion can then be made that the patient and family give the matter thought and consideration and return for a further interview after a period of months have elapsed. Should they decide to proceed with operation it is important:

1. To ensure that they appreciate the probable postoperative pain and discomfort.
2. To arrange an appropriate time for the procedure, designed to avoid as little absence from school as possible.
3. To explain the need for convalescence which will avoid contact sport for at least 6 weeks and with reference to some sports for 3 months.
4. To explain the technique which will be followed and specify the role of drain tubes and postoperative analgesic infusions [3]. There should be some discussion regarding blood transfusion although this is frequently not required.
5. To stress the need for and role of physiotherapy in the postoperative management.
6. To discuss at length the incision and specifically the unpredictability of the ultimate scar.

Such attention to detail is essential if the patient is to continue to feel confidence in the medical adviser and not to have any regrets regarding the decision to have a major operative procedure for a cosmetic disability.

In summary, therefore,

1. Frequently decision making is not difficult – this applies particularly to the mild degrees of deformity, on the one hand, and the severe deformities in the older child or adolescent on the other.
2. When there is doubt regarding the advisability of operation – a "wait and see policy" is warranted.
3. Many of the patients are in the adolescent age group – the special needs of the adolescent need to be understood and respected. Body self-image is of particular significance in this age group and may affect their thinking and their decision to request surgical correction.
4. Factors which specifically affect the decision to operate, or not to operate, other than age include the severity of the deformity, the attitude of the patient and of the parents and their attitude following the complete and adequate explanation of all aspects of the treatment which they will be given.

Surgical Options

Having made the decision to operate, the surgeon is in theory confronted with a variety of surgical possibilities. It is interesting to note that over 30 years ago

Koop [27] stated "There is less variation in recommended techniques than one might suppose. The different methods of management that are suggested, however, may indicate that no method is eminently satisfactory". On the other hand, there can be little doubt that satisfactory results can be obtained from different techniques but, to assess this, very long-term follow-up is essential particularly in the child and the early adolescent. As time passes the literature contains more and more references to "new" operations, but for the most part the variations in technique are very much variations in detail rather than principle.

The principles which have governed the author's surgical approach are as follows:

1. To accept the fact that there is no place for the "limited" operation as originally described by Brown [5] and referred to by Lester [29].
2. If possible to avoid operation in children under the age of 10–12 years. Even this age is regarded by some as being too young, but experience has shown that severe or moderately severe deformities in this age group can be successfully managed surgically with no increased risk of recurrence – despite the adolescent growth spurt which can be anticipated.

Despite the author's preference for operating in the preadolescent phase, there is no doubt that in our experience the majority of patients will present for surgery as adolescents; although this is in fact a reflection of the increasing concern of the adolescent for his or her physical image another very important factor is the increasing severity of deformity which occurs at this time. This is directly related to the adolescent growth spurt.

3. With the recognition of the many problems which occurred in the earlier years, we have come to the conclusion that an operative procedure is preferable to the use of a preformed, prefabricated prosthesis [31, 46]. We refer to the operative procedure as sternochondrioplasty.
4. Preoperative orientation of nursing staff and physiotherapy staff who will also be involved in the patient's management. This is essential if the postoperative course is to be as uncomplicated as possible; the nursing staff have a continuous role to play and therefore they must understand the background to the decision to operate, the planned procedure and the basis of the postoperative care. To facilitate this, admission to hospital should be at least 36 h before the time arranged for operation.

The surgical techniques available are well described in the literature and there is no doubt that a satisfactory end result may be obtained from several of these techniques including procedures without the use of internal fixation [15], procedures with such use, including the use of perichondrium as described by Fonkalsrud [12], fixation in various planes using various struts and splints [1, 34, 43], and sternal "turnover" [37, 47, 49]. An excellent summary of many of the operative procedures described was given by Humphreys [23] in 1974 and by Holcomb [19] in 1977. The author has progressed to the procedure to be described largely as a result of dissatisfaction with earlier procedures and recognition of the need for internal fixation in depression deformities and in many of the high-protrusion deformities. Our earliest experience at the Royal Children's Hospital, Melbourne, included fixation of the sternum using an external splint of the Jacob's ladder type (originally described by Brown [5] nearly 50 years ago); this was followed by a period when fixation other than by sternal suture following sternal osteotomy was not part of the operative programme and reliance was placed on operative correction and postoperative physiotherapy. Although many satisfactory results were obtained. Howard [22] pointed out that the recurrence rate was unacceptable and many were operated on for a second time. This second operation had as a major principle the use of a retrosternal subperiostial rib strut. A segment of the fifth rib was resected subperiostially and as a free graft was placed deep to the sternum at the level of the fourth costal cartilages to which it was fixed on both sides. Although satisfactory in Howard's hands, others did not find the procedure to their liking and one group of surgeons adopted the Rehbein [41] procedure. When Wesselhoeft [50] described his technique involving the use of an internal metal strut, the author decided to follow this technique with some modification and at about the same time was influenced by the teaching of Ravitch [40], and from this a technique has evolved and will be described. A guiding principle in the surgical correction of funnel chest has been the recognition that success essentially depends upon *adequate advancement of the sternum and its fixation in an appropriate position.*

Surgical Technique

If an eponymous title were to be given to the technique it could be the Myers modification of the Howard-Ravitch-Wesselhoeft procedure, although as pointed out by Wesselhoeft many others have advocated internal fixation by a variety of means.

The patient is postured in the supine position; it is acceptable to have the IV line in one or other arm but it is essential that both arms are placed by the side; if one or other arm is abducted to facilitate access by the anaesthetist, blood may "pool" in the axilla and increase the postoperative discomfort.

The incision is transverse from nipple line to nipple line and is centered over the level of the xiphisternal joint junction; some modification is possible in boys – but not in girls – in that the incision can be made a short distance above the level of the xiphisternal joint. In prepubertal girls a transverse incision at the xiphisternal joint level will prove to be satisfactory and when breast development occurs the scar will ultimately be sited in the inframammary groove and will be cosmetically ideal.

When the patient is a postpubertal female the incision should be in the inframammary groove and, to ensure that it is correctly sited, it should be marked with an appropriate pen in the ward with the patient standing up. If this is not done the incision placed in the inframammary groove with the patient lying on her back can result in the scar on the breasts themselves and not in the grooves below the breast. The consequences can be disastrous.

Having made the skin incision, this is carried through the underlying fascia and muscle mass to the chest wall and then superior and inferior musculocutaneous flaps are elevated; haemostasis is obtained by the use of the coagulation cautery, which is also used during the dissection to lessen the blood loss (in the majority of patients, with careful attention to detail blood transfusion will not be required; if the anaesthetist is happy with the techniques of operative hypotension this is an additional beneficial manoeuvre). The superior flap is elevated to a level decided preoperatively and assessment will have determined whether there will be a need to resect the second costal cartilage and/or perform sternal osteotomy above the level of the third costal cartilage. However high the need for operation on costal cartilages and sternum it is not necessary to use a longitudinal incision. The superior flap can be elevated to an adequate degree via a transverse incision.

More difficulty is experienced when the inferior musculocutaneous flap is elevated, necessitating dissection from the chest wall of the caudal portion of the pectoralis major, and the upper elements of the external oblique and the rectus abdominis muscles. It is expedient to reach an advanced point in the dissection of the lower flap before the xiphoid process is separated from its attachment to the main body of the sternum, separation which will usually necessitate the use of sharp bone cutters. It is preferable to divide the xiphisternal attachment at this stage and then ready access to the anterior mediastinum can be obtained at a later stage. The free xiphoid process is retracted inferiorly and this places on tension adjacent muscle fibres which can readily be divided. Dissection is carried inferiorly to the level of the costal margin and can usually be completed by blunt dissection.

To this point in the operation the technique is identical for depression and protrusion deformities and in many ways the techniques remain identical in that segments of the costal cartilages on both sides are now resected. The resection is performed in the subperichondrial plane; although a difficult plane to establish there are many advantages in preserving the perichondrium at this stage.

Funnel Chest

Segments of the third to the seventh costal cartilage will be resected but it is important only to resect a minimal segment of the fourth costal cartilages because at a later stage the retrosternal strut will be sutured to these cartilages. Occasionally it may be necessary to remove part of the second and/or eighth cartilage. The lateral end of each cartilage is preserved; our experience has shown that complete resection of the upper cartilages may be associated with an otherwise avoidable unsightly overgrowth of the second costal cartilages.

At this stage it may or not be possible to decide whether sternal osteotomy is necessary; opposing views are expressed in the very extensive literature on the subject regarding the necessity for osteotomy. The retrosternal strut is now introduced and to do this blunt dissection of the anterior mediastinum is performed

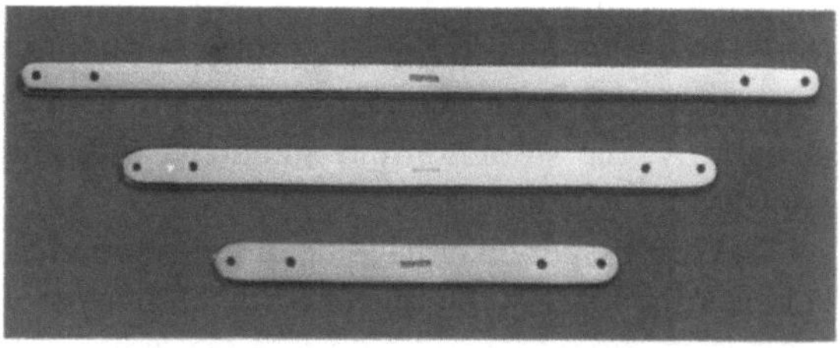

Fig. 4. Retrosternal steel struts (three sizes) used at the Royal Children's Hospital, Melbourne

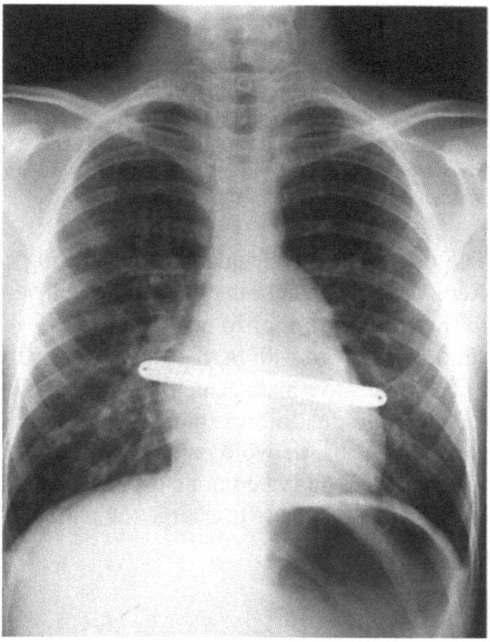

Fig. 5. Postoperative X-ray shows retrosternal strut

and on both sides the pleura is swept laterally (the right pleural cavity is not infrequently entered at this stage – this has not been a problem but it is essential for the anaesthetist to maintain complete expansion of the right lung and to ensure complete haemostasis to avoid the development of a right-sided haemothorax). A plane is developed between the sternum and its posterior periosteum at the level of the fourth costal cartilages and a stainless steel strut of appropriate length is introduced. (This is a modification of the procedure described by Wesselhoeft [50]) in 1982, who placed a strut transsternally and others (e.g. Sbokos [43]), who placed the strut behind the sternum leaving the posterior periostium intact.] The strut we use has blunt ends (Figs. 4, 5) with two holes at either and to enable it to be sutured to the costal cartilages on either side. Non-absorbable sutures are used for this purpose. This combined with its position in the subperiosteal plane provides adequate fixation.

If osteotomy is deemed necessary this is performed at an appropriate level; a triangular wedge of sternum is removed, thereby enabling the sternal depression to be corrected and, at the same time, if there is sternal rotation this too can be corrected. This is an anterior sternotomy with the apex of the wedge pointing posteriorly; the sternotomy is stabilized with anterior periosteal fixation (using polyglycolic acid sutures).

The soft tissues on either side of the sternum are divided to a point immediately below the level of the fourth costal cartilages; very careful attention to haemostasis is essential to avoid a postoperative haematoma or haemothorax. With reference to this point in the operation it is interesting to quote from Ravitch [40], who wrote

> The intercostal bundles are divided from the sternum while the sternum is elevated... a cut usually being made between the internal mammary vessels and the sternum. It astonishes me that a number of operators do not divide the intercostal bundles. Seeing how little the position of the sternum can be corrected until the sternum has been freed in this manner and observing how well the sternum comes forward after the intercostal bundles have been divided, I can only marvel that good results are achieved without this step.

The operation is concluded by introducing one or two drainage catheters of the Redi-vac type and closing the wound in layers. The muscles should be reattached to the chest wall prior to layered closure, which is completed with a subcuticular suture reinforced with Steri-strips. A pressure dressing is applied.

Postoperative management includes the use of an analgesic infusion [3, 10, 11, 42] and a gradual return to an upright position. Physiotherapy is commenced as early as possible to avoid pulmonary complications; the drain tube is removed on the 2nd or 3rd day when drainage has ceased. Early amublation is encouraged and it is usually possible to discharge the patient from hospital on or about the seventh postoperative day.

Pigeon Chest

The chest wall is exposed through a similar incision and, as with sternochondrioplasty for funnel chest, superior and inferior musculocutaneous flaps are elevated [20]. In the low protrusion deformity, following partial resection of the costal cartilages (second or third to seventh), the appearance of the chest wall is evaluated and the decision made regarding the need for sternal osteotomy and osteotomies of the ribs. If osteotomy of the sternum is necessary this is a simple open transverse osteotomy; osteotomies of several ribs are frequently required to avoid persisting protrusion of the costal cartilages relative to the sternum. Following these osteotomies correction is obtained by suturing the divided costal cartilage to the perichondrium medial to this or frequently to the lateral edge of the sternum. There is no need for internal fixation in the low protrusion type of deformity. The xiphoid process is reattached to the anterior surface of the lower end of the sternum and this provdes additional correction.

High-protrusion deformities are less common; a relatively large wedge osteotomy is performed at the apex of the deformity and stabilized with anterior periosteal sutures. Frequently there is a central depression in this group below the osteotomy and this will need correction by means of a retrosternal strut, the technique being identical to that described above for funnel chest.

In summary:

1. Operative sternochondrioplasty is the procedure of choice for the correction of both depression and protrusion deformities.
2. Although the principles of surgical treatment are similar in both groups, and in all patients, individual variations are required in keeping with the exact deformity present.
3. In funnel chest internal fixation of the advanced sternum is required.
4. The additional manoeuvre of dividing the soft tissues on either side of the lower sternum enhances the end result.
5. In the more frequently encountered pigeon chest ("low") deformity) internal fixation is not required. It may be necessary in the "high" deformity.
6. Careful attention to detail and anatomical closure will facilitate convalescence and the end result. Of particular importance is obliteration of dead space anterior to the sternum.
7. Despite careful attention to detail, the ultimate scar is unpredictable.

The Uncommon Varieties of Chest Wall Deformities

These can be listed as follows:

Deficiency Deformities

Reference has previously been made to this type of deformity and also to the excellent account of this condition given by Ravitch [40]. Operation is not required in the lesser degree of deficiency deformity; in those with a more severe deformity various operative procedures have been used and the technique include thoracoplasty utilizing the ribs and/or costal cartilages on the ipsilateral side, rib graft from the contralateral side and latisimus dorsi transplant [16, 17]. Many will also require some form of sternochondrioplasty when there is a significant deformity of the elements of the chest wall on the side opposite to the side of the deficiency.

Each patient will certainly need to be individualized with regard to:

1. Need for surgery
2. Timing of surgery
3. Optimal procedure
4. Additional procedures such as implantation mammoplasty or hand surgery

Cleft sternum

This rare condition may occur in isolation or may be associated either with true ectopia cordis or the pentalogy of Cantrell [7]. Mogilner [33] recently described one form of surgical management of cleft sternum.

Jeune's Syndrome (Asphyxiating Thoracic Dystrophy of the Newborn) [25, 26]

Synonyms for this condition include thoracic, pelvic, phalangeal dystrophy, Jeune thoracic dysplasia and infantile thoracic dystrophy. It is evident from the literature that this condition is rare and covers a wide spectrum from the "minor" form to the "major" form, a point well made by Ravitch [40], who has summarized much of the world experience.

Bizarre Rib Deformities

In the most severe form (Fig. 6), there is absence of many ribs and irregularity of others. The resulting paradox may lead to respiratory insufficiency or even respiratory failure. The patient whose X-ray is depicted in Fig. 6 was successfully managed using a Marlex prosthesis. He is awaiting surgery for the associated severe scoliosis.

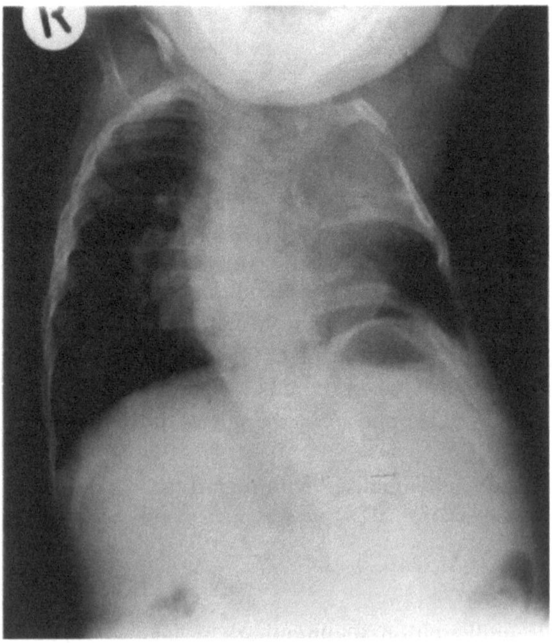

Fig. 6. Bizarre rib deformity

These are but a few of a miscellaneous group of abnormalities encountered in paediatric surgical practice. Limited abnormalities of cartilage and rib are frequently seen and rarely require any treatment other than reassurance. The rarity of the more severe deformities limits the experience of any one surgeon and faced with the unusual the surgeon is well advised to consult the literature and seek help from those who have had some experience in the field. An international register of the rarer of the anomalies would be helpful and could be organized by an appropriate national or international association.

Discussion

When one considers the extensive literature on the subject of chest wall deformities it is necessary to justify an additional article; the justification is that although the published articles, chapters and monographs provide an enormous amount of information regarding historical events of significance, types of deformity encountered in clinical practice and personal experience with management, they do not always specifically address the important issue of management of the individual patient and his or her family.

It is important to recognize that although a relatively simple classification is available recognizing the following three groups: (a) depression deformities, (b) protrusion deformities and (c) infrequently encountered deformities (including deficiency deformities), variants and combined forms are seen. Also with each group of deformities there is a spectrum of severity ranging from mild to severe. It follows that assessment of each patient must be individualized and therapeutic decisions made for the patient – not the deformity. The whole subject is emotive and assessment is frequently more subjective than objective; thus a deformity which may appear mild to the medical advisers may be severe in the eyes of child and parents. On the other hand attention may be drawn to a child's "deformity" as a result of a routine examination and they may have previously been unaware of any abnormality; unfortunate psychological consequences can follow.

Another important aspect relates to the fact that, although the majority of patients who present for assessment have a *primary* chest wall deformity, in a significant number the deformity is *secondary*. The need for accurate history taking and a complete physical examination is therefore twofold; firstly, it will be a basis for the subsequent discussion, and secondly it should enable underlying and secondly it should enable recognition of underlying disorders which have resulted in the deformity. At times these will be obvious, for example in patients with chronic asthma or congenital heart disease; in others the diagnosis may be less obvious as in some patients with Marfan's syndrome, but careful attention to detail should avoid such diagnoses being missed.

Fortunately most patients with chest wall deformity are otherwise completely normal and during the interview it is possible to stress this. In this way many fears can be allayed. Also, fortunately, in only a relatively small number of patients will surgery be considered – however, the number will reflect the referral pattern and in some situations only the more severe deformities may be referred, thus influencing the proportion of patients on whom surgery will be considered and/or performed.

Although opinions vary regarding the physiological significance of depression deformities, there is now sufficient data combined with many anecdotal experiences to be able to accept the fact that in some there is slight reduction in vital capacity and increased oxygen usage during breathing [14]. In our institution, Mead et al. [32] tested the hypothesis that such patients may have limitation in rib cage mobility but concluded that when a moderate deformity was present "there is no evidence to suggest limitation of rib cage mobility". Mead postulated that "it is possible that patients with more severe involvement may have rib cage restriction". Further pre- and postoperative studies are needed to study this hypothesis.

From clinical experience there can be no doubt that physiological disturbance is unusual and although some objective data are available the majority of patients are asymptomatic, and postoperative improvement in athletic performance is more likely to be of multifactorial origin. The same may well apply to the patient's general health and any decrease in the frequency of respiratory tract infections. In this context a well-conducted longitudinal trial with adequate data from normal controls is necessary. This should prove one way or the other whether improvement is related to or independent of the anatomical correction of the chest wall deformity.

The conclusion to be reached is that although investigation of cardiopulmonary function may show variations from the normal these are probably of little significance in most patients and can be ignored. In fact investigation other than a routine X-ray of the chest is unnecessary. With very few exceptions the only problem in the patient with a chest wall deformity is the cosmetic disability and its psychological implications and this will be the factor which influences therapeutic decisions. Operative correction is available for those who require it and although a variety of techniques have been described it is probable that different procedures will produce a satisfactory end result. It must be stressed, however, that very long-term follow-up is essential if the ultimate result is to be adequately evaluated.

The surgeon called upon to assess and manage a patient with chest wall deformity must have an open mind and regard each patient, and the family, as an individual. Total application to detail in the interview, in the transoperative management and in the follow-up is obligatory if a satisfactory end result is to be achieved.

References

1. Adkins PC, Blades B (1961) A stainless steel strut for correction of pectus excavatum. Surg Gynecol Obstet113 : 111
2. Bay V, Farthmann E, Naegele U (1970) Unoperated funnel chest in middle and advanced age: evaluation of indications for operation. J Pediatr Surg 5 : 606
3. Beasley SW, Tibballs J (1987) Efficacy and safety of continuous morphine infusion for postoperative analgaesia in the paediatric surgical ward. Aust NZ J Surg 57 : 233

4. Blickman JG, Rosen PR, Welch KJ, et al (1985) Pectus excavatum in children: pulmonary scintigraphy before and after corrective surgery. Radiology 167:781
5. Brown AL (1939) Pectus excavatum (funnel chest) J Thorac Surg 9:164
6. Cahill JL, Lees GM, Robertson HT (1984) A summary of preoperative and postoperative cardiorespiratory performance in patients undergoing pectus excavatum and carinatum repair. J Pediatr Surg 19:430
7. Cantrell JR, Haller JA, Ravitch MM (1958) A syndrome of congenital defects involving the abdominal wall, sternum, diaphragm, pericardium and heart. Surg Gynecol Obstet 107: 602
8. Castile RG, Staats BA, Westbrook PR (1982) Symptomatic pectus deformities of the chest. Am Rev Respir Dis 126:564
9. Currarino G, Silverman FN (1958) Premature obliteration of the sternal sutures and pigeon-breast deformity. Radiology 70:532
10. Dilworth NM (1988) Children in pain: an underprivileged group. Editorial. J Pediatr Surg 23:103
11. Dilworth NM, Mackellar A (1987) Pain relief for the pediatric surgical patient. J Pediatr Surg 22:264
12. Fonkalsrud EW, Follette D, Sarwat AK (1978) Pectus excavatum repair using autologous perichondrium for sternal support. Arch Surg 113:1433
13. Gattiken H, Buhlmann A (1966) Cardiopulmonary function and exercise tolerance in supine and sitting position in patients with pectus excavatum. Helv Med Acta 33:122
14. Gyllensward A, Irnell L, Michaellsson M, et al (1975) Pectus excavatum. A clinical study with longterm postoperative follow-up. Acta Paediatr Scand [Suppl] 255:1
15. Haller JA Jr, Shermeta DW, Teas JJ (1978) Correction of pectus excavatum without prosthesis or splints. Objective measurement of severity and management of asymmetrical deformities. Ann Thorac Surg 26:73
16. Haller JA Jr, Colombani PM, Miller D, et al (1984) Early reconstruction of Poland's syndrome using autologous rib grafts combined with a latissimus dorsi flap. J Pediatr Surg 19:423
17. Hester TR Jr, Bostwick J III. (1982) Poland's syndrome correction with latissimus muscle transposition. Plast Reconstr Surg 69:226
18. Hippocrates (1849) Genuine works, Sydenham Society
19. Holcomb GW Jr (1977) Surgical correction of pectus excavatum. J Pediatr Surg 12:295
20. Howard R (1958) Pigeon chest (protrusion deformity of the sternum) Med J Aust 2:664
21. Howard R (1959) Funnel chest: its effect on cardiac function. Arch Dis Child 34:5
22. Howard R (1978) Funnel chest: results and description of an improved operative technique. Med J Aust 2:134
23. Humpreys GH II, Jaretzki A III (1974) Operative correction of pectus excavatum. J Pediatr Surg 9:899
24. Jamieson EB (1937) Illustrations of regional anatomy, sect 5. Livingstone, Edinburgh
25. Jeune M, Carron R, Beraud C (1954) Polychondrodystrophie avec blocage thoracique d'evolution fatale. Pediatrie 9:390
26. Jeune M, Carron R, Beraud C (1955) Dystrophie thoracique asphyxiante de caractere familial. Arch Franc Pediatr 12:886
27. Koop CE (1956) The management of pectus excavatum. Surg Clin North Am 1627
28. Landtman B (1958) The heart in funnel chest. Pre and post operative studies of seventy cases. Ann Paediatr Fenn 4:181
29. Lester CW (1946) The surgical treatment of funnel chest. Ann Surg 123:1003
30. Lyons HA, Zuhdi MN, Kelly JJ (1955) Pectus excavatum ("funnel breast"). A cause of impaired ventricular distensibility as established by right ventricular pressure patterns. Am Heart J 50:921
31. Masson JK, Payne SW, Gonzalez JB (1970) Pectus excavatum: use of preformed prosthesis for correction in the adult. Plast Reconstr Surg 46:399
32. Mead J, Sly P, Le Soeuf P (1985) Rib cage mobility in pectus excavatum. Am Rev Respir Dis 132:1223

33. Mogilner J, Siplovich L, Barziv J, et al (1988) Surgical management of the cleft sternum. J Pediatr Surg 23:889
34. Naef AP (1976) The surgical treatment of pectus excavatum: an experience with 90 operations. Ann Thorac Surg 21:63
35. Pickard LR, Tepas JJ, Shermeta DW, et al (1978) Pectus carinatum: results of surgical therapy. J Pediatr Surg 14:228
36. Poland A (1841) Deficiency of the pectoral muscles. Guy's Hosp Rep VI:191
37. Pouliquen JC, Beneux J, Pasteyer J, et al (1973) Turning over of the sternal breast plate as a treatment for funnel chest. Report of 19 cases. Ann Chir Inf 14:245
38. Ravitch MM (1971) The form of congenital deformities of the chest and their treatment. Prog Pediatr Surg 3:1–12
39. Ravitch MM (1973) Discussion of "surgical correction of pectus carinatum (pigeon breast)." Article by Welch KJ and Voss A. J Pediatr Surg 8:666–667
40. Ravitch MM (1977) Congenital deformities of the chest wall and their operative correction. Saunders, Philadelphia
41. Rehbein F, Wernicke HH (1957) The operative treatment of the funnel chest. Arch Dis Child 32 (161):5–8
42. Rodgers BM, Webb CJ, Stergios D, et al (1988) Patient controlled analgaesia in pediatric surgery. J Pediatr Surg 23:259
43. Sbokos CG, McMillan IKR, Akins CW (1975) Surgical correction of pectus excavatum using a retrosternal bar. Thorax 30:40
44. Shamberger RC, Welch KJ (1988) Surgical correction of chondromanubrial deformity (Currarino Silverman Syndrome). J Pediatr Surg 23:319
45. Thomson J (1895) On a form of congenital thoracic deformity. Teratology II:1–12, Plates I–V
46. Vecchione TR (1978) Cosmetic correction of the mild or partially corrected pectus excavatum utilizing silastic implant. Ann Plast Surg 1:575
47. Wada J, Ideka K (1972) Clinical experience with 306 funnel chest operations. Int Surg 57:707
48. Welch KJ, Vos A (1973) Surgical correction of pectus cariantum. J Pediatr Surg 8:659
49. Wada J, Ikeda I, Ishida T, et al (1970) Results of 271 funnel chest operations. Ann Thorac Surg 10:526
50. Wesselhoeft CW Jr, De Luca FG (1982) A simplified approach to the repair of pediatric pectus deformities. Ann Thorac Surg 34:640

Unusual Problems in Oesophageal Surgery in Childhood

N. A. Myers

Summary

Unusual problems in oesophageal surgery in childhood include problems seen both frequently and infrequently. The former includes oesophageal atresia, peptic oesophagitis and corrosive oesophagitis; the latter includes such conditions as neonatal rupture of the oesophagus, explosive rupture of the oesophagus, achalasia of the cardia, pharyngo-oesophageal fibromatosis, nasogastric intubation stricture and stricture in the immunologically compromised patient. Examples of all of these conditions have been presented and reference has also been made to a wide variety of other conditions which have been reported in the literature. Because diagnostic delay is relatively common it is important for the paediatric surgeon carefully to evaluate the symptom of dysphagia when it is present and appreciate the fact that although organic disease in childhood is relatively uncommon there are many conditions which demand diagnosis and appropriate treatment.

Zusammenfassung

Sowohl bei häufigen als auch bei seltenen Erkrankungen gibt es in der Ösophaguschirurgie besondere Probleme. Die ersteren umfassen die Ösophagusatresie, peptische Ösophagitis und Ösophagusverätzungen, zu letzteren gehören Erkrankungen wie die explosive Ösophagusruptur, die Neugeborenenösophagusruptur, Kardiaachalasie, pharyngoösophageale Fibromatose, nasogastrische Intubationsstenose und Strikturen beim immunologisch gefährdeten Patienten. Beispiele aller dieser Erkrankungen werden präsentiert, und es wird Bezug genommen auf eine große Vielzahl anderer, über die in der Literatur berichtet wurde. Da es relativ häufig zu einer Verzögerung der Diagnose kommt, ist es für den Kinderchirurgen wichtig, das Symptom der eventuell auftretenden Dysphagie sorgfältig zu bewerten und die Tatsache zu berücksichtigen, daß es trotz relativer Seltenheit organischer Erkrankungen im Kindesalter viele pathologische Zustände gibt, die exakte Diagnostik und adäquate Behandlung erfordern.

Résumé

Les problèmes auxquels la chirurgie oesophagienne de l'enfant se voit confrontée sont autant le fait d'affections fréquentes que d'affections plus rares. Parmi les affections fréquentes, citons l'atrésie oesophagienne, l'oesophagite peptique et l'oesophagite caustique et parmi les affections rares la rupture de l'oesophage du nouveau-né, la rupture explosive de l'oesophage, le cardiospasme, la fibromatose pharyngo-oesophagienne, la sténose naso-gastrique d'intubation et la sténose chez un patient dont les défenses immunologiques sont affaiblies. Les auteurs présentent des exemples de chacune de ces affections et se réfèrent à un grand nombre d'autres affections traitées dans la littérature. Vu qu'il arrive fréquemment que le diagnostic soit posé avec quelque

Department of General Surgery, Royal Children's Hospital Melbourne, Flemington Road, Parkville 3052, Victoria, Australia.

Progress in Pediatric Surgery, Vol. 27
Myers and Angerpointner (Eds.)

retard, le chirurgien se doit d'évaluer avec soin le symptôme de dysphagie qui peut se présenter et tenir compte du fait que, bien que les affections organiques ne soient pas de règle chez les enfants, un grand nombre d'affections doivent être diagnostiquées et traitées.

Introduction

In the literature, as in clinical practice, oesophageal problems in childhood predominantly relate to oesophageal atresia, with or without tracheo-oesophageal fistula. This is undoubtedly appropriate because oesophageal atresia is a relatively common congenital anomaly, the figures quoted bearing testimony to this. Thus Haight [28] in 1957 suggested an incidence of 1:4500 births, Myers [52] in 1974 and Aberdeen and Myers [2] in 1979 a similar incidence, whereas Warren et al. [84] in 1979 placed the figure at 1:3000.

However, in certain patients with oesophageal atresia, unusual problems arise and, similarly, unusual problems arise in other frequently encountered conditions affecting the child's oesophagus, such as peptic oesophagitis and corrosive oesophagitis. In addition, infrequently, other diseases of the oesophagus are seen in childhood, examples including such conditions as neonatal rupture of the oesophagus, fibromatosis of the oesophagus and traumatic oesophageal pseudodiverticulum.

The purpose of this paper is to draw attention to the unusual problems seen in the oesophagus and hopefully to stimulate paediatricians, thoracic surgeons and paediatric surgeons to report their experiences. An international registry of such problems would be invaluable to those called upon to treat such unusual conditions and the suggestion is made that such a registry be organized.

Classification

From the above, it is evident that there are two broad groups [53] (Fig. 1) to be considered as being "unusual" oesophageal problems:

Group 1: unusual problems in frequently encountered conditions
Group 2: unusual problems in conditions seen infrequently

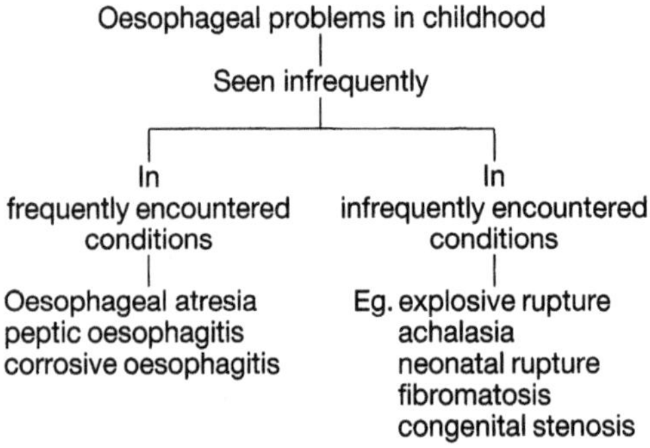

Fig. 1. Oesophageal problems in childhood: clinical classification

Group 1: Unusual Problems in Frequently Encountered Conditions

Oesophageal Atresia

Although the surgical anatomy in most babies with oesophageal atresia, with or without a tracheo-oesophageal fistula, is predictable, variants do occur (Kluth [42]). The following case reports illustrate one particular variant (cases 1, 2); an unusual method of effecting alimentary continuity in a baby with oesophageal atresia and distal fistula (case 3); unusual problems distal to the anastomosis (cases 4, 5), and an extreme example of staged management in a patient who had an intact upper oesophageal pouch for over 3½ years (case 6).

Case 1: Baby A
Baby A was born on 17 March 1972; excessive mucus was present with drooling, and the provisional diagnosis was oesophageal atresia. An orogastric tube was passed and reached a point 14 cm from the lips, and it was thought that this excluded the diagnosis. However, when fed, milk was regurgitated immediately and therefore a radiopaque study of the oesophagus was performed (Figs. 2, 3). Having confirmed the diagnosis of oesophageal atresia (excluding two conditions considered in the differential diagnosis, namely oesophageal stenosis and para-

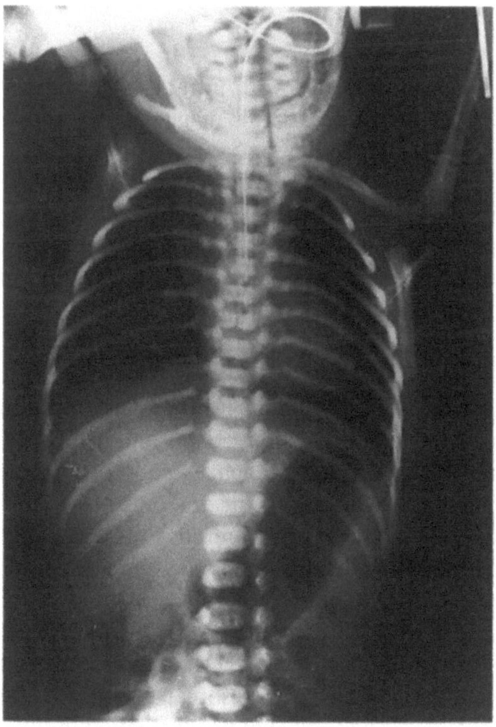

Fig. 2. Case 1: baby A. Oesophageal atresia with very low proximal segment (T6-7)

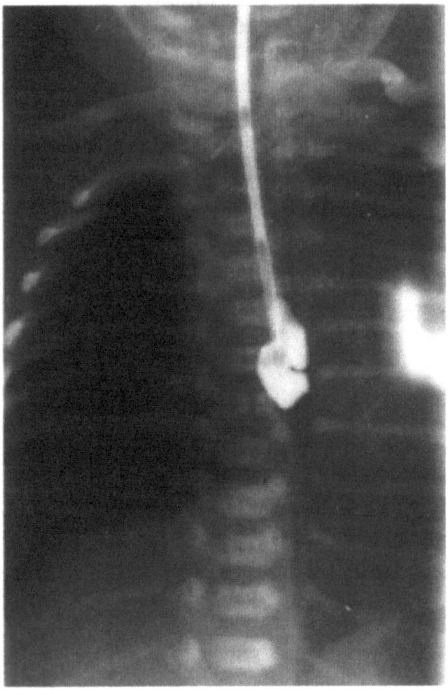

Fig. 3. Same case as Fig. 2: radiopaque study of upper pouch

oesophageal hernia with intrathoracic stomach), extrapleural right thoracotomy was performed and the diagnosis of oesophageal atresia with distal tracheo-oesophageal fistula confirmed. The unusual feature was the length of the upper pouch, which was combined with a common muscular sleeve to both segments. When first seen in the mediastinum, the oesophagus had a near-normal appearance. Quite extensive dissection was performed to enable end-to-end anastomosis be performed. The baby also had a complicated cardiac defect which led to his death on the seventh postoperative day.

Case 2: Baby B

Baby B was drooling mucus soon after birth on 15 September 1988. An orogastric tube met an obstruction 13 cm from the lips and a straight X-ray revealed an upper oesophageal pouch which extended to the level of the sixth thoracic vertebra (Fig. 4). At operation, the anatomy was identical to that described above but the surgical management differed; thus, after elucidating the situation, the tracheo-oesophageal fistula was divided and the lower oesophageal segment left in situ below the site of division, but resecting the mucosa from this segment by a stripping technique comparable to the technique used in the Soave procedure for Hirschsprung's disease. The septum between the two oesophageal segments was then divided to allow oesophageal continuity to be effected. The object of this manoeuvre was, by avoiding dissection in the oesophageal wall, to minimize post-

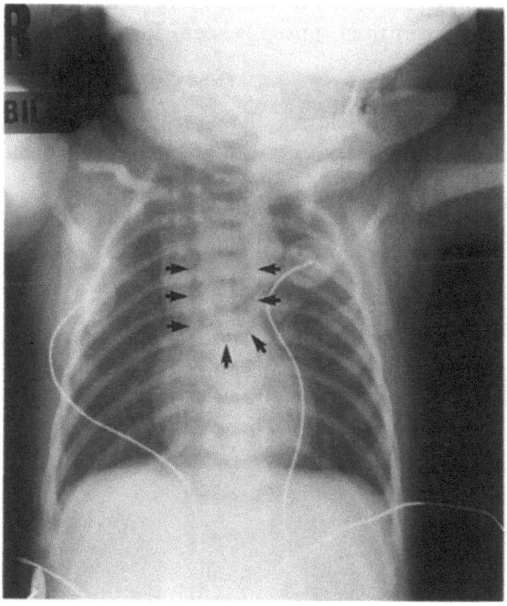

Fig. 4. Case 2: baby B. Oesophageal atresia; proximal pouch extending to T7

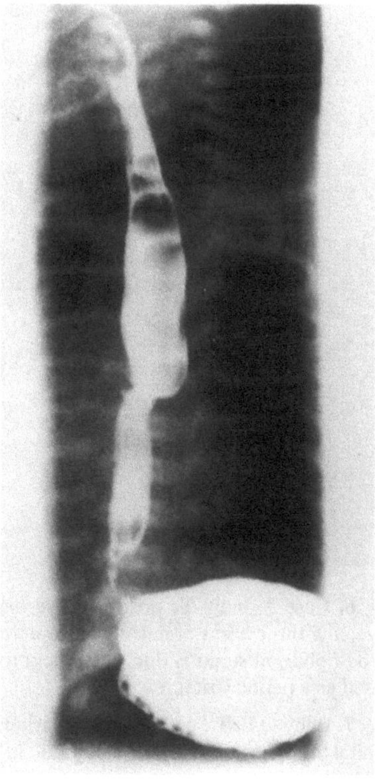

Fig. 5. Same case as Fig. 4: postoperative barium swallow showing low level of anastomosis

operative motility disturbance. The level of the anastomosis was clearly considerably lower than is usually seen (Fig. 5).

Comment

Reference to Kluth's "Atlas" [42] indicates that many variations of oesophageal atresia and/or tracheo-oesophageal fistula occur; the above represents only one of these variants but indicates the need for the surgeon operating on a baby with oesophageal atresia and a distal fistula to be familiar with this type of anomaly and plan the surgery accordingly.

Case 3: Baby Y

Thsi baby had some dysphagia following standard repair of oesophageal atresia with a distal trachea-oesophageal fistula; barium swallow (Fig. 6) revealed three

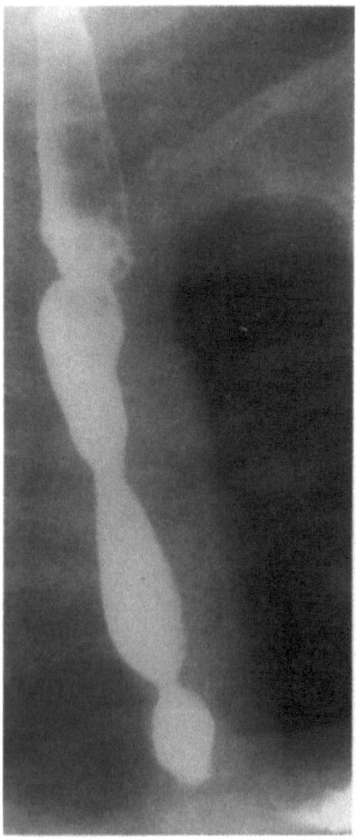

6

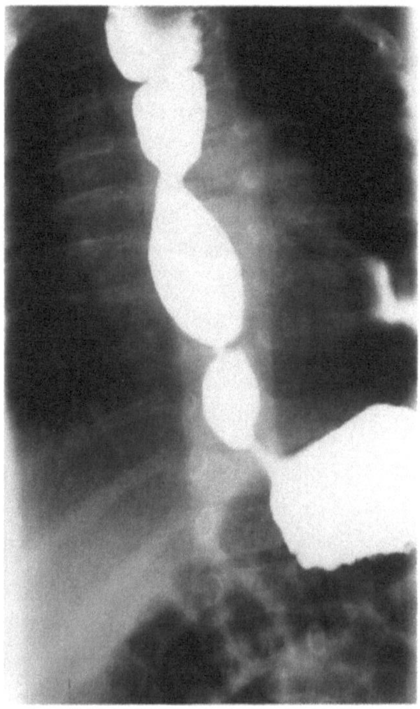

7

Fig. 6. Case 3: baby Y: postoperative barium swallow following repair of oesophageal atresia revealing three areas of narrowing – anastomotic stricture, mid-oesophageal stricture diagnosed as oesophageal stenosis due to tracheobronchial remnant and a stricture above the cardia diagnosed as a peptic stricture

Fig. 7. Baby C.L.B.: postoperative barium swallow revealing site of anastomosis above and congenital oesophageal stricture below due to a proven tracheobronchial remnant (the slight narrowing in the mid-oesophagus was inconstant and related to a "stripping" peristaltic wave)

areas of narrowing. Proximally the site of the anastomosis can be recognized; below this is a second narrowing which has been diagnosed as oesophageal stenosis due to a presumed tracheobronchial remnant and a third area of narrowing is present at the lower end of the oesophagus. This was attributed to a peptic stricture. As yet further surgery has not been performed.

Case 4: Baby B

This baby also had a standard repair of oesophageal atresia with a distal fistula; dysphagia commenced when solid foods were introduced into the diet. A barium study (Fig. 7) revealed inconsequential narrowing at the anastomotic site and a "tight" stricture in the lower third of the oesophagus. This latter was excised through a left thoracotomy and histologically was found to be a stricture due to a tracheobronchial remnant. A postoperative study of the oesophagus (Fig. 8) showed no residual narrowing at the site of resection and subsequently the clinical course has been completely satisfactory.

Comment

There are now several reports in the literature of congenital oesophageal stenosis due to a tracheobronchial remnant [3, 10, 17, 22, 37, 38, 44, 49, 58, 59, 60, 69, 73, 74, 80, 81] and there is a definite association with oesophageal atresia. Swallowing difficulties following repair of oesophageal atresia are usually due to a motility disorder with or without narrowing at the anastomotic site; however, these two cases illustrate that other factors may be involved and emphasize the necessity for at least one routine postoperative oesophagogram and later studies if the clinical situation warrants this. Strictures due to tracheobronchial remnants do not usually respond to dilatation and, if the symptoms are severe, resection of the stricture is indicated.

Case 5: Baby C

This baby, with oesophageal atresia and a distal tracheo-oesophageal fistula, was born following a gestational period of 30 weeks. The birth weight was 1200 g. The clinical course was complicated and stormy. At the initial operation, the tracheo-oesophageal fistula was divided and gastrostomy was performed with a view to staged anastomosis. The baby developed staphylococcal pneumonia and empyema, the organism being resistant to all standard antibiotics. Further attempts at oesophageal anastomosis failed and ultimately cervical oesophagostomy was performed. Over a period of months, multiple operative procedures on the lung were required, including lung resection on two occasions for a persisting broncho-pleural fistula, and subsequently for an acquired oesophago-bronchial fistula. Ultimately, right upper lobectomy was performed. In addition, severe tracheomalachia was present and tracheopexy was required. This was performed by a median sternotomy but wound disruption and sternal dehiscence followed. The baby survived this horrendous course and, with a gastrostomy and cervical oesophagostomy, thrived.

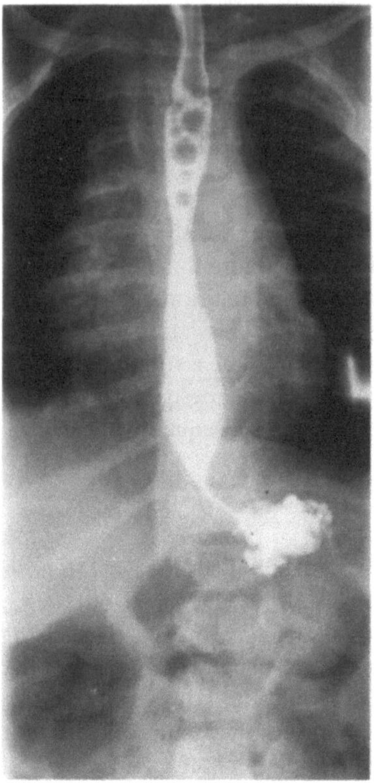

8

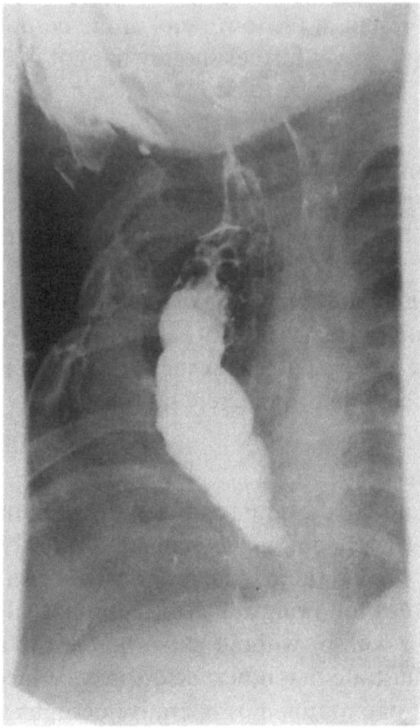

9

Fig. 8. Same case as Fig. 7: Barium swallow following resection of stricture (tracheobronchial remnant)

Fig. 9. Gastric transposition via the right pleural cavity: anteroposterior view

Faced with a decision as to the preferable method to establish alimentary continuity, it was obviously necessary to establish a conduit to the neck, and to do this would necessitate an approach via one of the four routes: (a) subcutaneous, (b) via the left pleural cavity, (c) anterior mediastinal and (d) via the right pleural cavity.

The first three of these possibilities were rejected for the following reasons – the subcutaneous route is cosmetically unacceptable and is now only of historic interest; the left lung provided the greater part of his pulmonary function and should not be compromised; and the anterior mediastinum was probably "frozen" following sternotomy and its postoperative complications. The posterior mediastinal route was not considered appropriate in view of the several previous operations on the lower oesophagus.

Having accepted the right pleural cavity as the course for the conduit, the decision was made to use the whole stomach, and therefore gastric transposition was performed combining the techniques as originally described by Ivor Lewis [46]

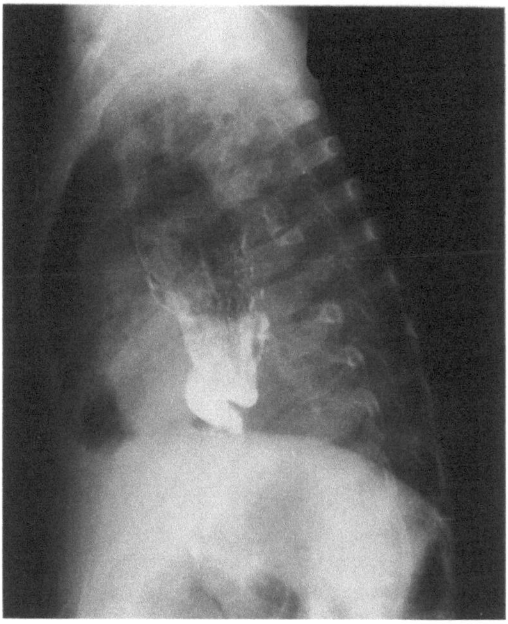

Fig. 10. Gastric transposition via the right pleural cavity: lateral view

and more recently modified by Spitz [75] for babies with a "long gap" oesophageal atresia. Laparotomy was performed and the stomach was mobilized; right thoracotomy was then performed and the lower oesophagus was mobilized (and later resected). The stomach was drawn up into the right pleural cavity and subsequently into the neck where in due course it was anastomosed to the cervical oesophagus. The situation is indicated in the X-ray studies (Figs. 9–11).

Comment

Expediency dictated the need for the above procedures. Although oesophageal replacement is required less and less in babies with oesophageal atresia, the surgeon must be familiar with a wide variety of techniques. Of these, the latest addition to the armamentarium is gastric transposition. The unusual aspect of the operative programme in this case report is that transposition was effected via the right pleural cavity.

Case 6: L.G.

Baby L.G. was born with oesophageal atresia and distal fistula. At the initial thoracotomy performed on the 1st day of life a long gap between the two oesophageal segments precluded anastomosis and therefore the fistula was divided, gastrostomy performed and the upper oesophageal pouch left in situ. She learned to regurgitate her saliva and a second thoracotomy was not performed until the age of 19 months. Again it was found impossible to achieve oesophageal anastomosis and again cervical oesophagostomy was not performed. The patient was

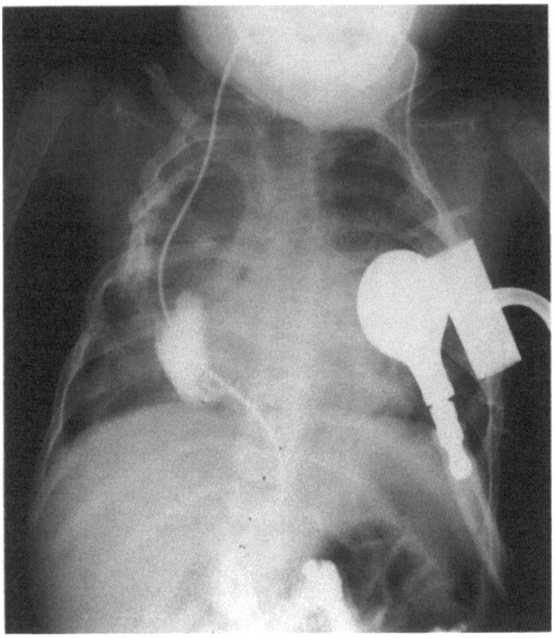

Fig. 11. Gastric transposition: pylorus at level of diaphragm

referred to the author at the age of 3½ years and a study (Fig. 12) showed a four-vertebra gap between the two oesophageal segments. At right thoracotomy it was found possible to anastomose the oesophagus and, although a stricture developed, ultimately the oesophagus had a satisfactory lumen (Fig. 13). She is now aged 19 years and is a university student; dysphagia is minimal.

Comment

This is an extreme example of staged management reminiscent of Humphreys patient born in 1935 and referred to by Ashcraft and Holder [4] and Myers [54].

Corrosive Oesophagitis

Corrosive burns of the oesophagus in childhood are almost invariably accidental rather than homicidal; nevertheless, very serious burns to the pharynx and/or oesophagus may occur, necessitating prolonged treatment and, in some, oesophageal replacement. Evaluation of the presence and severity of oesophageal burns [24, 29, 30] follows accepted lines today, and although treatment protocols vary it is generally accepted that the measures required include steroids, antibiotics and/or oesophageal dilatation.

Seen less frequently are corrosive burns of the stomach; these are particularly liable to occur following acid ingestion [76]. This may result in both corrosive oesophagitis and corrosive gastritis.

12 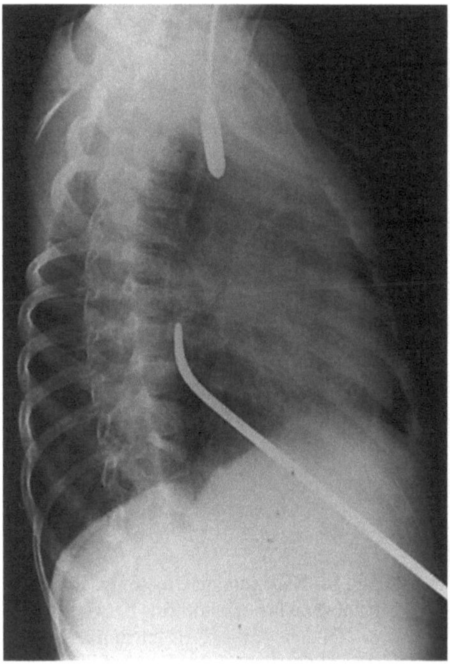

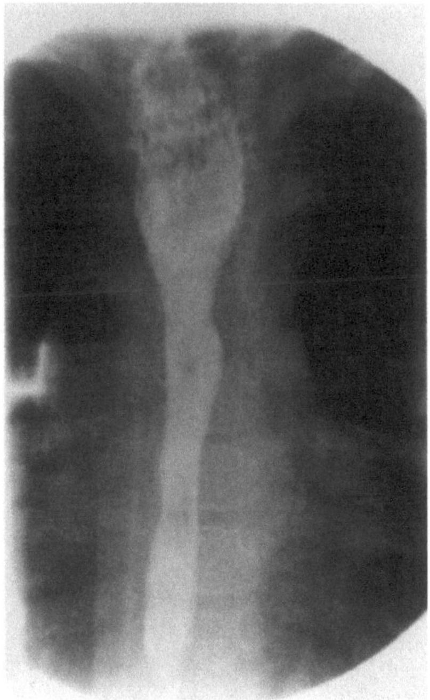 13

Fig. 12. Case 6: study with Bakes dilator in upper oesophageal segment and urethral sound (via gastrostomy) in lower oesophageal segment: four-vertebra gap between segments

Fig. 13. Same case as Fig. 12. Ultimate appearance of oesophagus following end-to-end anastomosis

Case Report

A male toddler, F.D., was aged 19 months when admitted to the Royal Children's Hospital, Melbourne, having swallowed soldering fluid which contained hydrochloric acid and zinc chloride. As anticipated, oesophagoscopy revealed severe corrosive oesophagitis and plans were made to commence the routine triple regime of treatment – steroids, antibiotics and daily bouginage.

Clinical examination indicated an intra-abdominal complication and laparotomy was required. At operation, the stomach, with the exception of the terminal 1–2 cm of the pyloric antrum, was found to be gangrenous and was little more than a shrivelled mass of tissue. Almost complete total gastrectomy was performed and in view of the boy's relatively poor general condition no attempt was made to restore alimentary continuity at this stage. In retrospect, this was probably a mistake. The lower end of the oesophagus was closed by suture and tube duodenostomy performed. Neither of these manoeuvres was succesful and salivary leak occurred from the lower end of the oesophagus and leak of duodenal contents from the duodenostomy. The decision was therefore made to restore alimentary continuity. This was effected by anastomosing the lower end of the oesophagus to the residual pyloric antrum immediately proximal to the pylorus

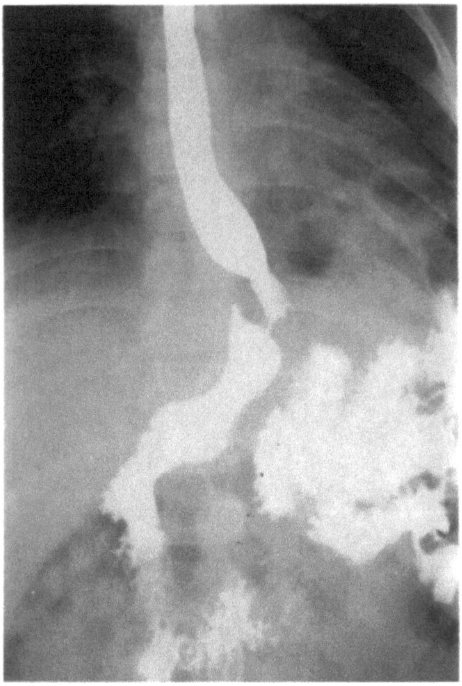

Fig. 14. Near total gastrectomy. Barium meal showing anastomosis between oesophagus and pyloric antrum. Also seen is position of duodenum following "Kocherization"

(Fig. 14). This proved to be successful, but at the age of 26 years severe alkaline oesophagitis has developed with poor response to appropriate medical treatment. Biliary diversion has been advised.

Comment

This case history illustrates the need to consider gastric involvement when corrosive ingestion occurs, particularly with acid ingestion. A method of restoring alimentary continuity involving Kocherization of the duodenum is described and was technically feasible in this particular patient. As pointed out by Steigmann and Dolehick [76] and Haller et al. [30], acid burns of the oesophagus produce coagulation necrosis which impedes deeper penetration and is more likely to cause damage to the stomach.

Peptic Oesophagitis

Peptic oesophagitis is almost invariably a consequence of gastro-oesophageal reflux, and in its most severe form results in a fibrous stricture of the oesophagus – the so-called peptic stricture. An unusual situation is finding a peptic stricture in the absence of demonstrable gastro-oesophageal reflux; if this occurs, it may well be an example of a true "congenital gastric-lined gullet".

15 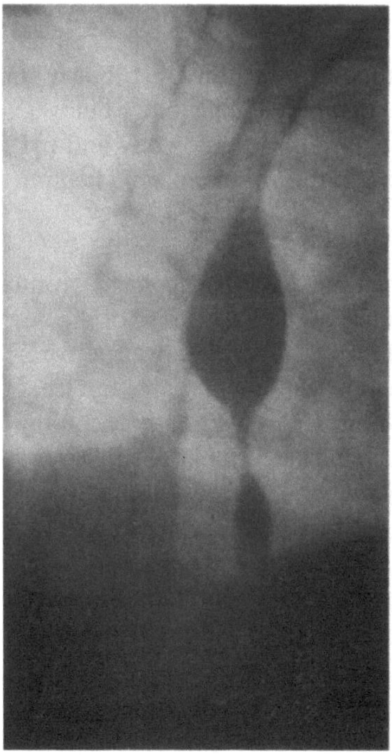

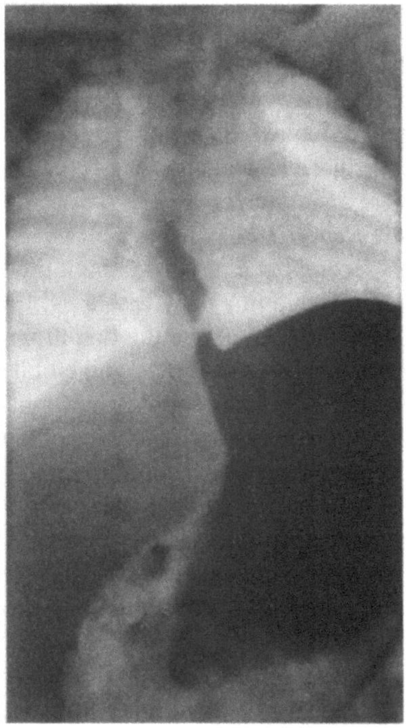 16

Fig. 15. Barium swallow in a 4 year old (case report 1) who presented with haematemesis and dysphagia. "Gastric-lined gullet" below stricture. No evidence of gastro-oesophageal reflux was demonstrated

Fig. 16. Barium swallow and meal (case report 2) revealing lower oesophageal stricture but not showing gastro-oesophageal reflux. A false diagnosis of congenital stricture was made

Case Report 1

A 4-year-old female child presented with haematemesis and dysphagia. Investigation revealed a stricture in the lower third of the oesophagus (Fig. 15); gastro-oesophageal reflux was not demonstrated. Oesophagoscopy did not reveal evidence of peptic oesophagitis above the stricture. The decision was made to perform thoracotomy and resect the stricture. At thoracotomy, the external appearance of the oesophagus above and below the stricture was normal; in retrospect, the decision to resect the stricture was incorrect (the operation was performed in 1974) and, today, attempts would be made to dilate the stricture, possibly by the technique of radial or balloon dilatation [6]. When the oesophagus was incised below the stricture, the mucosal lining had an obvious gastric appearance and, in keeping with the policy at that time [35], a limited resection of the oesophagus was performed and alimentary continuity restored via oesophagogastrostomy. The pathologist reported as follows:

the specimen consists of a tubular oesophagus with a central waist. It measures 4.5 × 3 × 1 cm. The upper ⅓ of the specimen is lined by oesophageal mucosa (squamous) and the lower ⅔ by gastric mucosa. Both are intact but beneath the squamous mucosa there are dense inflammatory infiltrations and significant submucosal fibrosis.

This report is perhaps of a little more than historical interest, but it emphasizes the need to establish more accurately the nature of the histology below an oesophageal stricture. With the introduction of fibre optic endoscopy and pH monitoring, a more logical and long-term solution to this problem could be anticipated.

Case Report 2
In a second patient seen at about the same time, gastro-oesophageal reflux was not demonstrated in a baby with a tight stricture of the lower third of the oesophagus, a short distance above the diaphragm (Fig. 16). Operation was performed with a provisional diagnosis of a congenital stricture and the plan was to resect the stricture and perform oesophago-oesophagostomy. However, at thoracotomy the presence of an intrathoracic loculus of stomach indicated that the stricture was peptic. Attempted pergastrostomy dilatation of the stricture was ultimately followed by disastrous perforation at the site of the stricture and in order to control the salivary leak a double-barrelled cervical oesophagostomy was performed, and this proved to be life-saving. At a later stage, alimentary continuity was effected utilizing the technique of oesophagogastrostomy, as described by Howard et al. [35].

Comment
The unusual feature in this patient was the method adopted to control the complication.

Group 2: Unusual Problems in Conditions Seen Infrequently

It is not possible to include all the unusual problems; the following are representative of some unusual experiences and, although anecdotal, they give some indication of the spectrum of the pathology seen in the oesophagus in patients in the paediatric age group.

Neonatal Rupture of the Oesophagus

Although uncommon, there are several references to this condition in the literature [1, 18, 82]. Kimura et al. [41] have also reported "esophageal perforation in a neonate associated with gastro-esophageal reflux".

The following case report describes our only experience [55] with neonatal rupture of the oesophagus.

Case Report
Baby S.M. was born at term with a birth weight of 2920 g. The pregnancy had been complicated by pre-eclampsia. During the first few hours of life the baby vomited some "brownish fluid", but her condition did not cause any concern until the age of 17 h when she was found to be in a state of collapse with cyanosis,

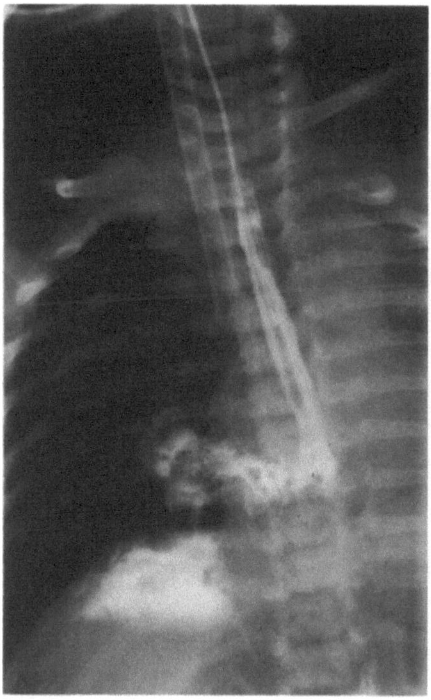

17

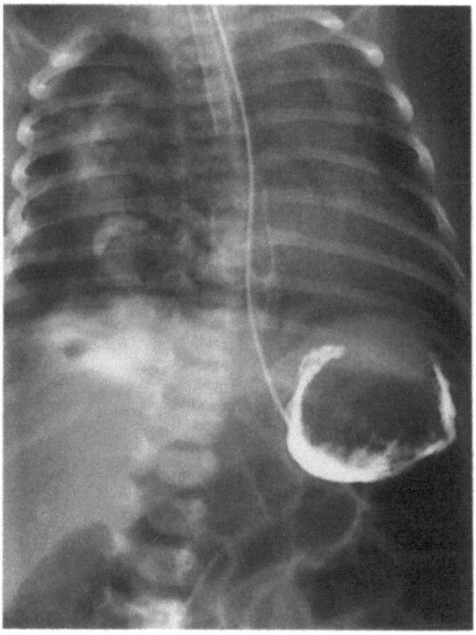

18

Fig. 17. Neonatal rupture of the oesophagus. X-ray showing endotracheal tube in situ. Residual right pneumothorax. Dye study of oesophagus with free escape of dye into right pleural cavity. (reproduced by kind permission of the *Australian Paediatric Journal*)

Fig. 18. Neonatal rupture of the oesophagus. X-ray showing residual dye in right pleural cavity and space-occupying blood clot in stomach outlined by dye. Nasogastric tube in situ

peripheral circulatory failure and a subnormal temperature. Examination revealed diminished air entry over the whole of the right side of the thorax and X-ray of the chest showed a right-sided tension pneumothorax. Tracheal intubation was necessary to control the respiratory failure; an intercostal catheter was then introduced into the right pleural cavity and this resulted in considerable escape of air followed by heavily blood stained fluid which contained mucus thought to resemble saliva. Simultaneously a nasogastric tube was passed and heavily blood stained fluid was aspirated from the stomach. It was estimated that the blood loss into the pleural cavity and the stomach was at least 100 ml and blood transfusion was commenced.

The nature of the fluid aspirated from the right pleural cavity led to the provisional diagnosis of ruptured oesophagus and further radiological studies confirmed the diagnosis. Radiopaque dye introduced into the mid-oesophagus via a naso-oesophageal tube immediately escaped into the right pleural cavity (Fig. 17). A catheter was then introduced into the stomach and further dye was introduced; this outlined a "space-occupying mass" which was interpreted as a blood clot (Fig. 18).

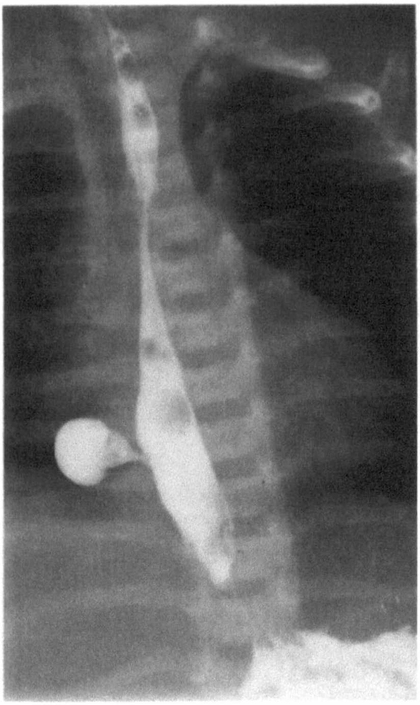

19

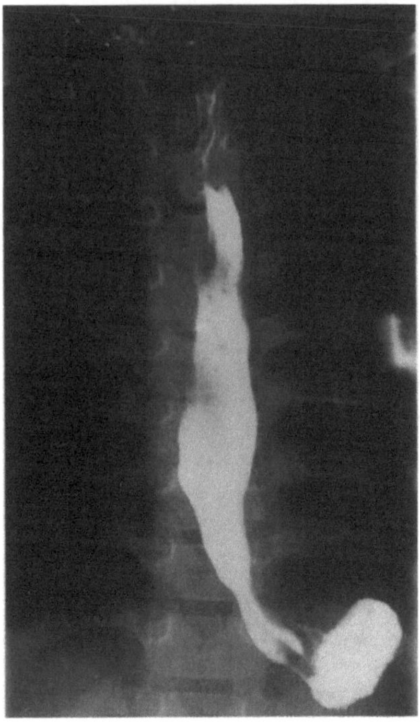

20

Fig. 19. Neonatal rupture of the oesophagus – small "pseudodiverticulum" following repair of oesophagus

Fig. 20. Neonatal rupture of oesophagus. Barium swallow revealing end result – normal oesophagus

Immediate operation was performed, taking the form of gastrostomy followed by thoracotomy through the right sixth intercostal space. On entering the pleural cavity a large volume of air and blood-stained salivary fluid escaped. A linear rupture of the oesophagus was present on the right side of the oesophagus a short distance above the diaphragm. This was 1.3 cm in length and at this site the mediastinal pleura was torn and the cellular tissues of the mediastinum were oedematous. The oesophageal rent was closed with interrupted silk sutures. There were some early postoperative problems and in particular recurrent pneumothorax, and a postoperative barium swallow revealed some leak from the site of the oesophageal rupture (Fig. 19).

This healed and a later barium swallow revealed a completely normal oesophagus (Fig. 20). Her subsequent progress was uneventful.

With the experience of this patient the following statement was made [50]. "The lesson to be learned from this patient is that when neonatal respiratory distress is present and an X-ray of the chest reveales a tension pneumothorax the possibility of rupture of the oesophagus should be considered; the index of suspicion should be greater if the right pleural cavity is involved.

21 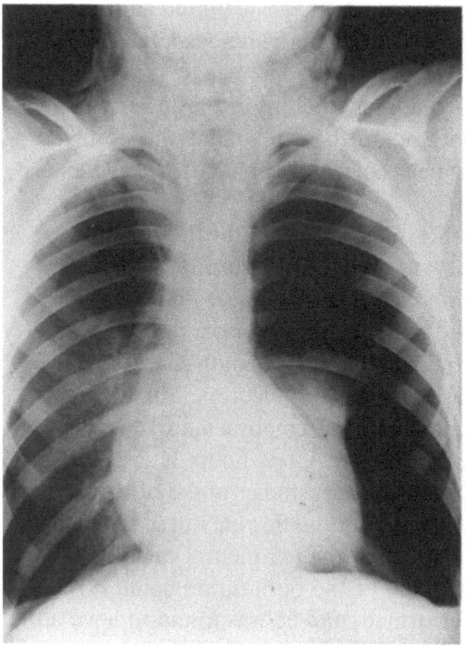

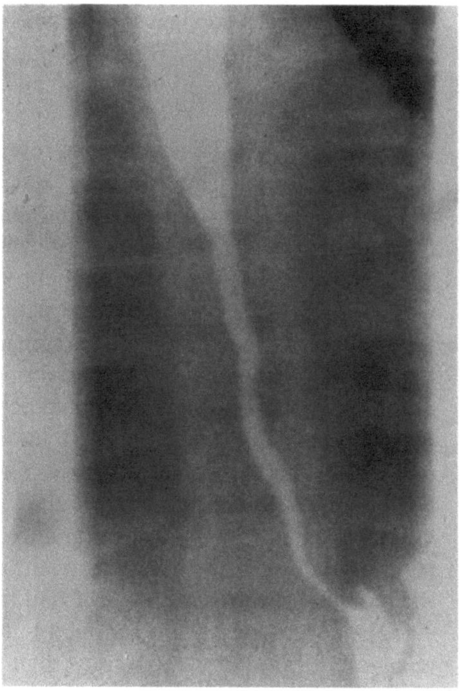 22

Fig. 21. Explosive rupture of the oesophagus: bilateral pneumothorax; surgical emphysema of neck

Fig. 22. Explosive rupture oesophagus. Post-repair stricture (this resolved spontaneously)

Explosive Rupture of the Oesophagus

There are rare anecdotal reports of the problems in the literature [34]. In 1972 Buntain and Lynn [11] reviewed the literature and reported a 3-year-old boy who had sustained "traumatic, pneumatic disruption of the esophagus" and referred to previous similar reports by Kerr et al. [40] and Randolph et al. [64]. We had a similar experience in 1965 and the details follow:

Case Report

On New Year's day M.G. presented with severe respiratory distress which occurred when he bit the inflated rubber inner tube of an old-fashioned tyre. Examination revealed gross surgical emphysema of the neck and signs indicative of bilateral pneumothorax. These diagnoses were confirmed at X-ray examination (Fig. 21). Bilateral intercostal drainage was instituted. Radiological evaluation of the oesophagus was then undertaken; escape of radiopaque dye from the oesophagus into the left pleural cavity indicated oesophageal disruption. Oesophagoscopy was performed and revealed an extensive rupture of the pharynx and oesophagus above the aortic arch; left thoracotomy was then performed and confirmed the diagnosis of ruptured oesophagus. There was marked mediastinal oedema and the oesophagus was extensively ruptured from the diaphragm below to the aortic arch above. This was repaired, pleural drainage instituted and gastrostomy performed. No attempt was made to repair the pharyngo-oesophageal rupture above the aortic arch.

Subsequent radiological studies revealed a long stricture of the lower part of the thoracic oesophagus (Fig. 22), but without further treatment this resolved completely and later evaluation indicated a near normal oesophagus. Subsequently, he did not have any residual dysphagia.

Some years later, a second patient with explosive rupture of the oesophagus was seen. In this second case, the patient was admitted to hospital with severe facial burns, but at the time of admission a clear-cut history was not available. Later it was elucidated that he had dropped a lighted match into a disused petrol drum which contained some residual petrol. Initially, major emphasis was on the thermal injury to his face, but with increasing respiratory distress, attention was focused on the chest, and an X-ray revealed surgical emphysema of the neck, pneumomediastinum and bilateral pleural effusions. A few hours later, he had developed a large left hydropneumothroax and contrast studies of the oesophagus revealed rupture of the oesophagus, the contrast material flowing out of the material into a large retrocardiac space and trickling into the left pleural cavity.

Oesophagoscopy was performed but the site of the perforation could not be recognized. Left thoracotomy was then performed, and he was found to have an empyema. The evidence showed that he had a mediastinal abscess which had ruptured into the left pleural cavity; the oesophagus was mobilized from the diaphragm below to the arch of the aorta above. It was intact. When a naso-oesophageal tube was passed from above, the tube appeared in the mediastinum, having escaped from the oesophagus at some point above the aortic arch. No further attempt was made to identify the site of oesophageal perforation because it was realized that it may have been cervical or thoracic, and it was thought that it was probably small. He developed a right empyema but a further X-ray examination of the oesophagus showed that this was intact, with no residual leak. The right empyema required formal drainage. He was fed by gastrostomy for 1 month and subsequently fed normally and has not had any further alimentary symptoms. There were two later problems – "tattooing" from the original burn and some tinnitus, no doubt a result of the explosive injury.

Achalasia of the Cardia

Although achalasia of the cardia occurs predominantly in adults, in many the symptoms date back to childhood and approximately 5% present before the age of 15 years [5]. As recently reported by Taylor and Myers [79], 20 children with achalasia of the cardia were seen at the Royal Children's Hospital, Melbourne, in the years 1953–1986. The youngest patient in our series was aged 4 days at the time of presentation and transthoracic Heller cardiomyotomy was performed at the age of 7 months: the case report follows.

23 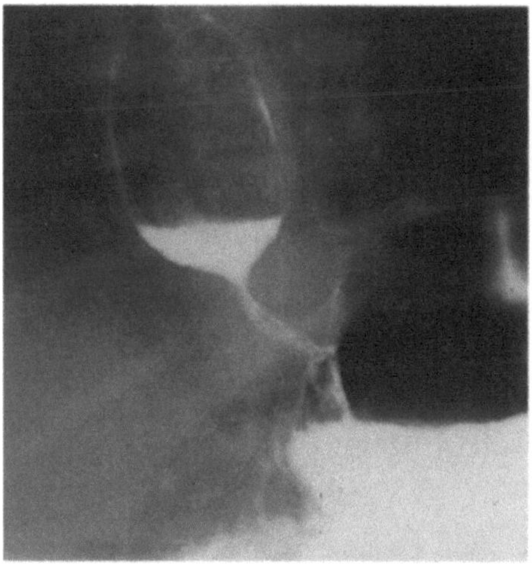 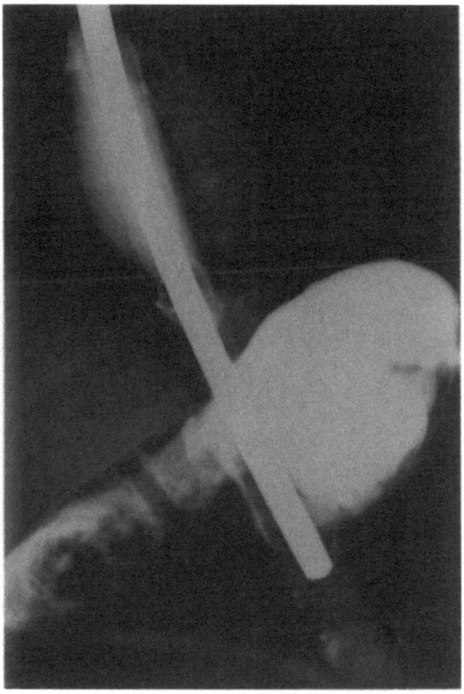 24

Fig. 23. Achalasia of the cardia. Barium swallow showing fluid level in oesophagus above cardiospasm

Fig. 24. Same case as Fig. 23. Bougie in situ confirmed oesophagoscopic evidence excluding stricture. (The study was performed before the introduction of manometry as a diagnostic technique)

Case Report

A female baby, J.P., was aged 4 days when she presented with cyanotic episodes during feeding. Initially, she was observed in hospital for 5 weeks, and at that time a barium swallow revealed oesophageal incoordination. With the administration of thicker milk feeds she improved, but there was persistent regurgitation of milk and at the age of 5 months she was readmitted to hospital having failed to thrive. A further barium swallow was performed and this revealed abnormal peristalsis in the upper oesophagus and findings in keeping with achalasia of the cardia (Figs. 23, 24). Heller cardiomyotomy was performed at the age of 7 months, following which her clinical progress was completely satisfactory and, many years later, a further barium swallow showed that there was no residual obstruction at the lower end of the oesophagus (Fig. 25).

Pharyngo-oesophageal Fibromatosis

The following case report illustrates the diagnostic and therapeutic difficulties encountered in a 3-year-old child with pharyngo-oesophageal occlusion which was ultimately diagnosed as fibromatosis of the oesophagus.

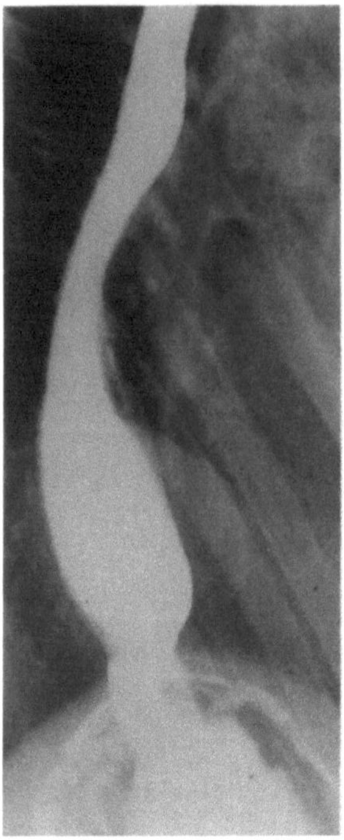
25

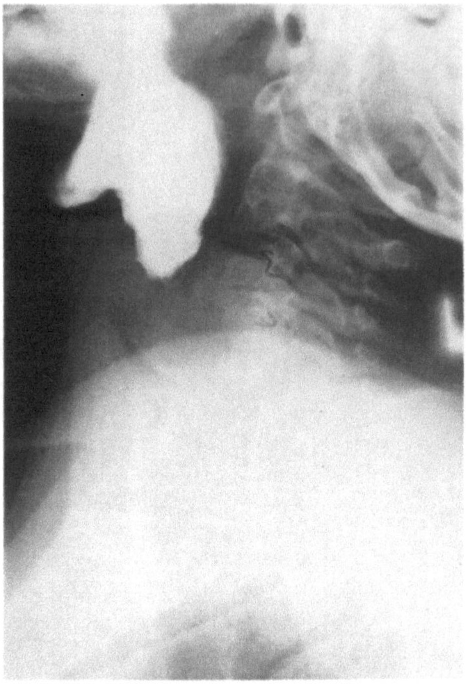
26

Fig. 25. Same case as Figs. 23 and 24: barium swallow 20 years following the Heller procedure

Fig. 26. Pharyngo-oesophageal fibromatosis: barium swallow revealing complete obstruction

Case Report

A 3-year-old girl, MD, presented with a history of progressive dysphagia over a period of several months. There was radiological and endoscopic evidence of gross obstruction at the pharyngo-oesophageal junction; biopsy revealed "fibrous tissue". Gastrostomy was required, and at a later stage a left cervical exploration was performed, but the only additional procedure at that time was a crico-pharyngeal myotomy. As this failed to produce any improvement, the child was referred to the Royal Children's Hospital, Melbourne. Further investigation revealed complete pharyngo-oesophageal occlusion (Fig. 26) and further biopsies were performed and reported as follows: "diagnosis: oesophagus: fibromatosis".

A further exploration of the neck was carried out; the pharynx was opened above the site of the occlusion and the oesophagus below, and these incisions were joined by a vertical limb traversing the site of the obstruction. The resultant defect in the pharyngo-oesophageal wall was sutured transversely, providing an excellent lumen. But, despite this and subsequent dilatations, complete obstruction recurred and persisted. Although dilatation was possible and although for some time a prosthetic plastic tube was left in situ, the obstruction remained unrelieved (Figs. 27, 28) and therefore a further operative procedure was performed. Through

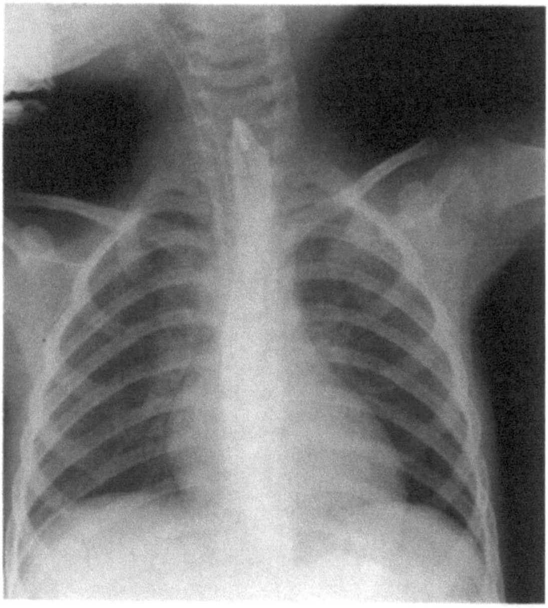

Fig. 27. Pharyngo-oesophageal fibromatosis: complete obstruction demonstrated from below via oesophageal tube introduced per gastrostomy stoma

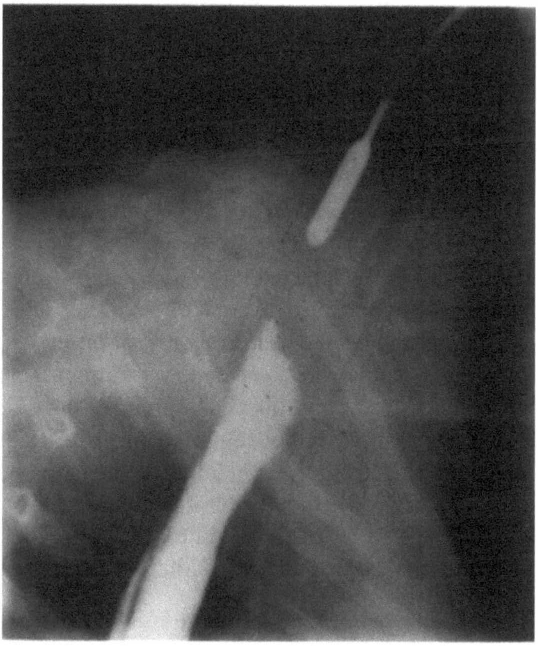

Fig. 28. Pharyngo-oesophageal fibromatosis: bougie in place above, separated from oesophagus below by fibromatosis mass

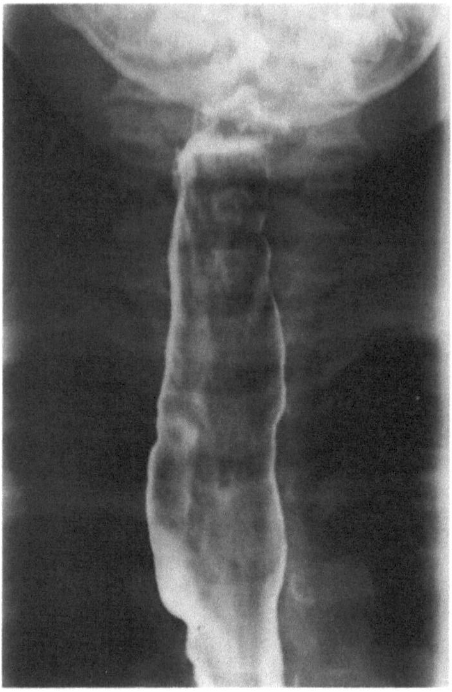

Fig. 29. Pharyngo-oesophageal fibromatosis: barium swallow following resection and anastomosis

a cervical approach, the pharynx above the obstructing mass was mobilized to the base of the skull above, and the oesophagus was mobilized in the posterior mediastinum below, to the level of the fifth thoracic vertebra. The obstructing mass was then resected; alimentary continuity was restored by anastomosing the mobilized oesophagus to the pharynx. The ultimate result is seen in Fig. 29.

Mid-oesophageal Stricture of Uncertain Aetiology

The X-ray study depicted in Fig. 30 demonstrates the findings in a 9-year-old boy who presented with a history of vomiting and dysphagia for solid foods. The symptoms had been of relatively recent onset. The patient was paraplegic and had previously had urinary diversion for neurogenic bladder. These neurological problems were a consequence of an intraspinal dermoid cyst, producing cord and root compression. Following a recent orthopaedic procedure on his foot, intractible vomiting occurred and, later, he developed the signs of oesophageal obstruction. A nasogastric tube had not been in situ for any length of time, and the X-ray which revealed a "tight" stricture did not reveal gastro-oesophageal reflux. The stricture was excised and the pathology report was as follows:

The specimen consists of a segment of oesophagus 2 cm in length. The lumen is narrow and admits a probe 0.4 cm in diameter. The mucosa is ulcerated and granular; the oesophageal wall

30 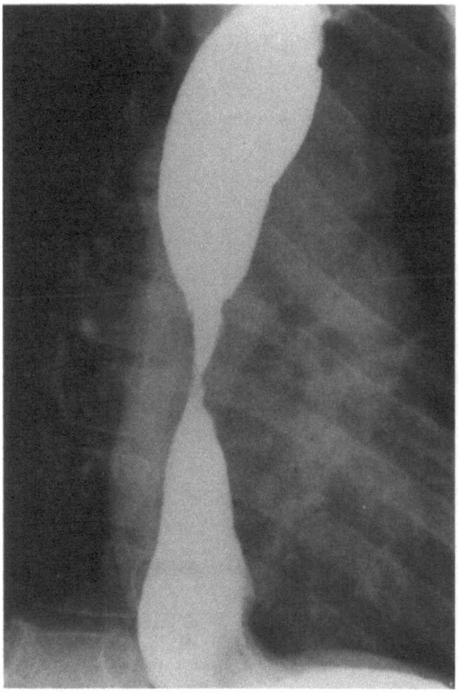 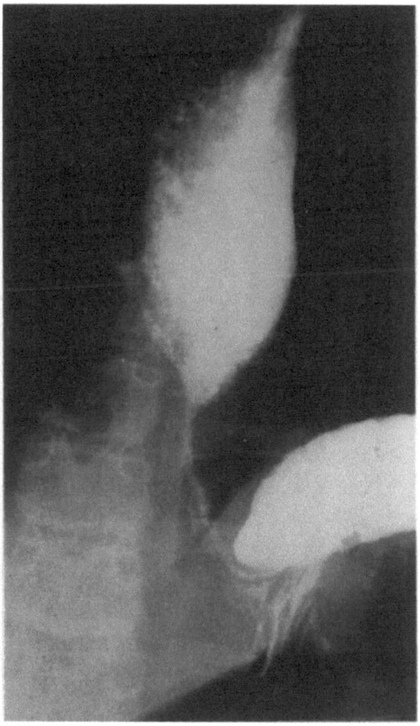 31

Fig. 30. Barium swallow demonstrating mid-oesophageal stricture of unknown aetiology

Fig. 31. Nasogastric intubation stricture

is thick and multiple sections prepared from the material show intact hyperplastic stratified squamous epithelium lining three quarters of the oesophageal surface. This ends abruptly at a zone of ulceration and dense inflammatory cell infiltration, which replaces the mucosa and has led to scarring of the submucosa. However, the underlying muscle layers appear intact, and show little abnormality apart from patchy foci of lymphocytic infiltration. No gastric mucosa is found. Diagnosis: oesophagus – ulceration with submucosal fibrosis.

Clearly, histological examination shed no light on the aetiology of the stricture. In retrospect, this stricture may have responded to the injection of steroids.

Nasogastric Intubation Stricture

This is an unusual condition which has been reported sporadically. The X-ray findings of such a patient are seen in Fig. 31. This was a barium swallow examination performed in an emaciated boy with gross intestinal dyskinesia; laparotomy had been performed, and a nasogastric tube was in situ pre- and postoperatively. At a later stage, dysphagia developed. Initially, it was thought that this may be another manifestation of dyskinesia, but investigation and oesophagoscopy revealed a fibrous stricture and led to a diagnosis of nasogastric intubation stricture. There was an excellent response to dilatation.

32 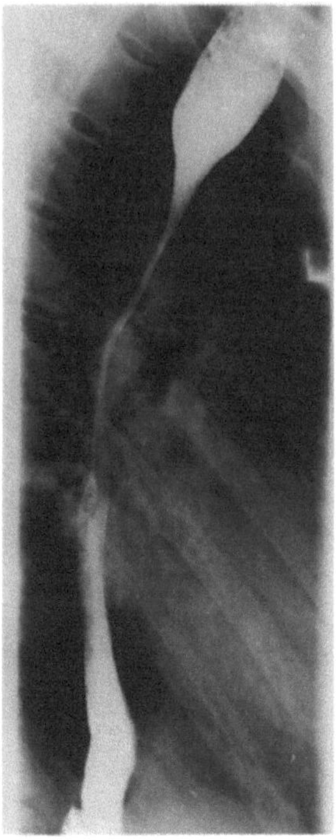 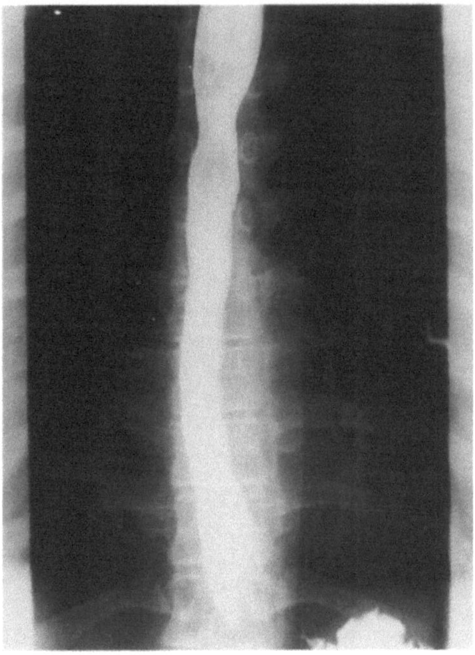 33

Fig. 32. Oesophageal stricture in immunologically compromised patient

Fig. 33. Same case as Fig. 32: response to programme of dilatation

Oesophageal Stenosis in the Immunologically Compromised Patient

Oesophagitis is a well-recognized complication in patients who are immunologically compromised [57]; the immunological deficiency may be congenital or acquired. The barium swallow of a patient with a congenital cause for immunological deficiency is depicted in Fig. 32. This boy had a variant of chronic granulomatous disease, and at one stage developed duodenitis and then a superior mesenteric artery syndrome. He became grossly emaciated, and when dysphagia ensued an anticipated finding on oesophagoscopy was oesophagitis. X-ray revealed a long stricture of the oesophagus (see Fig. 32) secondary to the oesophagitis. There was a very satisfactory response to dilatation (Fig. 33).

Discussion

It is evident that, although oesophageal atresia dominates the field of oesophageal surgery in childhood, there are many other oesophageal problems which confront paediatric surgeons. The unusual problems seen in clinical practice can broadly be divided into the two groups described in this article. The first group includes problems seen in oeosphageal atresia and other frequently encountered diseases such as peptic oesophagitis and corrosive oesophagitis. Selected examples have been used to illustrate this group but there are innumerable other examples which occur in large series of patients with oesophageal atresia, peptic oesophagitis or corrosive oesophagitis. The unusual aspects involve diagnosis as well as treatment; the former have been exemplified by the long upper pouch occasionally seen in babies with oesophageal atresia and also by reference to oesophageal stenosis due to tracheobronchial remnants below an oesophageal anastomosis. As time has passed oesophageal replacement has become less and less necessary in babies with oesophageal atresia; the case described was an unusual situation which demanded unusual methods and hence the decision to establish alimentary continuity by gastric transposition via the right pleural cavity.

With reference to corrosive oesophagitis there will always be anecdotal reports of unusual clinical situations and the recent popularity of electronic devices which need disc batteries [8, 9, 72] has been associated with ingestion of such batteries and the risk of severe oesophagitis. A further complication is the development of a tracheo-oesophageal fistula. There are also several anecdotal reports of acid burns of the oesophagus and stomach following ingestion of acid substances and although the emphasis may be on the gastric, rather than the oesophageal, involvement it is necessary to be aware of the complications of gastric perforation, gastric gangrene and prepyloric stricture.

Peptic oesophagitis is a serious complication of gastro-oesophageal reflux and may lead to fibrous stricture. Fortunately today oesophageal replacement is rarely required; such procedures as the Nissen fundoplication are effective and can be combined with appropriate management of a complicating stricture. The two cases reported in this article were selected as they identified two distinct problems; the first case report addresses the problem of the "Barrett" oesophagus and despite increasing experience there is still argument as to whether this may occasionally have a congenital basis. Although in the case reported gastro-oesophageal reflux was not demonstrated, techniques today (20 years later) may well have shown reflux. Regardless of this, treatment would be different today and would no doubt include appropriate management of the stricture and an antireflux operation at an appropriate level. The same applies with even greater force to the second case, which was also managed 20 years ago; one hopes that gastro-oesophageal reflux would have been demonstrated in this patient either by conventional radiological methods or newer methods of investigation such as pH monitoring or radionucleide evaluation. This case therefore demonstrates the danger of inadequate diagnosis of an oesophageal stricture; however, it also demonstrates the value of cervical oesophagostomy for salivary diversion under the circumstances which developed in this patient and perhaps in other situations.

One area which has not been addressed in this article involves ingested foreign bodies; these are a very frequent occurrence in childhood but not infrequently the manifestations may be unusual or atypical. One example of this in our experience is an aorto-oesophageal fistula in a 4-month-old baby which led to uncontrollable haemorrhage and death.

Of considerable interest are the patients described in the second group including those with neonatal rupture of the oesophagus, explosive rupture of the oesophagus, achalasia, pharyngo-oesophageal fibromatosis and stricture resulting from immunological compromise. A wide variety of pathologies are represented by these patients; many other conditions are seen rarely and the literature includes examples of the following:

1. Traumatic oesophageal pseudodiverticulum [7, 14, 20, 43, 85]
2. Congenital cricopharyngeal achalasia [45]
3. Congenital cystic dysplasia of the oesophagus [83]
4. Congenital diverticulum [47, 71]
5. Body brace oesophagitis [62]
7. Inflammatory oesophagogastric polyps [86]

Oesophageal strictures and/or oesophagitis have been reported in dystrophic epidermolysis bullosa [23, 32], Stevens-Johnson syndrome [36], dermatomyositis [70] and scleroderma. Miscellaneous tumours have been reported including hamartoma [19], leiomyoma [56] and rhabdomyoma [61]. Dysphagia has also been attributed to ectopic gastric mucosa in the cervical esophagus [48, 63, 65].

Much more could be written about unusual problems in oesophageal surgery in childhood; thus, with reference to achalasia, there are reports of other very young patients [21] and also its association with the Riley-Day syndrome [12, 66, 68] and treatment [77]. With reference to Barrett's oesophagus and possible surgical treatment, there have been many contributions, including those of Cooper et al. [15], Dahms and Rothstein [16], Hennessy [33] and Clark and Woodward [13]. Duplication cysts are neither common nor rare; there are innumerable descriptions of such cysts and their variations in the literature, including those of Gans et al. [25], Harmannd et al. [31], Jaubert de Beaujeau and Chavrier [39] and Robison et al. [67]. Various forms of aberrant rests, with or without oesophageal atresia, have been reported [26, 65] and congenital oesophageal stricture with lack of submucosa [78].

Not infrequently, there is diagnostic delay in children with oesophageal disease and frequently the delay relates to the fact that swallowing difficulties in infants and children are more often than not apparent rather than real. However, there are several organic causes for dysphagia in childhood and before the symptoms are incorrectly attributed to immaturity or emotional disturbance or both consideration must always be given to the possibility that there is an organic basis. Apart from conditions described in this article the possibility of a neurological disorder must always be considered.

The paediatric surgeon must therefore be aware that there is a wide spectrum of oesophageal disease in childhood, must be familiar with diagnostic techniques and his therapeutic armamentarium must include endoscopy and various forms of oesophageal dilatation, oesophageal resection and anastomosis and, where indicated, oesophageal replacement.

Acknowledgements. The author gratefully acknowledges the help given by the very efficient staff of the J. W. Grieve Library of the Royal Children's Hospital, Melbourne, and of the Department of Radiology. He also wishes to place on record his great appreciation of the secretarial help provided by Mrs. Judith Hayes, Mrs. Elizabeth Vorrath and Mrs. Robyn Da Silva. The Educational Resources Centre of the Royal Children's Hospital provided the usual efficient help with the production of the figures, and details regarding these were prepared by Mrs. Robyn Da Silva.

References

1. Aaronson IA, Cywes S, Louw JH (1975) Spontaneous esophageal rupture in the newborn. J Pediatr Surg 10:459
2. Aberdeen E, Myers NA (1979) The esophagus. In: Ravitch MM, Welch KJ, Benson CD, Aberdeen E, Randolph JG (eds) Paediatric surgery, 3rd edn. Yearbook Medical, Chicago, p 446
3. Anderson CM, Burke V (1975) Congenital oesophageal stenosis. In: Anderson CM, Burke V (eds) Paediatric gastroenterology. Blackwell, Oxford
4. Ashcraft KW, Holder TM (1969) The story of esophageal atresia and tracheoesophageal fistula. Surgery 65:332
5. Azizkhan RG, Tapper D, Eraklis A (1980) Achalasia in childhood: a 20 year experience. J Pediatr Surg 15:452
6. Ball WS, Strife JL, Rosenkrantz J (1984) Esophageal strictures in childhood. Treatment by balloon dilatation. Radiology 150:263
7. Blair GK, Filler RM, Theodorescu D (1987) Neonatal pharyngoesophageal perforation mimicking esophageal atresia: clues to diagnosis. J Pediatr Surg 22:770
8. Blatnik DS (1977) Swallowed battery causes fatal burn. JAMA 238:381
9. Blatnik DS, Toohill RJ, Lehman RH (1977) Fatal complication from an alkaline battery foreign body in the esophagus. Ann Otol Rhinol Laryngol 86:611
10. Briceno LI, Grases PJ, Gallego S (1981) Tracheo-bronchial and pancreatic remnants causing esophageal stenosis. J Pediatr Surg 16:731
11. Buntain WL, Lynn HB (1972) Traumatic pneumatic disruption of the esophagus. J Thorac Cardiovasc Surg 63:553
12. Burke V (1966) Familial dysautonomia. Aust Pediatr J 2:58
13. Clarke JM, Woodmard ER (1968) Transthroacic fundoplication for hiatal hernia and short esophagus in a 3 year old child: case report. Surgery 64:858
14. Cohen RC, Myers NA (1987) Traumatic oesophageal pseudodiverticulum. Aust Paediatr J 23:125
15. Cooper JE, Spitz L, Wilkins BM (1987) Barrett's esophagus in children: a histological and histo-chemical study of 11 cases. J Pediatr Surg 22:191
16. Dahms BB, Rothstein FC (1984) Barrett's esophagus in children: a consequence of chronic gastroesophageal reflux. Gastroenterology 86:138
17. Deeraniya AK (1974) Congenital oesophageal stenosis due to tracheobronchial remnants. Thorax 29:720
18. Desargher G, Bayart M (1972) Spontaneous performation of the lower esophagus in a newborn baby. Ann Chir Inf 13:17
19. Dieter RA Jr, Riker WL, Holinger P (1970) Pedunculated esophageal hamartoma in a child. A case report. J Thorac Cardiovasc Surg 59:851
20. Ducharme JC, Bertrand R, Debie J (1971) Perforation of the pharynx in the newborn: a condition mimicking esophageal atresia. Can Med Assoc J 104:785
21. Eaton H (1972) Achalasia of the cardia in a 3 month old infant treated successfully by a modified Heller's operation. Aust NZ J Surg 41:240
22. Fonkalsrud EW (1972) Esophageal stenosis due to tracheo bronchial remnant. Am J Surg 124:101
23. Fonkalsrud EW, Ament ME (1977) Surgical management of esophageal stricture due to recessive dystrophic epidermolysis bullosa. J Pediatr Surg 12:221

24. Fyfe AH, Auldist AW (1984) Corrosive ingestion in children. Z Kinderchir 39: 229
25. Gans SL, Lackey DA, Zuckerbraun L (1968) Duplications of the cervical esophagus in infants and children. Surgery 63: 849
26. Goldman RL, Ban JL (1972) Chondroepithelial choristoma (tracheobronchial rest) of the esophagus associated with esophageal atresia. Report of an unusual case. J Thorac Cardiovasc Surg 63: 318
27. Gryboski J, Kocoshis SA, Seashore JH, et al (1978) "Body-brace" esophagitis. A complication of kypho-scoliosis surgery. Lancet II: 449
28. Haight C (1957) Some observations on esophageal atresia and tracheo-esophageal fistulas of congenital origin. J Thorac Surg 34: 141
29. Haller JA Jr (1979) Corrosive strictures of the esophagus. In: Ravitch MM, Welch KJ, Benson CD, Aberdeen E, Randolph JE (eds) Pediatric Yearbook Medical, Chicago, p 472
30. Haller JA Jr, Gibbs-Andrews H, White JJ (1971) Pathophysiology and management of acute corrosive burns of the esophagus: results of treatment in 285 children. J Pediatr Surg 6: 578
31. Harmannd D, Grosdider J, Hoefferl JC (1981) Multiple bronchogenic cyst of the esophagus. Am J Gastroenterol 75: 321
32. Harmel RP (1986) Esophagela replacement in two siblings with epidermolysis bullosa. J Pediatr Surg 21: 175
33. Hennessy TPJ (1985) Barrett's oesophagus. Br J Surg 72: 336
34. Holadday WJ (1959) Rupture of esophagus by compressed air. N Engl J Med 261: 1071
35. Howard R, Myers NA, Stokes K (1976) Peptic structure of the oesophagus. The role of oesophago-gastrostomy. Aust NZJ Surg 46: 26
36. Howell CE, Mansberger JA, Parrish RA (1987) Esophageal stricture secondary to Stevens Johnson syndrome. J Pediatr Surg 22: 994
37. Ibrahim NBN, Sandy RJ (1981) Congenital oesophageal stenosis caused by tracheobronchial structures in the oesophageal wall. Thorax 36: 465
38. Ishida M, Tsuchida Y, Saito S, et al (1969) Congenital oesophageal stenosis due to tracheobronchial remnants. J Pediatr Surg 4: 339
39. Jaubert de Beaujeu M, Chavrier Y (1974) Digestive duplication: two intramural oesophageal cysts. Ann Chir Inf 15: 15
40. Kerr HH, Sloan H, O'Brien CE (1953) Rupture of the esophagus by compressed air: case report. Surgery 33: 417
41. Kimura K, Okasora T, Eto T, et al (1984) Esophageal perforation in a neonate associated with gastroesophageal reflux. J Pediatr Surg 19: 191
42. Kluth D (1976) Atlas of esophageal atresia. J Pediatr Surg 11: 901
43. Krasna IH, Rosenfeld D, Benjamin BE (1987) Esophageal perforation in the neonate. An emerging problem in the newborn nursery. J Pediatr Surg 22: 784
44. Kumar R (1962) A case of congenital esophageal stricture due to a cartilaginous ring. Br J Surg 49: 533
45. Lernau OZ, Sherzer E, Mogie P, et al (1984) Congenital cricopharyngeal achalasia treated by dilatations. J Pediatr Surg 19: 202
46. Lewis I (1946) The surgical treatment of carcinoma of the oesophagus. Br J Surg 34: 18
47. MacKellar A, Kennedy JC (1972) Congenital diverticulum of the pharynx simulating esophageal atresia. J Pediatr Surg 7: 408
48. Miles-Fox EH (1957) Ectopic gastric mucosa in the cervical esophagus. A possible cause of dysphagia. J Laryngol Otol 71: 419
49. Moyson FR (1970) Congenital esophageal stenosis and cervical tracheo-esophageal fistula. Ann Chir Inf 11: 179
50. Myers NA (1972) Neo-natal rupture of the oesophagus. Ann Chir Inf 13: 213
51. Myers NA (1973) Dysphagia in childhood. Aust NZ J Surg 42: 365
52. Myers NA (1974) Oesophageal astresia: the epitomy of modern surgery. Ann R Coll Surg Engl 54: 277
53. Myers NA (1975) Unusual problems in the surgery of the oesophagus in childhood. Proceedings Annual Meeting of Japanese Association of Pediatric Surgeons

54. Myers NA (1986) The history of oesophageal atresia and tracheo-oesophageal fistula, 1670–1984. Prog Pediatr Surg 20:106
55. Myers NA, Hiller HE (1973) Neonatal rupture of the oesophagus. The radiological diagnosis of a cause of acute respiratory distress in neonates. Aust Paediatr J 9:106
56. Nahmad M, Clatworthy HW Jr (1973) Leiomyoma of the entire esophagus. J Pediatr Surg 8:829
57. Newburger PE, Cassady JR, Jaffe N (1978) Esophagitis due to Adriamycin and radiation therapy for childhood malignancy. Cancer 42:417
58. Nihoul-Fekete C, De Backer A, Lortat-Jacob S, et al (1987) Congenital esophageal stenosis. Pediatr Surg Int 2:86
59. Nishina T, Tsuchida Y, Saito S (1981) Congenital esophageal stenosis due to tracheobronchial remnants and its associated anomalies. J Pediatr Surg 16:190
60. Ohkawa H, Takahasi Y, Hoshino Y, et al (1975) Lower esophageal stenosis in association with tracheobronchial remnants. J Pediatr Surg 10:453
61. Pai GK, Pai PK, Kamath SM (1987) Adult rhabdomyoma of the esophagus. J Pediatr Surg 22:991
62. Picus D, Frank PH (1981) Eosinophilic esophagitis. Am J Radiol 136:1001
63. Powell RW, Luck SR (1988) Cervical esophageal obstruction by ectopic gastric mucosa. J Pediatr Surg 23:632
64. Randolph H, Melick DW, Grant AR (1967) Perforation of the esophagus from external trauma or blast injuries. Dis Chest 51:121
65. Rector LE, Connerley ML (1941) Aberrant mucosa in the esophagus in infants and in children. Arch Pathol 31:285
66. Riley CM, Day RL, Greeley DM, et al (1970) Central autonomic dysfunction with defective lacrimation. Report of 5 cases. Pediatrics 3:468
67. Robison J, Paulina PM, Sherer LA, et al (1987) Multiple esophageal duplication cyst. J Thorac Cardiovasc Surg 94:144
68. Santel L (1970) Megaesophagus in two cases of familial dysautonomia. Riv Chir Pediatr 12:511
69. Scherer LR, Grosfeld J (1986) Congenital esophageal stenosis and esophageal diaphragm. In: Ashcraft KW, Halder TM (eds) Pediatric esophageal surgery. Grune and Stratton, Orlando, p 56
70. Schullinger JN, Jacobs JC, Berdon WE (1985) Diagnosis and management of gastrointestinal perforations in childhood in dermatomyositis with particular reference to perforations of the duodenum. J Pediatr Surg 20:521
71. Sepe S, Fischetti E, Pisciotta R, et al (1980) Congenital pharyngeal esophageal diverticulum in the newborn. Chir Pediatr 21:57
72. Sigalet D, Lees E (1988) Tracheoesophageal injury secondary to disc battery ingestion. J Pediatr Surg 23:996
73. Sneed WF, La Garde DC, Kogutt MS, et al (1979) Esophageal stenosis due to cartilaginous tracheo-bronchial remnant. J Pediatr Surg 14:786
74. Spitz L (1973) Congenital esophageal stenosis distal to associated esophageal atresia. J Pediatr Surg 8:973
75. Spitz L (1984) Gastric transposition via the mediastinal route. J Pediatr Surg 19:149
76. Steigmann F, Dolehick RA (1956) Corrosive acid gastritis. N Engl J Med 254:981
77. Tachovsky TJ, Lynn HA, Ellis FH (1968) The surgical approach to esophageal achalasia in children. J Pediatr Surg 3:226
78. Takayanagi O, Li K, Komi N (1975) Congenital esophageal stenosis with lack of the submucosa. J Pediatr Surg 10:425
79. Taylor RG, Myers NA (1988) Achalasia of the cardia in children. A retrospective review of 20 cases. Pediatr Surg Int (in press)
80. Thomason MA, Gay BB (1987) Esophageal stenosis with esophageal atresia. Pediatr Radiol 17:197
81. Todani T, Watanabe Y, Mizuguchi T, et al (1984) Congenital esophageal stenosis due to fibromuscular thickening. Z Kinderchir 39:11

82. Tolstedt GE, Tudor RB (1968) Esophagopleural fistula in a newborn infant. Arch Surg 97:780
83. Traversa FP, Nibbi F, Bossu M (1970) Congestive cystic dysplasia of the esophagus and stomas. Riv Chir Pediatr 12:212
84. Warren J, Evans K, Carter CO (1979) Offspring of patients with tracheo-oesophageal fistula. J Med Genet 16:338
85. Wells SD, Leonidas JC, Conkle D, et al (1974) Traumatic prevertebral pharyngoesophageal pseudodiverticulum in the newborn infant. J Pediatr Surg 9:217
86. Zitsman JL, Schullinger JN, Berdon NE (1988) Inflammatory esophago-gastric polyps: resolution following antireflux surgery. J Pediatr Surg 23:1016

Magnetic Resonance Imaging as a New Diagnostic Criterion in Paediatric Airway Obstruction

U. Hofmann[1], D. Hofmann[2], T. Vogl[3], C. Wilimzig[3], and K. Mantel[1]

Summary

Magnetic resonance imaging of the trachea was performed in 21 children with congenital or acquired narrowing of the trachea or main bronchi. Diagnosis included aortic arch anomalities, innominate artery compression, pulmonary artery compression and tracheomalacia. All patients were examined after bronchoscopy. The demonstration of the trachea and the surrounding tissue and vessels on MR images enables the cause of tracheal compression and the degree and location of collapse to be evaluated. MRI is a modality well suited to characterizing tracheal narrowing without employing ionizing radiation or intravenous contrast medium. All MRI examinations were carried out with the patient under general anaesthesia so as not to risk pulmonary deterioration during sedation. In the cases presented MRI is the diagnostic step of choice after tracheobronchoscopy and broadens the diagnostic potential in extrinsic tracheal or bronchial stenosis in paediatric patients.

Zusammenfassung

Magnetresonanzuntersuchungen (MRI) der Trachea wurden bei 21 Kindern mit angeborenen oder erworbenen Stenosen der Trachea oder der Hauptbronchien durchgeführt. Die Diagnosen umfaßten Aortenbogenanomalien, Truncus-brachiocephalicus-Kompressionen, A.-pulmonalis-Kompressionen und Tracheomalazie. Alle Patienten wurden der Untersuchung nach vorausgegangener Bronchoskopie unterzogen. Die Darstellung der Trachea, des umgebenden Gewebes und der großen Gefäße im MRI erlaubt die Diagnose der Ursache des Trachealkollapses. MRI ist eine geeignete Technik zur Charakterisierung der Trachealkompression ohne Anwendung ionisierender Strahlung oder intravenöser Kontrastmittel. Alle MRI-Untersuchungen wurden unter Vollnarkose durchgeführt, um die Gefahr einer pulmonalen Verschlechterung durch Sedierung auszuschalten. In den beschriebenen Fällen war MRI die diagnostische Methode der Wahl nach Tracheobronchoskopie und erweiterte das diagnostische Spektrum bei Tracheal- und Bronchusstenosen bei Kindern.

Résumé

L'imagerie par résonance magnétique (IRM) ou résonance magnétique nucléaire a été utilisée pour obtenir des images de la trachée dans le cas de 21 enfants présentant un rétrécissement con-

[1]Department of Paediatric Anaesthesia, Dr. von Haunersches Kinderspital, University of Munich, D-8000 Munich (W), FRG.
[2]Department of Paediatric Surgery, Dr. von Haunersches Kinderspital, University of Munich, D-8000 Munich (W), FRG.
[3]Department of Radiology, Klinikum Großhadern, University of Munich, D-8000 Munich (W), FRG.

Progress in Pediatric Surgery, Vol. 27
Myers and Angerpointner (Eds.)

génital ou acquis de la trachée ou des bronches principales. On diagnostiqua des anomalies de l'arc aortique, des compressions de l'artère pulmonaire, d'autres artères et des trachéomalacies primitives. Tous les patients furent examinés après bronchoscopie. Les images de la trachée et des tissus adjacents, obtenues par résonance magnétique électronique, permettent d'évaluer la cause de la compression trachéale et le degré et la localisation du collapsus. Cette technique permet de distinguer un rétrécissement de la trachée sans avoir recours à la radiation ionisante et à l'injection intraveineuse d'un produit de contraste. Tous les examens effectués par résonance magnétique ont été pratiqués sous anesthésie générale afin de ne pas risquer une détérioration pulmonaire durant la sédation. Dans les cas présentés, l'imagerie par résonance magnétique est la technique diagnostique de choix après trachéo-broncoscopie et vient compléter avantageusement les possibilités diagnostiques des sténoses trachéales ou bronchiques en pédiatrie.

Introduction

In paediatric patients compression of trachea and main bronchi are often responsible for stridor and recurrent pulmonary infections, which need further clarification. Thus it is important to use capable diagnostic methods to demonstrate the cause of stenosis. In cases where compression of the airway is present in bronchoscopy only degree and location of collapse can be evaluated; it may be difficult, however, to determine the aetiology of tracheal narrowing. Until recently in these cases angiotracheography was the method of choice to secure definite diagnosis. As this procedure is quite invasive, since October 1987 in these cases bronchoscopy in our hospital has been followed by magnetic resonance imaging (MRI) of the thorax. MRI offers a direct and multiplanar imaging method of the airways and surrounding tissues especially the heart and the big vessels and has the added advantage of requiring neither intravascular contrast medium nor X-ray exposure. The aim of the study was to prove the diagnostic value of MRI examination in paediatric airway obstruction.

Materials and Methods

From October 1987 to December 1988 bronchoscopy was performed in 525 children, and compression of trachea or main bronchi was diagnosed in 49 children. All of these had presented with recurrent pulmonary infections, stridor or apnoeic spells. In 21 patients an MRI examination was performed to clarify the cause of compression. Average age was 12.3 months. In 28 children no MRI investigation was carried out. Average age was 11.2 months. In nine patients stenosis of less than 50% was found and therapy was not necessary, so we saw no indication for further investigation. In 12 children cardiac catheterization had been already performed because of a known cardiac abnormality and in bronchoscopy only the degree of tracheal narrowing was evaluated. The other seven children had been sent to our hospital for ambulant bronchoscopy; we recommended on MRI investigation, but have no information about further history.

Magnetic resonance imaging was performed with a 1.0 T Magnetom (Siemens) using multisectional, ECG-gated single-echo sequences. The patients were imaged in a 25-cm-diameter head coil. In order to maintain a satisfactory signal-to-noise ratio a minimal-section thickness of 4 mm was chosen. The number of sections depend on the extent of the anatomical region to be examined as determined by bronchoscopy. By overlapping a second sequence after shifting the slice position by one-half of the slice thickness, we were able to obtain better anatomical detail than with contiguous slices. The slices were obtained in sagittal and transaxial orientation. The transaxial slices were obtained from the level of the hypopharynx to the lower mediastinum. The duration of MRI examination was about 1 h.

All MRI examinations were performed with the patient under general anaesthesia (halothane, oxygen, nitrous oxide) and controlled ventilation with a Servo ventilator 900 D (Siemens). Monitoring included ECG, oscillatory blood pressure and monitoring of ventilation (minute volume, airway pressures, oxygen concentration, respiratory rate). To avoid motion artefacts we chose a short inspiration time of 20% and a long exspiration time of 80%. The resulting pictures show as cumulative effect the expiratory phase. The tubus tip was positioned immediately below the glottis, so that there was no distension of the stenosis by the endotracheal tube.

Results

From October 1987 to December 1988 bronchoscopy in 49 children led to suspected vascular compression of the large airways. In 21 children MRI of the thorax was performed. They were divided into four groups according to diagnosis:

1. In four dilation of the pulmonary artery due to pulmonary hypertension caused severe compression mainly of the left-stem bronchus. Partial agenesis of the right lung was found in two children, complex vitium cordis in one and in one child the pulmonary hypertension was caused by bronchopulmonary dysplasia grade IV. In none of these patients were further invasive diagnostic procedures necessary, and therapy was symptomatic. The last case in this group is described as follows:

Case 1. The 7-month-old boy had been a premature baby born in the 25th week of gestation. He had a grade IV bronchopulmonary dysplasia and suspected pulmonary hypertension. A prolonged expiration and recurrent atelectasis on the left side were indications for bronchoscopy. On laryngotracheoscopy small granulomas of the vocal cords were found on both sides, due to long-term ventilatory therapy. In addition, pulsatile compression of the bifurcation with almost total obstruction of the left-stem bronchus and 60% stenosis of the right-stem bronchus was found (Fig. 1a). On MRI, dilation of the pulmonary artery was found with compression mainly of the left-stem bronchus (Fig. 1b, c). The child was treated with oxygen therapy with an improvement in the pulmonary problems. Bronchoscopy 2 weeks later showed a significant improvement, with only 50% compression of both stem bronchi.

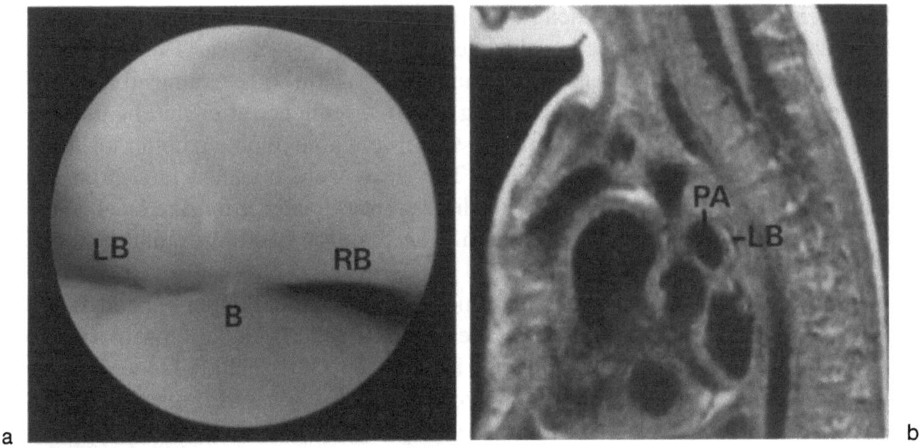

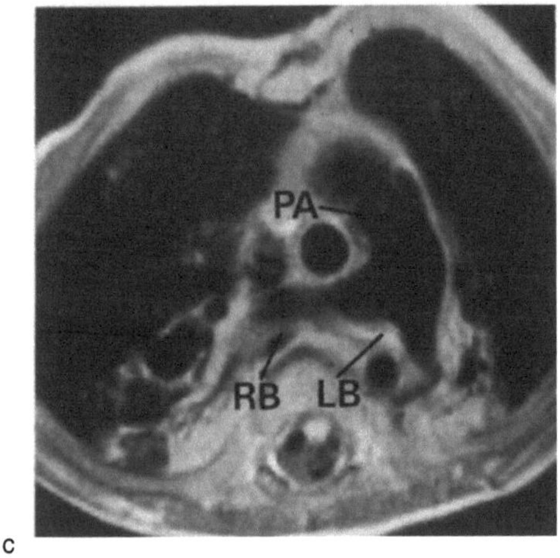

Fig. 1a–c. Case 1: tracheal compression by dilated pulmonary artery due to pulmonary hypertension. **a** Bronchoscopic findings before treatment: view of the tracheal bifurcation *(B)* with subtotal compression of the left main bronchus *(LB)* and 50% compression of the right-stem bronchus *(RB)*. **b, c** MRI findings: sagittal MR image (**b**) shows in paramedian planes compression of the left-stem bronchus *(LB)* by the dilated pulmonary artery *(PA)*. In the transaxial plane (**c**) can be seen the dilated pulmonary artery *(PA)* and the compressed main bronchi *(RB, LB)*. In the left-stem bronchus *(LB)* no lumen is visible

2. In three children MRI showed that the tracheal narrowing was caused by aortic arch anomalies. One had a right descending thoracic aorta and a markedly dilated arch crossing above the right-stem bronchus and compressing the lower trachea. The other two patients had a right aortic arch with a normal ascending and descending thoracic aorta. The arch crossed above the right main bronchus dorsal of trachea and oesophagus displacing and compressing them. In all cases diagnosis was possible by MRI, and in two patients angiography was also performed preoperatively to confirm the diagnosis. Operation verified MRI findings in all cases. One typical case is described:

Case 2. A 5-year-old girl had suffered from stridor and recurrent pulmonary infections since birth. On bronchoscopy pulsatile compression of the lower trachea with inflammatory changes was seen (Fig. 2a). MRI (Fig. 2b, c) showed the right

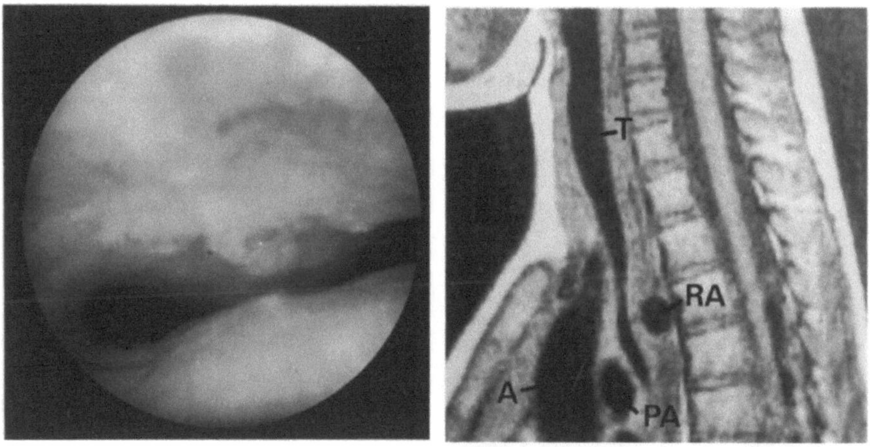

a b

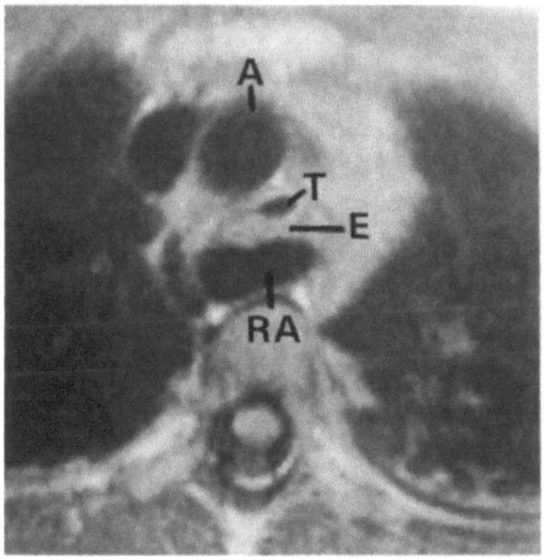

c

Fig. 2a–c. Case 2: tracheal compression by double aortic arch. **a** Bronchoscopic findings before operation: compression of the distal trachea from ventral and dorsal, with the mucosa showing inflammatory changes. **b, c** MRI shows in sagittal view (**b**) the compression of the trachea *(T)* from ventral by the ascending aorta *(A)* and dorsal by the right aortic arch *(RA)*. The pulmonary artery *(PA)* crosses the trachea at the bifurcation, but causes no compression. In transaxial slices (**c**) 2 cm above the tracheal bifurcation the vascular compression *(A, RA)* of the oesophagus *(E)* and trachea *(T)* can be seen

aortic arch crossing dorsal to the trachea and esophagus, compressing the trachea from the back. A hypoplastic left aortic arch could also be identified. After dissection of the hypoplastic left aortic arch the child was grossly asymptomatic; there was mild stridor only with exertion. This was explained by the bronchoscopic finding 3 months after the operation where malacia of the distal trachea was still present.

3. In 11 patients MRI identified innominate artery compression as the reason for respiratory problems, and in 3 children atresia of the esophagus had been operated on. All patients had been admitted to hospital because of severe stridor, recurrent pulmonary infections and apnoeic spells. In MRI investigation the course of the innominate artery was easily shown in transaxial planes. In addition the transaxial plane allowed the best evaluation of the adjacent structures, their location and relationships. Sagittal planes were best in demonstrating the site and

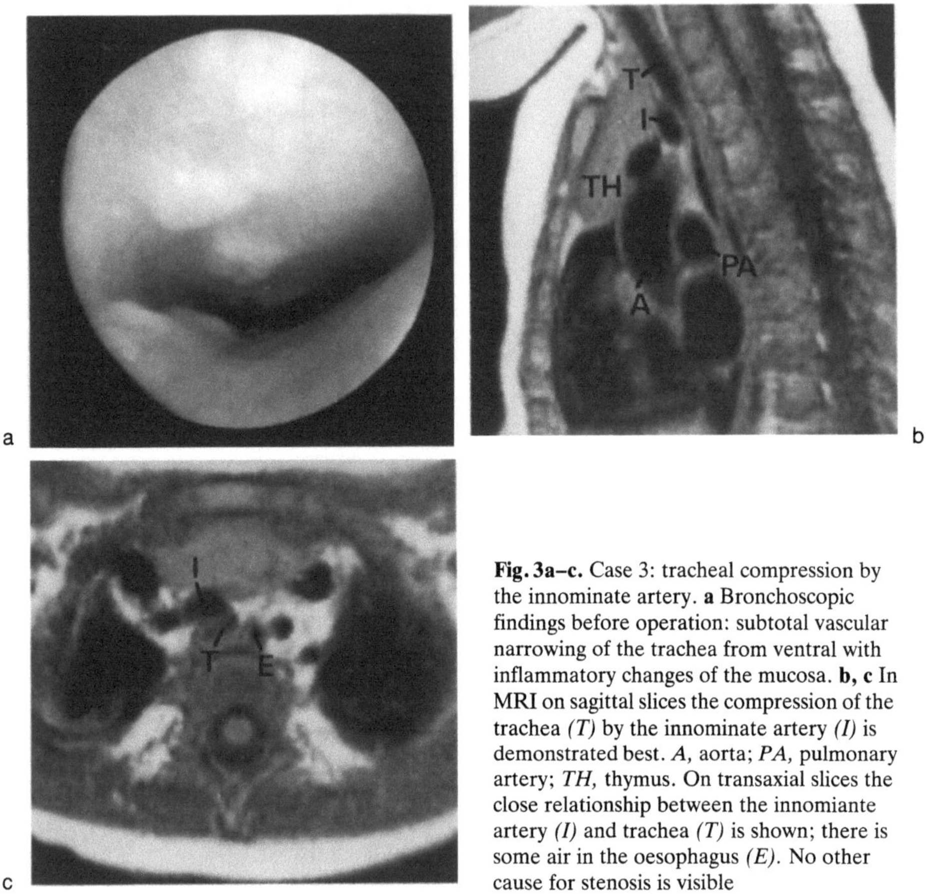

Fig. 3a–c. Case 3: tracheal compression by the innominate artery. **a** Bronchoscopic findings before operation: subtotal vascular narrowing of the trachea from ventral with inflammatory changes of the mucosa. **b, c** In MRI on sagittal slices the compression of the trachea *(T)* by the innominate artery *(I)* is demonstrated best. *A*, aorta; *PA*, pulmonary artery; *TH*, thymus. On transaxial slices the close relationship between the innomiante artery *(I)* and trachea *(T)* is shown; there is some air in the oesophagus *(E)*. No other cause for stenosis is visible

extent of tracheal compression. In none of the cases were further preoperative examinations necessary. In all patients aortopexy was carried out, and in all patients postoperative clinical condition improved. The case presented below shows a typical course:

Case 3. A 6-month-old boy was admitted to our hospital because of apnoeic spells, recurrent pulmonary infections, expiratory stridor and a barking cough. High-kV X-ray of the trachea showed a collapse of the distal trachea and oesophagography showed no pathological findings. Laryngotracheoscopy showed an 80% pulsatile narrowing of the lower trachea from ventral (Fig. 3a). In MRI (Fig. 3b, c) the close anatomical relationship between the innominate artery and the trachea could be demonstrated. Thus the innominate artery could be identified as the cause of the tracheal compression. Aortopexy was performed; postoperatively the child was without symptoms. Tracheoscopy 3 months later showed no remaining stenosis.

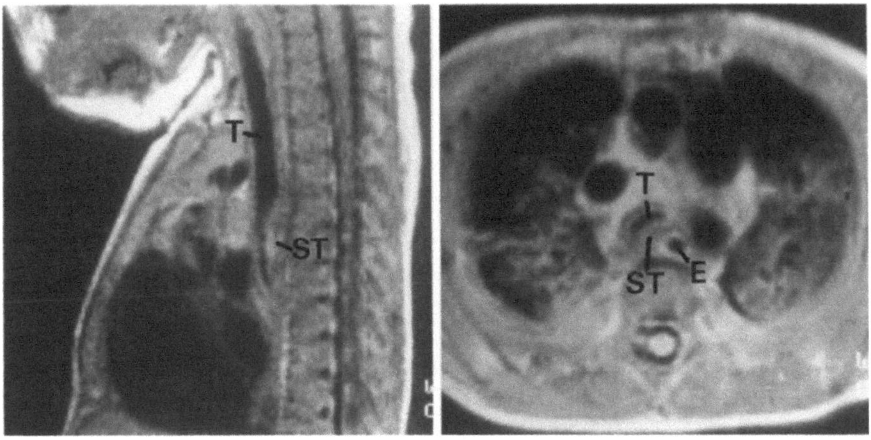

a b

Fig. 4a, b Case 4: tracheal narrowing by scar tissue after repair of oesophageal atresia. In MRI neither in sagittal (**b**) nor in transaxial (**c**) slices is there a vascular cause for the distal tracheal stenosis. On a sagittal view the impression from dorsal is shown. The transaxial plane demonstrates the tracheal *(T)* narrowing from dorsal and the location of the oesophagus *(E)*. Between the trachea and oesophagus additional tissue *(ST)* after repair of the oesophageal atresia is found (scar tissue)

4. In three children MRI verified tracheal or bronchial compression, but there was no sign of involvement of vessels. Complex cardiac or vascular abnormalities were excluded. The cause rather was tracheomalacia due to tracheitis and in one case scar tissue after correction of atresia of the oesophagus. This patient is described as follows:

Case 4. A 6-month-old boy with Down's syndrome had undergone repair of atresia of the oesophagus after birth. Postoperatively clinical course was complicated by recurrent pulmonary infections and atelectasis, thus requiring repeated intubation and prolonged ventilatory support. Because of innominate artery compression of the trachea aortopexy was performed at the age of 6 months. Afterwards bronchoscopy showed severe stenosis of the lower trachea by dorsal compression. Therefore MRI examination was carried out (Fig. 4a, b). No vessel could be identified compressing the trachea. Stenosis, however, was caused by scar tissue between the oesophagus and lower trachea after operative dissection of the tracheo-oesophageal fistula. Thus only conservative treatment was possible.

Discussion

Trachel stenosis in paediatric patients typically presents with respiratory distress, wheezing and stridor [1–7]. Two main groups have to be differentiated:

1. Intrinsic stenosis of the airways caused by inflammation, malformations, tumours, foreigns bodies or injuries. This group is reliably diagnosed by bronchoscopy.

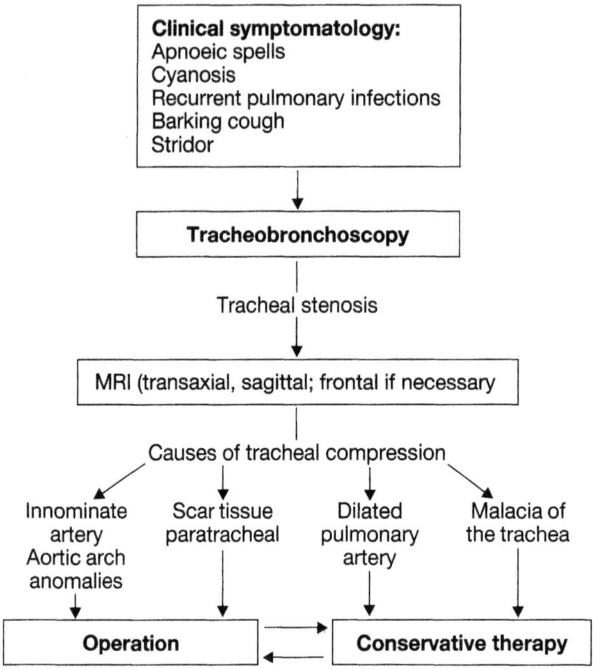

Fig. 5. Flow chart of diagnostic steps in paediatric airway obstruction

2. Extrinsic stenosis of the airways caused by the great vessels, tumours or malacia of the tracheal cartilage. In these cases bronchoscopy can only evaluate the degree of tracheal or bronchial narrowing, but not the definite cause of stenosis. To date tracheobronchoscopy has been followed in these cases by combined aorto-tracheography, ultrafast computed tomography (CT) or conventional CT.

However, performing combined aortotracheography in infants with respiratory difficulties is dangerous, because it may cause deterioration of pulmonary function; on the other hand, it shows the direct course of the vessels and their relationship to the airways [11]. Ultrafast CT has the advantage of speed [8], therefore requires no sedation and is capable of recording dynamic changes. Conventional CT has its main indication when mediastinal tumours are suspected. The major disadvantage of all these diagnostic modalities is the use of ionizing radiation and contrast medium. As a new diagnostic modality we tested the use of MRI in paediatric airway compression. MRI has a very high soft tissue contrast and is able to identify a wide range of disorders in the mediastinum. The blood vessels and heart are extremely well visualized without the use of any contrast agents and provide excellent anatomical detail [9]. The possibility of positioning different planes, in our examination regimen transaxial and sagittal, enables the cause of tracheal compression and the degree and location of collapse to be evaluated. In all patients diagnosis was made by MRI examination.

In our patients we distinguished four groups.

The *first* group included children with pulmonary hypertension. In these childen the MRI examination was performed to exclude complex malformations of the big vessels. In two of the three patients congenital hypo- or aplasia of one lung was present and so additional malformations of the intrathoracal vessels had to be excluded. In both cases MRI was capable of showing normal vascular structures except the far above normal size of the pulmonary artery which compressed the left main bronchus at the tracheal bifurcation. It was difficult to show the position of the compressed stem bronchi, because of its small size and if compressed the low air signal was missing. But the combination of bronchoscopy and MRI findings in all patients was enough for a satisfactory diagnosis.

The *second* group in our study were patients with anomalies of the aortic arch. In these cases the tracheal stenosis and surrounding vessels were well shown in the transaxial planes. Sagittal planes allowed the abnormal course of the aortic arch to be evalucated. In all cases diagnosis was verified with MRI. In two cases catheterization of the heart was performed, but uncovered no additional malformations. Diagnosis in all cases was confirmed by surgery, and the hypoplastic aortic arch was dissected in all patients.

In the *third* group the innominate artery was the cause of tracheal compression. In all cases tracheal narrowing by the innominate artery was best shown on the sagittal slices. In transaxial planes the course of the innominate artery and the aortic arch as well as surrounding tissues were shown best. No anatomical abnormality could be shown except tracheal narrowing. Innominate artery compression is the commonest cause of tracheal narrowing in early childhood [10]. As Döhlemann et al. [11] demonstrated, it is caused by the specific mediastinal anatomy in small infants and usually has no relevance as the cause of tracheal stenosis in children older than 3 years. To date no definite reason for the compression has been identified. In some patients tracheomalacia has been supposed to be an additional factor, as it is found in children after repair of oesophageal atresia. These findings correspond to those of Fletcher et al. [12], who performed MRI in children with suspected tracheal stenoses of the innominate artery and found impression of the trachea but no anatomical abnormalities in the course of the innominate artery.

In the *fourth* group of children no vascular compression of the trachea could be found. Nevertheless MRI was helpful in providing a diagnosis. In patients with suspected tracheomalacia, thickening of the tracheal wall due to inflammatory changes can hint at the diagnosis, but the main information from MRI was that there were no anatomical structures causing tracheal narrowing.

In this study we preferred general anaesthesia for keeping the infants motionless during the examination, which is regarded as the main disadvantage of this method. Sedation is also described in the literature [12], but has its risks [13]. In children with severe pulmonary problems as in this study, general anaesthesia in our opinion is the procedure of choice, because control of respiration is always provided.

Magnetic resonance imaging showed in this study that it can serve as a diagnostic modality after tracheobronchoscopy (Fig. 5) with a high reliability for providing a definite diagnosis in paediatric airway compression without the use of ionizing radiation or intravenous contrast medium.

References

1. Berdon WE, Baker DH, Borduik J, Mellins R (1969) Innominate artery compression of the trachea in infants with stridor and apnea. Radiology 92:272–278
2. Schwartz MZ, Filler RM (1980) Tracheal compression as a cause of apnea following repair of tracheoesophageal fistula: treatment by aortopexy. J Pediatr Surg 15:845–848
3. Sotomayor JL, Godinez RI, Bordon S, Wilmott RW (1986) Large-airway collapse due to acquired tracheobronchomalacia in infancy. Am J Dis Child 140:367–371
4. Döhlemann C, Mantel K, Dusch T, Bühlmeyer K (1978) Trachealkompression durch den Truncus brachiocephalicus. Herz 3:126–132
5. Bradham RR, Sealy WC, Young G (1968) Respiratory distress associated with anomalies of the aortic arch. Surg Gynecol Obstet: 9–14
6. Joseph PM, Berdon WE, Baker DH, Slovis TL, Haller JO (1976) Upper airway obstruction in infants and small children. Radiology 121:143–148
7. Filler RM, Rossello RJ, Lebowitz RL (1976) Life threatening anoxic spells caused by tracheal compression after repair of esophageal atresia: correction by surgery. J Pediatr Surg 11:739–748
8. Brasch RC, Gould RG, Gooding CA, Ringertz HG, Lipton MJ (1987) Upper airway obstruction in infants and children: evaluation with ultrafast CT. Radiology 165:459–466
9. Cohen MD (1986) Pediatric magnetic resonance imaging. Saunders, Philadelphia
10. Welz A, Reichert B, Weinhold C, Überfuhr P, Mantel K, Döhlemann C, Hecker W (1984) Innominate artery compression of the trachea in infancy and childhood: is surgical therapy justified? Thorac Cardiovasc Surg 32:85–88
11. Döhlemann C, Mantel K, Dusch T, Bühlmeyer K (1978) Trachealkompression durch den Truncus brachiocephalicus. Herz 3:126–132
12. Fletcher BD, Cohn RC (1989) Tracheal compression and the innominate artery: MR evaluation in infants. Radiology 170:103–107
13. Mitchell AA, Louik C, Lacouture P, Slone D, Goldman P, Shapiro S (1982) Risks to children from computed tomographic scan premedication. JAMA 17:2385–2388

Tracheal Stenosis by Innominate Artery Compression in Infants: Surgical Treatment in 35 Cases

T. Schuster, W. Ch. Hecker, E. Ring-Mrozik, K. Mantel, and T. Vogl

Summary

This is a report on 35 cases of innominate artery compression of the trachea and its surgical correction by means of aortotruncopexy. Diagnostic procedures of choice were tracheoscopy and magnetic resonance imaging, which offers representative images of inspiration and expiration, shows the anatomical relations between aortic arch and trachea and reveals the extent of tracheal compression. Surgical treatment is indicated if narrowing of the tracheal lumen exceeds 70%. By fixation of the aortic arch and the proximal innominate artery to the back of the sternum, tracheal compression is relieved. There was no unsuccessful operation in the 35 children. One late death occurred from cardiac failure, unrelated to tracheal compression.

Zusammenfassung

Es wird über 35 Kinder mit Trachealstenose durch Truncus-brachiocephalicus-Kompression sowie deren operative Korrektur berichtet. Die diagnostischen Methoden der Wahl waren Tracheoskopie und Magnetic Resonance Imaging (MRI); diese Verfahren lieferten repräsentative Bilder von In- und Exspiration, von den anatomischen Beziehungen zwischen Aortenbogen und Trachea und dem Ausmaß der Trachealkompression. Die chirurgische Korrektur ist indiziert, wenn die Einengung des Tracheallumens 70% übersteigt. Durch Fixation des Aortenbogens und des proximalen Truncus brachiocephalicus an die Rückseite des Sternums wird die Trachealkompression beseitigt. Ein Therapieversager wurde bei den 35 Kindern nicht beobachtet. Ein später auftretender Todesfall durch Herzversagen stand nicht in Zusammenhang mit der Trachealkompression.

Résumé

Il est question de 35 cas de trachéosténoses dues à une compression de l'artère brachiocéphalique et de leur correction chirurgicale. Les méthodes de choix pour le diagnostic étaient la trachéoscopie et l'imagerie par résonance magnétique qui permet d'obtenir des images précises de l'inspiration et l'expiration, mettant en lumière les rapports anatomiques entre l'arc aortique et la trachée et révèlant également l'ampleur de la compression de la trachée. Un traitement chirurgical s'impose si le rétrécissement de la lumière de la trachée excède 70%. En fixant l'arc aortique et le tronc brachiocéphalique à l'arrière du sternum, on met fin à la compression de la trachée. Toutes les interventions pratiquées dans le cas des 35 enfants ont été couronnées de succès. Ultérieurement, un décès est survenu, dû à une défaillance cardiaque, sans rapport avec la compression de la trachée.

Paediatric Surgical Clinic, University Children's Hospital of Munich, Lindwurmstraße 4, D-8000 München 2, (W) FRG.

Progress in Pediatric Surgery, Vol. 27
Myers and Angerpointner (Eds.)

In 1945, Mercer [15] described severe respiratory distress symptoms in a child who had been previously operated on for oesophageal atresia by Haight [11]: dyspnoea with stridor, particularly during feeding or shortly thereafter, followed by cyanotic attacks and bradycardia.

The same symptoms were described by Gross and Neuhauser in 1948 [10] in a child without oesophageal atresia; they were relieved by hyperextension of the head. Lateral projection tracheography revealed definite narrowing of the distal third of the trachea, caused by external compression of the anterior tracheal wall. At operation, the innominate artery was found to be adjacent to the trachea. Tracheal compression was relieved by fixation of the vessel to the back of the sternum.

Our knowledge on the syndrome today, 40 years after the first description of innominate artery compression of the trachea and its successful surgical correction by aortopexy, is summarized in the following.

Pathology and Pathogenesis

Compression of a Malacic Trachea

It is thought that a malacic trachea is compressed by a normal innominate artery [17, 19]. In half of the patients we have operated on for innominate artery compression of the trachea, we found that tracheal narrowing extended proximally and distally from the main compression point by the vessel, even down to the left main bronchus. There was no difference between children who had been operated on for oesophageal atresia and those who had not.

In more than 50% of the children with oesophageal atresia the posterior tracheal wall also bulged into the lumen. Wailoo and Emmery [24] found abnormal shape and number of the cartilaginous rings of the trachea in 75% of 40 children with tracheo-oesophageal fistula; this caused abnormal widening of the posterior wall. On a transverse section of a normal trachea, the ratio between the cartilaginous and membranous parts is 4.5:1. In a malacic trachea, however, the ratio is only 2:1 [2]. Nakazato et al. [18] carried out autopsies on 28 patients with oesophageal atresia and tracheo-oesophageal fistula and concluded that pathologic tracheal innervation might possibly be responsible for pathologic ciliary movements, tracheal gland secretion and flaccidity of the posterior tracheal wall. Caldera [4] reported on 27 children with oesophageal atresia, nine of whom developed symptoms of tracheal compression by the innominate artery. Tracheoscopy revealed a collapse of the whole distal trachea, mainly during inspiration, without circumscript tracheal compression.

Sixteen of the 35 children in our series underwent angiography. An abnormal origin of the innominate artery, described as a variant of moderate degree, was seen in one case only. In the 15 patients of Moes et al. [16] who had angiography and aortopexy, the innominate artery arose from the aortic arch either in front of or to the left of the trachea on antero-posterior projection. This was in accordance with the normal anatomical situation as described by Strife et al. [22] angiographically in 96% of 172 patients and by Remy et al. [19] in 98% of 118 infants without respiratory problems.

Feeding and Respiratory Distress

The relation between feeding and attacks of respiratory distress can be explained by the fact that the trachea, compressed anteriorly by the innominate artery, is additionally obstructed from behind by a bolus passing through the oesophagus (Fig. 1) [20].

It has also been supposed that the passage of a bolus triggers a reflex, mediated by the vagal nerve. Thus, apnoea would be a reflectory event initiated by irritation of the compressed area of the trachea [9].

Herbst et al. [13] assume that micro-aspiration and oesophagitis due to gastro-oesophageal reflux are responsible for laryngospasm, followed by stridor and apnoeic spells. Bargy et al. [1], for instance, reported on six children with innominate artery compression syndrome who became free of symptoms following surgical correction of the gastro-oesophageal reflux.

Stabilization of the Trachea with Growth

In the framework of growth during the first half of the 2nd year of life, the skeleton of the collapsing trachea stabilizes. This is evidenced by the disappearance of the stridoric, barking cough attacks, which we call "oesophageal cough" in chil-

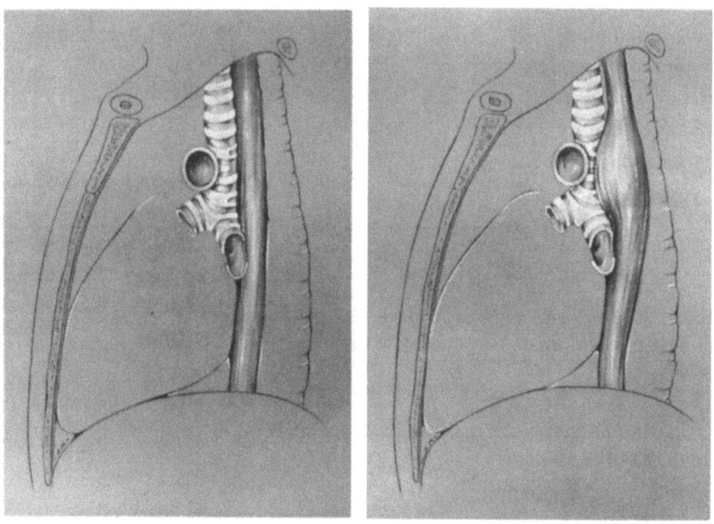

a b

Fig. 1. a Tracheal compression by the innominate artery and the aortic arch. **b** Food bolus passing through the oesophagus and effecting nearly total tracheal obstruction

dren with operated oesophageal atresia. Moreover, the innominate artery moves away from the trachea within the first 2 years of life [7]. Thus it is well established that the innominate artery compression syndrome can resolve spontaneously, and the question therefore arises of which patients have to be operated on and which can be managed expectantly or conservatively.

Symptoms

The main symptom of our 35 children operated on by aortotruncopexy were as follows: Thirty-one presented with noisy respiration, mainly inspiratory and expiratory stridor (89%), 24 with apnoeic spells (69%) and about half exhibited bradycardia and cyanotic attacks, recurrent bronchopulmonary infections and the characteristic barking cough. Half of the children showed these symptoms during feeding or shortly thereafter (Table 1).

The severity of the syndrome depends on the remaining tracheal lumen as defined endoscopically, as well as on the age at onset of symptoms [2].

In all our cases there was 70%–90% narrowing of the tracheal lumen. Twenty-four of the 35 children (67%) presented with symptoms as early as the first 2 months of life, seven (20%) in the 3rd to 5th months, and four (13%) during the 6th to 13th months (Table 2).

Table 1. Tracheal compression by the innominate artery: incidence of symptoms (n = 35)

Symptom	n	%	Symptoms	n	%
Apnoeic spells	24	(69)	Symptoms occurring during or shortly after feeding	18	(51)
Noisy respiration	31	(89)	Bradykardia	17	(49)
Inspiratory/expiratory stridor	22	(63)	Cyanotic attacks	23	(60)
Mainly inspiratory	6	(20)	Recurrent bronchopulmonary infections	17	(49)
Mainly expiratory	3	(9)	Spontaneous hyperextension of the head	9	(26)
Barking cough	17	(49)			
Dysphagia	8	(23)			

Table 2. Tracheal compression by the innominate artery: time of onset of symptoms (n = 35)

Time n		%
Up to end of 2nd month	24	(67)
During 3rd to 5th months	7	(20)
During 6th to 13th months	4	(13)
Total	35	(100)

Differential Diagnosis

Differential diagnoses range from cardiac, cerebral and metabolic disorders to bronchopulmonary disorders of other origin, particularly in those children operated on for esophageal atresia or tracheo-oesophageal fistula. Postoperative complications such as atelectases, pneumonia, aspiration and laryngospasm should also be kept in mind. Furthermore, recurrence of a tracheo-oesophageal fistula, hypertrophy of granulation tissue at the site of a former fistula, a foreign body and a food bolus in the oesophagus all come into question, as do anastomotic stricture after repair of an oesophageal atresia and gastro-oesophageal reflux. Yet another form of tracheal stenosis is subglottic stenosis following long-term intubation. Pulsatile tracheal compressions require exclusion of anomalies of the great vessels, such as double aortic arch, aberrant left pulmonary artery, right aortic arch and aberrant origin of the innominate artery. We have seen two children with double aortic arch who presented with symptoms the same as those caused by innominate artery compression of the trachea. The diagnosis was established by means of esophagography and tracheography [6].

Diagnosis

Various investigations may be necessary according differential diagnosis: ECG, long-term EEG, polygraphic examinations (i.e. simultaneous recording of ECG, EEG, abdominal movements and nasal air flow during respiration), transcutaneous PO_2 measurement or pulse oximetry, brain ultrasound, cardiac ultrasound, 24-h pH-metry, oesophagography, endoscopy, chest X-ray and investigations to exclude certain metabolic diseases.

The specific diagnosis of innominate artery compression of the trachea is established by tracheoscopy and MRI. In doubtful cases combined angiotracheography may be necessary.

Tracheoscopy, which was performed in all cases (Table 3), revealed the typical pulsatile tracheal stenosis with 70%–90% narrowing of the distal tracheal lumen

Table 3. Tracheal compression by the innominate artery: diagnostic procedures (n = 35)

Procedure	Number performed	Diagnosis established	
		n	%
Tracheoscopy	35	35	100
Combined angiotracheography	16	12	74
Tracheal X-ray	17	14	82
Cardiac ultrasound	11	0	0
CT	2	1	50
MRI	12	10	83

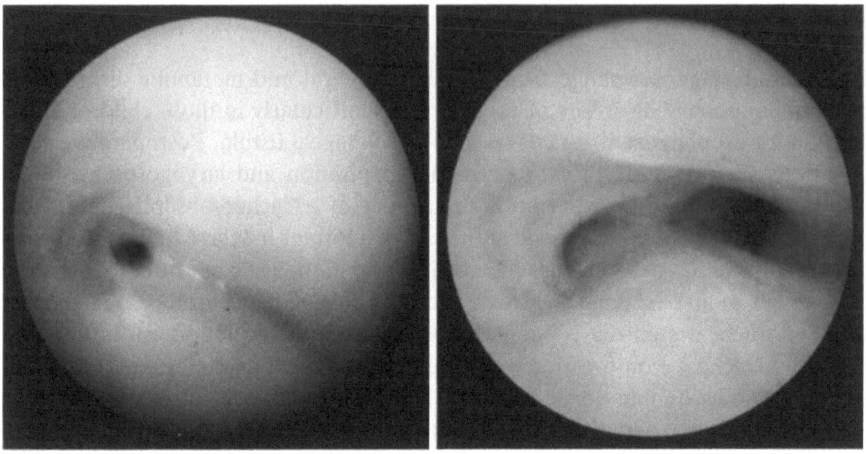

a b

Fig. 2a Tracheoscopy: right anterior compression of the distal trachea. **b** Same case after aortotruncopexy: almost normal lumen of the trachea. Note the bulging dorsal wall and the absence of the horseshoe shape of the malacic cartilages

(Fig. 2). Combined angiotracheography, which was carried out in 16 cases, established the diagnosis of innominate artery compression syndrome in 14 instances. Other examinations, such as chest X-ray, echocardiography or CT, were not found to be useful.

We are now of the opinion that MRI, carried out after tracheoscopy, is the most decisive diagnostic tool, since it demonstrates the relations between the innominate artery and the trachea very clearly (Fig. 3) [23]. The diagnosis was established in 10 of our 12 patients in whom MRI was carried out. Body plethysmography is being used with increasing frequency to confirm the diagnosis and to assess postoperative pulmonary function in infants [26].

Surgical Management

In our opinion, the indications for surgery are the following:

1. Life-threatening anoxic spells
2. Tracheal narrowing in excess of 70% and recurrent bronchopulmonary infection
3. Evidence that symptomatic tracheal stenosis is due to compression by the innominate artery or the aortic arch

Different surgical approaches to the aortic arch and the innominate artery are described in the literature (Table 4). Besides sternotomy [5], left- or right-sided thoracotomy is used to provide access for aortotruncopexy [10, 14, 20]. Blair et al.

[3] combined aortotruncopexy with splinting of the flaccid trachea by implantation of a semirigid Marlex-Silastic sleeve. Hartl [12] performed a sternotomy and wrapped the vessels with lyophilized dura before doing aortopexy. Spitz [21] recommended left-sided thoracotomy and attached a Dacron patch to the anterior surface of the aortic arch before performing aortopexy.

We prefer a right-sided thoracotomy in the third intercostal space after longitudinal skin and muscle incision in the median axillary line, thus achieving easy access to the aortic arch and the innominate artery. This approach leaves only an inconspicious scar.

In detail, our surgical procedure is as follows: A longitudinal skin incision is made in the median axillary line on the right side, followed by thoracotomy in the third intercostal space. After resection of a part of the right thymic lobe, the upper pericardium is opened to expose the aortic arch and the origin of the innominate artery.

Then, using a periosteal needle, five to seven nonresorbable 5×0 Prolene stitches are placed in the anterior wall of the aortic arch and the origin of the innominate artery, running through the sternum to its anterior surface. All stitches are tied so that the aortic arch and the innominate artery are pulled toward the back of the sternum (Fig. 4). The pericardium is left open, a thoracic drainage tube is put in place and the thoracotomy is closed in the usual way.

Patients and Results

From 1976 to 1989, aortotruncopexy was performed in 35 children at our institution. All patients showed clinical and endoscopic evidence of innominate artery tracheal compression syndrome.

Sixteen children had formerly undergone repair of oesophagela fistula and tracheo-oesophageal fistula (14 with oesophageal atresia of Vogt type IIIB, 2 with Vogt type IIIA).

Depending on the onset of compression symptoms (see Table 2), 13 infants (37%) were operated on up to the 4th month of life, 15 (43%) between the 5th and the 8th month, and the remaining 7 patients (20%) between the 8th and the 15th month of life (Table 5).

In all children positive results could be achieved. Twenty-seven children (77%) were free of symptoms immediately after surgery or within 2 weeks postoperatively (Table 6).

Three patients (9%) temporarily developed apnoeic spells again. In all three severe tracheomalacia of nearly the whole trachea was present, and all formerly had repair of an oesophageal atresia. Two of these additionally had a mucosal fold at the site of the former tracheo-oesophageal fistula, and one suffered additionally from severe subglottic tracheal stenosis secondary to long-term intubation.

The remaining five children showed remarkable relief of their symptoms, having no apnoeic spells postoperatively; they did, however, display stridor during

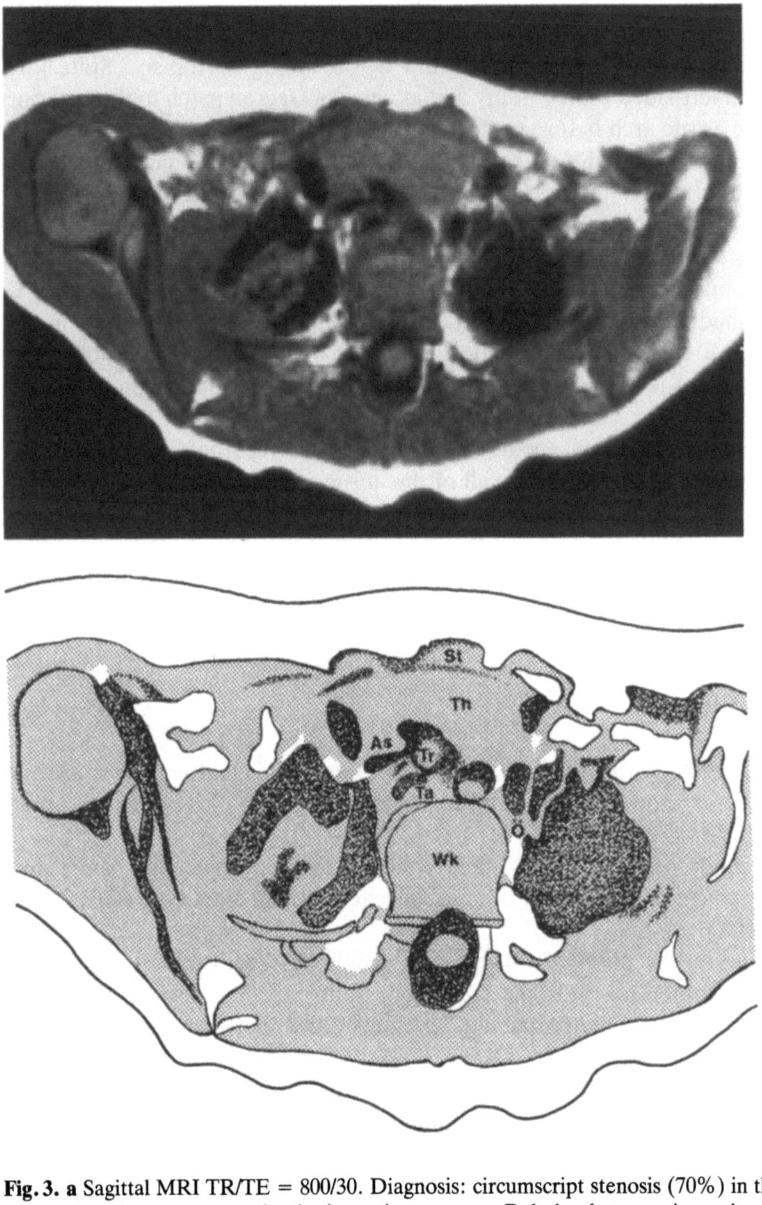

a

Fig. 3. a Sagittal MRI TR/TE = 800/30. Diagnosis: circumscript stenosis (70%) in the middle of the trachea due to compression by innominate artery. Relation between innominate artery and trachea can be clearly seen. *St,* sternum; *Th,* thymus; *Tr,* innominate artery; *Ta,* trachea. **b** Transverse MRI at level of upper thoracic aperture, same case. The trachea is rescent-shaped due to the compression. *St,* sternum; *Th,* thymus; *Tr,* innominate artery; *Ta,* trachea; *As,* subclavian artery; *Ö,* oesophagus; *Wk,* vertebral body

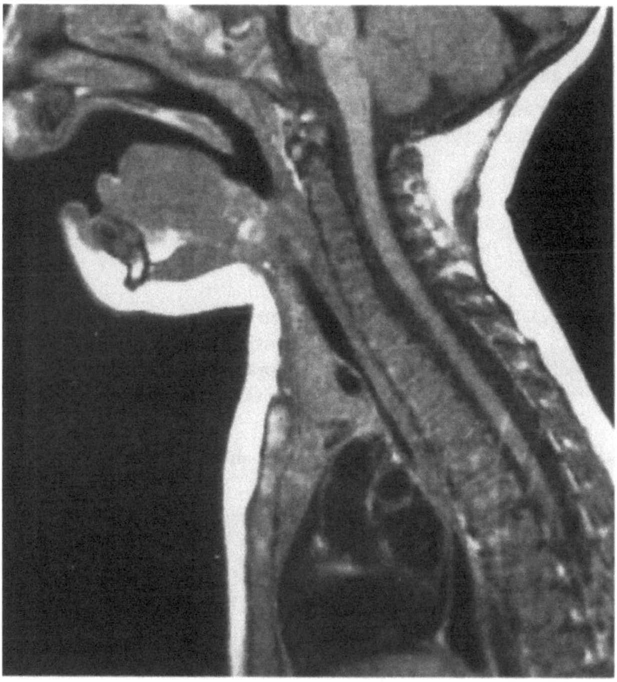

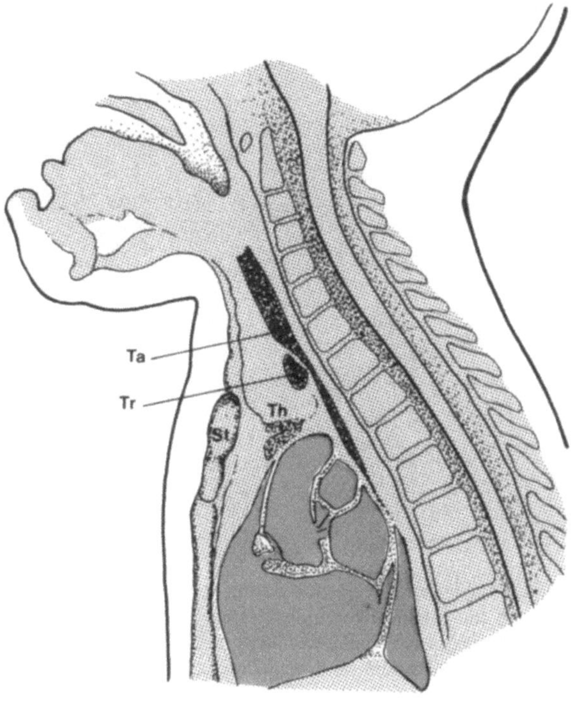

Fig. 3b

b

Table 4. Tracheal compression by the innominate artery: surgical approach and procedures

Author(s)	Year	Approach	Procedure
Gross and Neuhauser [10]	1948	Left lateroventral thoracotomy	Aortotruncopexy
Schwartz and Filler [20]	1980	Left lateroventral thoracotomy	Aortotruncopexy
Hartl [12]	1977	Sternotomy	Lyophilized dura sleeve around vessel, aortotruncopexy
Cohen [5]	1981	Sternotomy	Aortotruncopexy, possibly with pexy of common carotid artery
Blair et al. [3]	1986	Left anterior thoracotomy, possibly lateroposterior thoracotomy, right cervical incision, sternotomy	Aortotruncopexy, external airway splinting by attachment of a semi-rigid cylindrical Marlex-mesh sleeve
Spitz [21]	1986	Left anterior thoracotomy	Aortic Dacron patch, aortotruncopexy
Kiely et al. [14]	1987	Left anterior thoracotomy	Aortotruncopexy, possibly with tracheopexy
Hecker and colleagues	1989	Right lateroventral thoracotomy, longitudinal skin incision in median axillary line	Aortotruncopexy

a

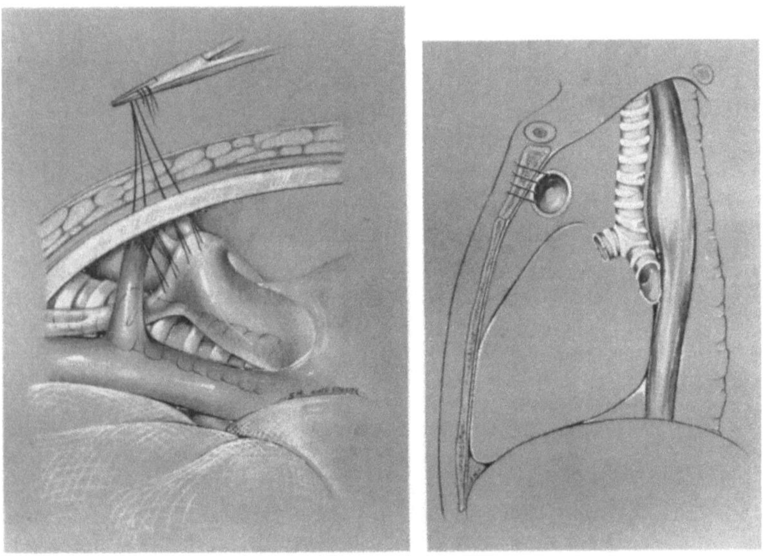

b

Fig. 4. a Aortotruncopexy, view during operation: sutures placed at the anterior wall of the aortic arch and the origin of the innominate artery run through the sternum to its anterior surface. **b** Aortotruncopexy completed. The sutures pull the aortic arch and the innominate artery toward the back of the sternum, thus relieving tracheal compression. A food bolus does not compress the trachea

Table 5. Tracheal compression by the innominate artery: age at aortotruncopexy ($n = 35$)

Age	n	%
Up to 4 months	13	(37)
3–5 months	15	(43)
9–15 months	7	(20)
Total	35	(100)

Table 6. Tracheal compression by the innominate artery: results of aortotruncopexy ($n = 35$)

Result	n	%
"Excellent" (immediately free of all symptoms)	27	(77)
"Good" (almost free of symptoms, stridor when excited)	5	(14)[a]
"Poor" (temporary apnoeic spells, all after repair of oesophageal atresia)	3	(9)[b]

[a] One extensive tracheomalacia, tracheal splinting with a rib; one bronchomalacia, lung aplasia, colonic interposition after oesophageal atresia; one subglottic tracheal stenosis secondary to long-term intubation after oesophageal atresia, laryngoplasty later; two residual stenoses (10%)

[b] One extended tracheomalacia, stenosis of right intermediate bronchus, dorsal mucosal fold, trisomy 21, cor pulmonale, shock lung, died later from cardiac failure; one extensive tracheomalacia and stenosis of right main bronchus, dorsal mucosal fold, subglottic circular tracheal stenosis (80%); one extensive tracheomalacia, residual stenosis (50%)

effort and on excitement. In one case, tracheomalacia was so severe that tracheal stenting became necessary later on. In another case tracheomalacia extended to a single main bronchus (lung aplasia), and an oesophageal atresia had been treated by colonic interposition. One child developed subglottic stenosis secondary to long-term intubation and is therefore not free of respiratory symptoms. The last two patients showed slight narrowing of the distal trachea postoperatively on endoscopy (see Table 6).

Postoperative Complications

We encountered intraoperative damage with subsequent palsy of the phrenic nerve, the complication most often described in the literature [8, 25], in four instances (11%). Nine children (26%) developed pleural effusions postoperatively, and seven inflammatory bronchopulmonary processes (20%).

Temporary atelectases were seen in 16 cases (46%), and respiratory insufficiency could be controlled by oscillatory ventilation in one child postoperatively. There were no early deaths in the series, but one child later died from cardiac failure unrelated to the condition that had prompted surgery (trisomy 21).

Conclusions

Aortotruncopexy is a suitable procedure for treatment of the innominate artery compression syndrome of the trachea.

It is emphasized by many authors that "excellent" results, i.e., promt relief of symptoms postoperatively, can be achieved in 70%–80% of cases [2, 3, 5, 14, 16, 17, 20]. On the basis of our own experience and the results reported in the literature, "good" results, i.e., temporary noisy respiration, are obtained in another 15%–28%. In the patients who still had apneic spells after aortotruncopexy, extensive tracheomalacia and additional pathological changes of the tracheobronchial tree were observed. Those children had already developed bronchopulmonary complications following repair of an oesophageal atresia [3, 14, 16].

The indications for surgery are based on the predominantly life-threatening character of the symptoms – apnoeic spells and bradycardia – and on cyanotic attacks, recurrent bronchopulmonary infections with retention of mucus, and endoscopically proven narrowing of the tracheal lumen, which exceeded 70% in all our cases. MRI reveals the causal relation between the innominate artery and the tracheal stenosis [23].

Particularly in children who develop respiratory problems after repair of an oesophageal atresia, tracheal compression by the innominate artery must be taken into account, and timely tracheobronchoscopy is required.

Our own investigations revealed that 59% of such children who survived then presented with bronchopulmonary complaints, and 17% of these patients required aortotruncopexy. Similar figures were reported by Bargy et al. [1].

Lung function tests should be performed routinely in children with oesophageal atresia as well as before and after aortotruncopexy for follow-up and assessment of tracheal instability and tracheal stenosis respectively.

References

1. Bargy F, Manach Y, Wakim A (1984) Tracheomalacia in esophageal atresia. Chir Pediatr 25:261–264
2. Benjamin B, Cohen D, Glasson M (1976) Tracheomalacia in association with tracheo-esophageal fistula. Surgery 79:504–508
3. Blair GK, Cohen R, Filler RM (1986) Treatment of tracheomalacia: eight years experience. J Pediatr Surg 21:781–785
4. Caldera R (1978) Tracheal compression as a cause of respiratory symptoms after repair of esophageal atresia. Arch Dis Child 53:761–764
5. Cohen D (1981) Tracheopexy – aortotracheal suspension for severe tracheomalacia. Aust Pediatr J 17:117–121
6. Daum R, Hecker WCh (1965) Beitrag zur Operationstechnik beim sog. vasculären Ring (doppelter Aortenbogen). Chirurg 36:510–512
7. Döhlemann C, Mantel K, Dusch T, Bühlmeyer K (1978) Trachealkompression durch den Truncus brachiocephalicus. Herz 3:126–132
8. Ekkelkamp S, Voss A, Moormann-Voestermanns EEM, Krul E (1986) Treatment of paroxysmal dyspnoea after operative correction of oesophageal atresia. Acta Paedochir Hellen 1:41–44

9. Fearon B, Shortreed R (1963) Tracheobronchial compression by cardiovascular anomalies. Ann Otol Rhinol Laryngol 72:949–969
10. Gross RE, Neuhauser EBD (1948) Compression of the trachea by an anomalous innominate artery. An operation for its relief. Am J Dis Child 75:570–574
11. Haight C (1944) Congenital atresia of the esophagus and tracheoesophageal fistula. Reconstruction of esophageal continuity by primary anastomosis. Ann Surg 120:623–655
12. Hartl M (1977) Congenitaler Stridor durch Anomalien des Aortenbogens. Z Kinderchir 22:232–240
13. Herbst JJ, Minton A, Book D (1979) Gastroesophageal reflux causing respiratory distress and apnea in newborn infants. J Pediatr 95:736–768
14. Kiely EM, Spitz L, Brereton R (1987) Management of tracheomalacia by aortopexy. Pediatr Surg Int 2:13–15
15. Mercer RD (1945) Laryngeal stridor with temporary cardiac and respiratory arrest. A complication of congenital esophageal atresia with tracheoesophageal fistula. Am J Dis Child 70:336–338
16. Moes C, Izukawa T, Trusler G (1975) Innominate artery compression of the trachea. Arch Otolaryngol 101:733–738
17. Mustard R, Bayliss C, Fearson B (1969) Tracheal compression by the innominate artery in children. Ann Thor Surg 8:313–319
18. Nakazato Y, Wells TR, Landing BH (1986) Abnormal tracheal innervation in patients with esophageal atresia and tracheo-esophageal fistula. Study of intrinsic tracheal nerve plexus by a microdissection technique. J Pediatr Surg 21:838–844
19. Remy J, Dupuis C, Breviere GM (1974) Etude anatomo-radioligique de "L'anomalie de naissance" du tronc arterial brachio-cephalique. Arch Franc Pediatr 31:641–655
20. Schwartz MZ, Filler RM (1980) Tracheal compression as a cause of apnoe following repair of tracheo-esophageal fistula. Treatment by aortopexy. J Pediatr Surg 15:842–848
21. Spitz L (1986) Dacron patch aortopexy. Progr Pediatr Surg 19:117–119
22. Strife J, Baumel AS, Dunbar JS (1981) Tracheal compression by the innominate artery in infancy and childhood. Radiology 139:73–75
23. Vogl T, Wilimzig C, Hofmann U, Hofmann D, Hecker WCh, Lissner J (1989) Wertigkeit der KST der Thorax bei congenitalen Trachealstenosen. Fortschr Röntgenstr 151:428–433
24. Wailoo MP, Emmery JM (1979) The trachea in children with tracheoesophagela fistula. Histopathology 3:329–338
25. Welz A, Reichert B, Weinhold C, Überfuhr P, Mantel K, Döhlemann C (1984) Innominate artery compression of the trachea in infancy and childhood: is surgical therapy justified? Thorac Cardiovasc Surg 32:85–88
26. Wenig BI, Allan LA (1984) Innominate artery compression of the trachea. Bull N Y Acad Med 60:525–531

Indication and Results of Thoracic Surgical Procedures in Premature Infants

E. Ring-Mrozik, W. Ch. Hecker, C. Hutterer, and D. Hofmann

Summary

This analysis concerns three groups of malformations: Congenital diaphragmatic hernia, patent ductus arteriosus, and oesophageal atresia. We registered a total mortality rate for all congenital diaphragmatic hernias and defects of 28.5%; the rate in full-term neonates was 27.6% and in premature infants 33.6%.

Of 65 infants with a patent ductus arteriosus and a birth weight less than 1500 g, 14 died (21.5%). In most cases death was caused by sepsis.

Among the 159 patients with oesophageal atresia who were treated in our hospital, 58 were premature infants. During the last 20 years, the total mortality rate among our patients was 28.9%. We had a mortality rate of 44.8% in premature infants and of 19.8% in full-term neonates.

An analysis of the last 10 years showed a survival rate of 97% in healthy infants (group A in Waterston's classification). In group C, the most disadvantageous group (premature infants, severe anomalies), the rate was 61%.

Zusammenfassung

Die vorliegende Analyse behandelt 3 Gruppen von Fehlbildungen: die kongenitale Zwerchfellhernie, den offenen Ductus arteriosis und die Ösophagusatresia.

Bei der kongenitalen Zwerchfellhernie betrug die Gesamtletalität 28,5%, 27,6% bei reifgeborenen Kindern und 33,6% bei Frühgeborenen; 14 Kinder von 65 mit einem offenen Ductus arteriosus und einem Geburtsgewicht unter 1500 g verstarben (21,5%). Häufigste Todesursache war eine Sepsis. Unter den 159 behandelten Kindern mit einer Ösophagusatresia waren 58 Frühgeborene. Die Gesamtletalität während der letzten 20 Jahre betrug 28,9% (44,8% bei Frühgeborenen und 19,8% bei Reifgeborenen). Eine Analyse der letzten 10 Jahre ergab eine Überlebensrate von 97% bei Kindern ohne begleitende Fehlbildungen (Gruppe A der Waterston-Klassifikation). In der ungünstigsten Gruppe C (Frühgeborene, schwere begleitende Fehlbildungen) betrug die Überlebensrate 61%.

Résumé

Cette étude traite de trois groupes de malformations: la diaphragmatocèle congénitale, la persistance du canal artériel et l'atrésie de l'oesophage.

En ce qui concerne les cas de diaphragmatocèle congénitale, la mortalité totale fut de 28,5% chez les enfants nés à terme et de 33,6% chez les prématurés. Quatorze des 65 enfants, pesant moins de 1500 g à la naissance et présentant une persistance du canal artériel sont décédés (soit

Department of Pediatric Surgery, Dr. von Haunersches Kinderspital of the University of Munich, Lindwurmstraße 4, D-8000 Munich 2 (W), FRG.

Progress in Pediatric Surgery, Vol. 27
Myers and Angerpointner (Eds.)

21,5%). La cause de décès la plus fréquente était la septicémie. Parmi les 159 enfants présentant une atrésie de l'oesophage traités dans notre clinique, il y avait 58 prématurés. La mortalité totale au cours des 20 dernières années s'éleva à 28,9%, dont 44,8% chez les prématurés et 19,8% chez les enfants nés à terme. L'analyse des 10 dernières années indique un taux de survie de 97% chez les enfants ne présentant pas d'autres anomalies (groupe A de la classification de Waterston). Parmi le groupe le plus désavantagé, le groupe C, constitué de prématurés présentant de graves anomalies d'un autre ordre, le taux de survie était de 61%.

Introduction

Up to 1988, 8% of all aseptic operations in the Munich paediatric surgical hospital were thoracic surgical procedures. In the year 1988, we had a total of 6728 aseptic operations, and of these 531 were thoracic surgical procedures. Also in 1988, the number of surgical interventions in the neonatal period amounted to 22% – more than double the usual percentage.

Because of the progress in neonatology, it is increasingly possible to perform an operation quickly when the necessity can be foreseen, and we can now save the lives of premature and extremely immature infants with a birth weight of less than 1000 g.

We studied three groups of malformations: congenital diaphragmatic hernia and defect, patent ductus arteriosus and oesophageal atresia.

Results

Analysis of the *diaphragmatic malformations* in newborns demonstrated a mortality rate of 16% in premature infants. The total mortality rate (Table 1) of all 112 patients with diaphragmatic hernia or defect who underwent surgery during the last 10 years, was 28.5%. The difference in mortality rate between full-term neonates (27.6%) and premature infants with a birth weight of less than 2500 (33.3%) was 6%.

The main problem with the therapy in infants with diaphragmatic hernias or defects is not prematurity but pulmonary hypoplasia. This is caused by the organs of the abdominal tract penetrating the thorax, by the relatively poor development of the lungs and by postoperative pneumothoraces. In a considerable proportion of cases these is hypoplasia of the lung on the contralateral side as well. To date, it is not known whether this is caused by a mechanical disorder in development, induced by the defective part, or if it is a disorder of the whole development of the lungs. Of the 112 patients, 53 (47.3%) developed a pneumothorax on the contralateral side, or secondarily on the side of the disorder (Table 2). In full-term neonates, a pneumothorax developed in 44% of cases, and in preterm infants, we had clearly higher incidence of 61%. The mortality rate of patients with diaphragmatic hernia, after a pneumothorax occurred was 57.1% in full-term neonates and 63.6% in premature infants. Hence, 42.9% of the full-term neonates hernia or defect survived after a pneumothorax had occurred. The respiratory distress syn-

Table 1. Results of the surgical treatment of diaphragmatic hernia and defects from 1969 to 1989

Birthweight (g)	No. of cases	%	No. of deaths	%
≥ 2500	94	83.9	26	27.6
< 2500	18	16.0	6	33.3
Total	112	100	32	28.5

Table 2. Pneumothorax in patients with diaphragmatic hernias and defects from 1969 to 1989

Birth weight (g)	No. of cases	Pneumo-thorax	%	No. of deaths	%
> 2500	94	42	44	24	57.1
< 2500	18	11	61	7	63.6
Total	112	53	47.3	31	58.4

drome is, of course, a determining factor. Postoperative pneumothoraces, especially on the contralateral side, are due to forced respiration and a shift of the mediastinum. Because the hypoplastic lung is unable to expand postoperatively, an "empty cavity" remains in this hemithorax. A mediastinal shift to this side is induced by resorption of the air or by suction drainage followed secondarily by overexpansion of the contralateral lung. The result is emphysema with a disruption of alveoli which may be followed by pneumothorax.

The postoperative pneumothorax is the main reason for the severe secondary, mostly progressive, respiratory insufficiency (Fig. 1). In addition to Joppić [6] recommendations, we suggest taking the following precautions: Avoid and com-

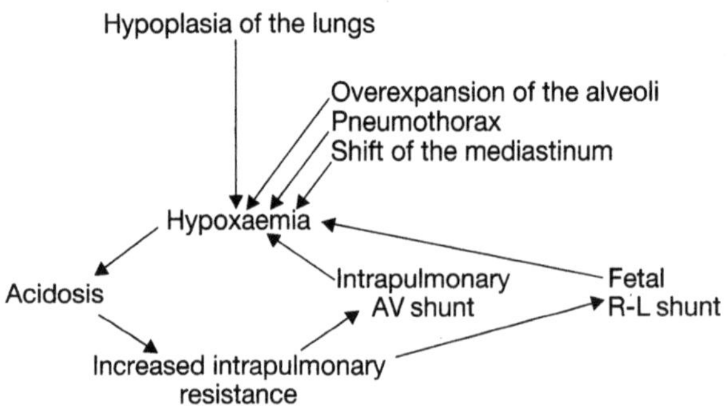

Fig. 1. The progressive respiratory insufficiency in patients with diaphragmatic hernia and defects. (From [6])

pensate for all kinds of ventilation with negative airway pressure in the diseased and repaired side. The mediastinum must be stabilized in the midline, if necessary, by the application of air insufflation to the repaired side of the thorax under X-ray control. Additionally, administration of an alpha-blocker to constrict the ductus arteriosus and dilate the pulmonal alveoli, improves peripheral circulation. If necessary, there must be low-pressure, high-frequency or oscillatory ventilation, and, if possible, extracorporal membrane oxygenation (ECMO). In the literature, there are no detailed statistical analyses concerning the influence of prematurity on the mortality of patients with diaphragmatic hernia, but there are reports on the fatal influence of the pneumothorax. Raffensperger et al. [9] from Chicago and Ramenowsky [10] from Boston conducted experimental investigations on this problem. They concluded that the mediastinum has to be stabilized in the midline under all circumstances. In the studies conducted by Gibson and Fonkalsrud [3], only two out of nine patients survived with a postoperative pneumothorax, and none of five newborns survived with a preoperative pneumothorax.

Today, neonatologists are able to save the lives of extremely premature infants with a birth weight of as little as 500 g. In this case, complications occur as a result of *patent ductus arteriosus (PDA)*. The clinical signs are reduced renal output with increased creatinine, enlarged abdomen, and poorer oxygenation (higher ventila-

Table 3. Indication for ligation of the ductus arteriosus in preterm infants

Site	Indication
Renal tract	Decreased renal output, decreased flow and renal arteries, increased creatinine
Abdominal tract	Absent diastolic flow or diastolic backflow in the mesenteric arteries
Heart	Increased cardiac output
Cerebrum	No diastolic flow or diastolic backflow in cerebral arteries

Table 4. Causes of death following ligation of the patent ductus arteriosus in neonates with a birth weight of less than 1500 g

Cause of death	No. of patients
Bronchopulmonary dysplasia	2
Posthaemorrhagic hydrocephalus	1
Sepsis	8
Renal failure	2
Bleeding disorders	1
Total	14

Table 5. Mortality rate in patients with ligation of ductus arteriosus and birthweight less than 1500 g

Reference	Year	Rate (%)
Gay et al. [2]	1973	34
Lippmann et al. [7]	1976	37.5
Salomon et al. [11]	1979	32
Zerella et al. [15]	1983	25
Wagner et al. [13]	1984	23
Hubbard et al. [5]	1986	23
Singer et al. [12]	1986	27
Present study		21.5

tion pressure and higher oxygen concentration are necessary). The decisive investigation to determine the necessity for ligation of the ductus arteriosus is Doppler scanning. This reveals a decreased flow in the renal artery, an absent or reversed diastolic flow of the mesenteric vessels, an increase of the cardiac output, and an absent or reversed diastolic flow in the cerebral arteries (Table 3).

This study includes 65 patients with a PDA and birth weight less than 1500 g. Of these patients, 14 died (21.5%). In eight patients (57.1%) death was primarily caused by sepsis (Table 4). One survivor had a birth weight of only 530 g. In the literature, reported mortality rates for infants with a birth weight less than 1500 g and a PDA are between 21% and 37% (Table 5).

The operative technique for *oesophageal atresia* is quite demanding. The anaesthesia is complex, and the pre- and postoperative support – depending on the type of anomaly – is highly problematical. Since 1969, in the Dr. von Haunersches Kinderspital in Munich, 159 newborns with oesophageal atresia have been treated. For our study, we put all variations of oesophageal atresia in one group. The total mortality rate of these 159 infants was 28.9% (Table 6). In premature infants we had a fatality rate of 44.8%. Thus, the risk factor for premature infants is almost twice as high as in full-term neonates. Besides prematurity, associated anomalies and pneumonia are equally important factors. According to Waterston's classification [14] from 1969 to 1989 we had a mortality rate of 8.6% in group A (the most advantageous group), 33.3% in group B and 61.5% in group C (Table 6).

The improvement in treatment of oesophageal atresia is quite evident over the last 20 years. The most significant improvement is the decrease in mortality in group C, from 100% 10 years ago to 29% in recent years. This is clearly the result of improved pre- and postoperative management. Nowadays, the survival chances for full-term neonates with oesophageal atresia without pneumonia or associated anomalies (group A, the most favourable group in Waterston's classification) is

Table 6. Results of surgical treatment of patients with oesophageal atresia from 1969 to 1989 according to **a** birth weight and **b** Waterston's classification

	No. of cases	No. of deaths	%
a Birthweight			
> 2500	101	20	19.8
< 2500	58	26	44.8
b Waterston's classification			
A	58	5	8.6
B	75	25	33.3
C	26	16	61.5
Total	159	46	28.9

Table 7. Severe anomalies associated with oesophageal atresia in 36 patients

Anomaly	%
Charge syndrome	25
Vitium cordis	37.5
Hydrocephalus	25
Trisomy 21	12.5

97%. In group C, the most unfavourable group – patients with prematurity, pneumonia and associated anomalies – the survival rate is 71% now, compared to 0% at the beginning of the 1970s.

The following analysis illustrates the influence of grave associated anomalies on survival of patients with oesophageal atresia. Out of 159 patients, 88 (55.3%) had such anomalies. Out of 46 patients who died, 36 (78.3%) had malformations (Table 7), vitium cordis being the most common (37.5%).

The results of surgical treatment of oesophageal atresia published by Louhimo and Lindahl [8] and by Abrahamson and Schandling [1] show a survival rate of 100% in groups A and B. In our department, we expect further improvement in the survival rate of our patients to be achieved by the following means: (1) preventive measures to avoid prematurity, (2) improvement in prenatal diagnosis and (3) routine examinations of the oesophageal tract with a nasogastric tube in all neonates to detect any anomaly. Observing these principles, it should be possible to perform any necessary surgery immediately.

Conclusion

Our analysis indicates that optimal surgical treatment of premature infants, among them extremely premature infants with a birth weight less than 1000 g, is not just a question of operative procedures; rather, success depends on progress made in neonatology and intensive care, with which every paediatric surgeon should be familiar.

References

1. Abrahamson J, Schandling B (1972) Esophageal atresia in the underweight baby. J Pediatr Surg 7:608
2. Gay JH, Daily WJR, Meyer BHP, Trump DS, Cloud DT, Molthan ME (1973) Ligation of the patent ductus arteriosus in premature infants: report of 45 cases. J Pediatr Surg 8(5): 677–683
3. Gibson C, Fonkalsrud EW (1983) Iatrogenic pneumothorax and mortality in congenital diaphragmatic hernia. J Pediatr Surg 18:555–559
4. Hecker WCh (1985) Postoperativer Pneumothorax nach Eingriffen wegen Zwerchfellhernien und -defekten. Chirurg 56:319–321
5. Hubbard C, Rucker WR, Realyvasquez ZF, Sperling DR (1986) Ligation of the patent ductus arteriosus in newborn respiratroy failure. J Pediatr Surg 21:3–5
6. Joppich I, Lochbühler A (1984) Kongenitale Zwerchfellhernien und -defekte. Lect Congress Pediatr Surg Bochum
7. Lippmann M, Nelson RJ, Emmanouilides GC, Diskin J, Thibeault DW (1976) Ligation of patent ductus arteriosus in premature infants. Br J Anaesth 48:365–369
8. Lohimo J, Lindahl H (1983) Esophageal atresia. J Pediatr Surg 18:217–229
9. Raffensperger JG, Luck SR, Inwood RJ, Gora P, Hunt CE (1979) The effect of overdistension of the lung on pulmonary function in beagle puppies. J Pediatr Surg 14:757–760
10. Ramenofsky ML (1979) The effects of intrapleural pressure on respiratory insufficiency. J Pediatr Surg 14:750–756

11. Salomon NW, Anderson RM, Copeland JC, Allen HD, Goldberg SJ, Sahn DJ (1979) A rational approach to ligation of patent ductus arteriosus in the neonate. Chest 75:671–674
12. Singer H, Deeg KH, Richter K, Bundscherer FJ, Rein JG (1986) Operative Behandlung des offenen Ductus arteriosus Botalli beim Frühgeborenen. Monatsschr Kinderheilkd 134:480–484
13. Wagner HR, Ellison RC, Ziercer S (1984) Surgical closure of patent ductus arteriosus in 268 preterm infants. J Thorac Cardiovasc Surg 87:870–875
14. Waterston DJ, Bonham Carter RE, Aberdeen E (1962) Esophageal atresia. Lancet I:819–822
15. Zerella JT, Spies RJ, Deaver DC, Dailry JR, Haple DLE, Trump DS (1983) Indomethacin versus immediate ligation in the treatment of 82 newborns with patent ductus arteriosus. J Pediatr Surg 18:835–841

Subject Index

MIX
Papier aus verantwortungsvollen Quellen
Paper from responsible sources
FSC® C105338

If you have any concerns about our products,
you can contact us on
ProductSafety@springernature.com

In case Publisher is established outside the EU,
the EU authorized representative is:
Springer Nature Customer Service Center GmbH
Europaplatz 3, 69115 Heidelberg, Germany

Printed by Libri Plureos GmbH
in Hamburg, Germany